Recent Advances in
HEMATOLOGY-4

Recent Advances in
HEMATOLOGY-4

Authors

Ishani Gupta MD (Pathology)
Assistant Professor
Department of Pathology
All India Institute of Medical Sciences Vijaypur
Jammu, J&K, India

Shivani Gandhi MD (Pathology)
Assistant Professor
Department of Pathology
All India Institute of Medical Sciences Vijaypur
Jammu, J&K, India

Reetika Menia DNB (Pathology)
Assistant Professor
Department of Pathology
All India Institute of Medical Sciences Vijaypur
Jammu, J&K, India

Foreword

Pranab Dey

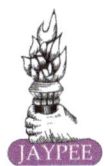

JAYPEE BROTHERS MEDICAL PUBLISHERS
The Health Sciences Publisher
New Delhi | London

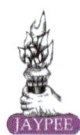 **Jaypee Brothers Medical Publishers (P) Ltd**

Headquarters
EMCA House
23/23-B, Ansari Road, Daryaganj
New Delhi 110 002, India
Landline: +91-11-23272143
+91-11-23272703, +91-11-23282021
+91-11-23245672
E-mail: jaypee@jaypeebrothers.com

Corporate Office
Jaypee Brothers Medical Publishers (P) Ltd
4838/24, Ansari Road, Daryaganj
New Delhi 110 002, India
Phone: +91-11-43574357
Fax: +91-11-43574314
E-mail: jaypee@jaypeebrothers.com

Overseas Office
JP Medical Ltd.
83, Victoria Street, London
SW1H 0HW (UK)
Phone: +44-20 3170 8910
Fax: +44(0)20 3008 6180
E-mail: info@jpmedpub.com

EU GPSR Authorised Representative
LOGOS EUROPE, 9 rue Nicolas Poussin
17000, LA ROCHELLE, France
Phone: +33 (0) 6 67 93 73 78
Email: Contact@logos europe.eu

Website: www.jaypeebrothers.com
Website: www.jaypeedigital.com

© 2024, Jaypee Brothers Medical Publishers

The views and opinions expressed in this book are solely those of the original contributor(s)/author(s) and do not necessarily represent those of editor(s) or publisher of the book.

All rights reserved. No part of this publication may be reproduced, stored or transmitted in any form or by any means, electronic, mechanical, photocopying, recording or otherwise, without the prior permission in writing of the publishers.

All brand names and product names used in this book are trade names, service marks, trademarks or registered trademarks of their respective owners. The publisher is not associated with any product or vendor mentioned in this book.

Medical knowledge and practice change constantly. This book is designed to provide accurate, authoritative information about the subject matter in question. However, readers are advised to check the most current information available on procedures included and check information from the manufacturer of each product to be administered, to verify the recommended dose, formula, method and duration of administration, adverse effects and contraindications. It is the responsibility of the practitioner to take all appropriate safety precautions. Neither the publisher nor the author(s)/editor(s) assume any liability for any injury and/or damage to persons or property arising from or related to use of material in this book.

This book is sold on the understanding that the publisher is not engaged in providing professional medical services. If such advice or services are required, the services of a competent medical professional should be sought.

Every effort has been made where necessary to contact holders of copyright to obtain permission to reproduce copyright material. If any have been inadvertently overlooked, the publisher will be pleased to make the necessary arrangements at the first opportunity.

Inquiries for bulk sales may be solicited at: jaypee@jaypeebrothers.com

Recent Advances in Hematology-4 / Ishani Gupta, Shivani Gandhi, Reetika Menia

First Edition: 2024

ISBN: 978-93-5696-583-6

Contributors

Aarushi Chopra MD (Pathology)
Consultant Pathologist
Basant Sahney Hospital
Telangana, Hyderabad, India

Aby Abraham MD DM
Professor and Head
Department of Clinical Haematology
Christian Medical College
Vellore, Tamil Nadu, India

Afshan Atta MD (Pathology)
Consultant Hematopathologist
Dr Qadri's Hematology Center and
Clinical Laboratory
Srinagar, J&K, India

Ambreen Beigh MD (Pathology)
Assistant Professor
Department of Pathology
Government Medical College
Srinagar, J&K, India

Anshu Palta MD (Pathology)
Professor
Department of Pathology
Government Medical College and
Hospital
Chandigarh, India

Aparna Bhardwaj MD (Pathology)
Professor
Department of Pathology
In-Charge, Blood Bank
Shri Guru Ram Rai Institute of
Medical and Health Science
Dehradun, Uttarakhand, India

Brijesh Thakur MD (Pathology)
Professor, Department of Pathology
Shri Guru Ram Rai Institute of
Medical and Health Science
Dehradun, Uttarakhand, India

Gaurav Raturi MD (Transfusion Medicine)
Associate Professor
Department of Transfusion Medicine
Shri Guru Ram Rai Institute of
Medical and Health Science
Dehradun, Uttarakhand, India

Harish Chandra MD (Pathology)
Professor
Department of Pathology and
Laboratory Medicine
All India Institute of Medical Sciences
Rishikesh, Uttarakhand, India

Jyotsna Suri MD (Pathology)
Professor, Department of Pathology
Government Medical College
Jammu, J&K, India

Karthik Rengaraj MD DNB MRCP (UK)
Senior Postgraduate Registrar
Department of Clinical Haematology
Christian Medical College
Vellore, Tamil Nadu, India

Manveen Kaur MD (Pathology)
Assistant Professor
Department of Pathology
Government Medical College
and Hospital
Chandigarh, India

Contributors

Nimisha Sharma MD (Pathology)
Assistant Professor
Department of Pathology
Govind Ballabh Pant Hospital
and PGIMER
New Delhi, India

Nuzhat Samoon MD (Pathology)
DipRCPath
Assistant Professor
Department of Pathology
Government Medical College
Srinagar, J&K, India

Reetika Menia DNB (Pathology)
Assistant Professor
Department of Pathology
All India Institute of Medical
Sciences Vijaypur
Jammu, J&K, India

Sana Umar MD (Pathology) Dip FRCPath
Assistant Professor
Department of Pathology
Government Doon Medical College
and Hospital
Dehradun, Uttarakhand, India

Sanjay Kaushik MD (Pathology)
Professor
Department of Pathology
Shri Guru Ram Rai Institute of
Medical and Health Science
Dehradun, Uttarakhand, India

Saqib Ahmed MD (Pathology)
Assistant Professor
Department of Pathology
Shri Guru Ram Rai Institute of
Medical and Health Science
Dehradun, Uttarakhand, India

Snigdha Petwal MD (Pathology)
Assistant Professor
Department of Pathology
Government Doon Medical College
Dehradun, Uttarakhand, India

Sudha Sharma MD DNB (Pathology)
Assistant Professor
Department of Pathology
Dr Yashwant Singh Parmar
Government Medical College
(YSPGMC)
Nahan, Himachal Pradesh, India

Sumayya Shah MD (Pathology)
Consultant Pathologist
Srinagar, J&K, India

Summyia Farooq MD (Pathology)
Assistant Professor
Department of Pathology
Government Medical College
Srinagar, J&K, India

Surbhi Mahajan MD (Pathology)
Assistant Professor
Department of Pathology
Government Medical College,
Kathua, J&K, India

Swati Arora MD (Pathology)
Lecturer
Department of Pathology
Government Medical College
Jammu, J&K, India

Uday Prakash Kulkarni MD DM
Assistant Professor
Department of Clinical Haematology
Christian Medical College
Vellore, Tamil Nadu, India

Foreword

It is my pleasure to introduce the book *"Recent Advances in Hematology-4"*. Hematology is a rapidly growing area, and therefore it is important to keep pace with the advancement in this subject. The authors of this book have taken the most difficult task in this setting. The book describes the frontiers of hematology such as gene therapy, genetic profiling, and micro-RNA. It also highlights the pathogenesis of various hematological disorders. The chapters are carefully chosen to cover the major areas of hematology. I strongly believe that this book will be a good asset to students and medical practitioners.

Pranab Dey MD FRCPath
Ex-Professor of Cytology
Postgraduate Institute of Medical Education
and Research, Chandigarh, India

Preface

Welcome to "*Recent Advances in Hematology-4*," a comprehensive book that explores the latest developments and breakthroughs in the field of hematology. This book is a testament to the remarkable progress made in our understanding of blood and its components, the diagnosis and management of blood disorders, and the development of novel therapies.

Hematology is a dynamic and ever-evolving discipline that plays a pivotal role in healthcare. It encompasses the study of blood, blood-forming tissues, and disorders related to the blood, from anemia, leukemia to clotting disorders and rare hematologic conditions. With the advent of new technologies, diagnostic tools, and therapeutic interventions, hematology has witnessed significant advancements in recent years.

Our aim in compiling this book is to provide the healthcare professionals, researchers, students, and anyone interested in hematology with a comprehensive resource that reflects the current state of the field. This book has been divided into various sections, each dedicated to a specific aspect of hematology, from the basic science underpinning blood cell formation to the clinical management of hematologic disorders.

In the following pages, you will find contributions from experts in the field, sharing their insights, research findings, and clinical experiences. Topics covered include the molecular basis of blood disorders, cutting-edge diagnostic techniques, therapeutic advancements, and emerging trends in hematology research.

As editors of this book, we are grateful to the contributing authors for their valuable contributions and expertise. We hope that this book serves as a valuable reference for practitioners, educators, and students, facilitating a deeper understanding of the complexities and nuances within hematology. Whether you are a seasoned hematologist, a medical student, or a healthcare professional from a related field, "*Recent Advances in Hematology-4*" is designed to provide you with the latest knowledge and insights that will contribute to better patient care and further advancements in the field.

We would like to extend our gratitude to the readers for choosing this book as a resource to stay updated on the rapidly evolving field of hematology. We hope that you find the content both informative and inspiring, sparking new ideas and collaborations that will ultimately contribute to improved patient outcomes.

We also want to express our appreciation to the publishers for their support and dedication to bringing this book to fruition. Their commitment to the dissemination of knowledge is instrumental in advancing the field of hematology.

We look forward to the continued progress and innovation in hematology and the positive impact it will have on the lives of patients. We hope that *Recent Advances in Hematology* plays a role in facilitating this progress and inspiring the next generation of hematologists and researchers.

Ishani Gupta
Shivani Gandhi
Reetika Menia

Acknowledgments

We extend our heartfelt appreciation to the esteemed institutions and individuals whose invaluable contributions and unwavering support have been instrumental in the realization of this book *Recent Advances in Hematology-4*.

Our deepest gratitude is directed toward the prestigious All India Institute of Medical Sciences (AIIMS) Jammu (J&K), an institution renowned for its dedication to excellence in healthcare and medical education. AIIMS has provided the fertile ground from which this project has grown, fostering an environment that values innovation and knowledge advancement.

We wish to express our profound thanks to our Executive Director and CEO, Professor (Dr) Shakti Kumar Gupta, whose visionary leadership and wholehearted encouragement have been a constant source of inspiration. Under your guidance, we have found the motivation to pursue this endeavor and strive for excellence.

Our acknowledgments extend to the Medical Superintendent and Dean Research, Lt Gen (Dr) Sunil Kant, SM, VSM (Retd) or facilitating the resources and support necessary for the successful completion of this book. Your commitment to enhancing the academic and research environment at AIIMS has been pivotal to our progress.

We also wish to express our appreciation to our seniors, colleagues and fellow researchers whose contributions, insights, and collaboration have greatly enriched the content of this book. Your collective expertise has added depth and substance to the discussions contained within its pages.

A special thank you goes to the contributors of the chapters whose dedication and expertise have been crucial in shaping the content and perspectives presented in this book.

Finally, we are indebted to our families, friends, and loved ones for their unwavering patience and encouragement during the challenging journey of creating this book.

We are extremely thankful to Shri Jitendar P Vij (Group Chairman), Mr Ankit Vij (Managing Director), Mr MS Mani (Group President), Ms Chetna Malhotra (Senior Director—Professional Publishing, Marketing, and Business Development), Ms Pooja Bhandari (Director—Production), and Mr Akhilesh Saxena (Publishing Coordinator), M/s Jaypee Brothers Medical Publishers (P) Ltd, New Delhi, India, for constant encouragement.

This book is a testament to the collective effort of an institution, its leaders, faculty, and students, and the collaborative spirit that drives us all toward the advancement of knowledge.

Ishani Gupta
Shivani Gandhi
Reetika Menia

Contents

1. **ER Blood Group** — 1
   Nimisha Sharma, Reetika Menia

2. **Precursor Myeloid Neoplasms: Recent Insights** — 10
   Jyotsna Suri

3. **Gene Therapy in Hematological Diseases** — 16
   Summyia Farooq, Nuzhat Samoon

4. **Role of Flow Cytometry in Transfusion Medicine** — 48
   Aparna Bhardwaj, Gaurav Raturi, Sanjay Kaushik, Saqib Ahmed

5. **Hematological Changes Associated with COVID-19 Infections** — 58
   Aarushi Chopra

6. **Mature T- and NK-cell Neoplasms: Updates on Molecular Genetic Features** — 80
   Sudha Sharma

7. **Pediatric Leukemias: Recent Updates** — 96
   Sumayya Shah, Afshan Atta

8. **CAR-T Cell in the Treatment of Hematological Malignancies** — 118
   Karthik Rengaraj, Uday Prakash Kulkarni, Aby Abraham

9. **Role of MicroRNA in the Pathogenesis of Plasma Cell Dyscrasias** — 136
   Manveen Kaur, Anshu Palta

10. **Genomic Profiling for Clinical Decision-making in Hematological Malignancies** — 154
    Harish Chandra

11. **Hereditary Hemorrhagic Telangiectasia/Osler–Weber–Rendu Syndrome** — 176
    Nuzhat Samoon, Ambreen Beigh

12. Pathogenesis of Chemotherapy and Cancer-induced
    Anemia: Recent Updates ... 184
    Snigdha Petwal, Sana Umar

13. Anemia in CKD—Pathophysiology and Recent
    Updates in Treatment Strategy ... 199
    Brijesh Thakur

14. Tumor-like Lesions Associated with B-cell Predominance ... 210
    Surbhi Mahajan, Swati Arora

Index ... *225*

CHAPTER 1

ER Blood Group

Nimisha Sharma, Reetika Menia

■ INTRODUCTION

In the early 1980, a significant breakthrough occurred in the field of blood group categorization with the discovery of the estrogen receptor (ER) antigen.[1] This discovery was a pivotal moment that laid the foundation for further exploration. Subsequently, scholars from the NHS Blood and Transplant organization embarked on an extensive investigation, aiming to understand the implications of this newly identified ER blood group.[2] The first ER antigen, called Er^a, was described by Daniels et al. in 1982.[3] Six years later, Hamilton et al.[4] described an antithetical antigen, Er^b that was detected in the serum of an Er (a+ b–) woman who had no common red blood cell (RBC) alloantibodies and had given birth to a child with a positive direct antiglobulin test (DAT).[5] Initially, this novel blood group was distinguished through serological analysis of RBCs. It revealed the presence of high- and low-frequency antigens, designated as Er^a, Er^b, and Er3 (Er a–b–), which raised intriguing questions.[6] Over three decades ago, these antigenic markers had already left their mark in the scientific literature, creating an enigma that was about to be unraveled.

As the investigation advanced, it harnessed cutting-edge methodologies that enabled the simultaneous examination of DNA sequences responsible for gene coding. Within this genetic framework, researchers made a breakthrough discovery.[7] They pinpointed distinct genetic alterations in the gene responsible for encoding the PIEZO1 protein.[8] These genetic modifications resulted in the production of a modified version of the PIEZO1 protein, which became evident on the cellular surfaces of the individuals under investigation.

This discovery marked a critical turning point and raised fundamental questions about the relationship between PIEZO1 and the newly identified Er antigens. To establish this connection, including the identification of two novel high-incidence antigens named Er4 and Er5, the investigators turned to gene editing techniques. The process involved the precise removal and subsequent reintroduction of the PIEZO1 protein in an immortalized cell line developed in the Bristol region.[9] Through this meticulously designed experimental approach, the researchers successfully demonstrated the binding of alloantibodies to Er antigens. This pivotal experiment provided the concrete evidence needed to confirm the indispensable role of PIEZO1 in the expression of Er antigens.

HISTORICAL BACKGROUND

Tracing the Roots of the ER Blood Group and ER Antigens

Understanding the significance of the ER blood group and its associated antigens, such as Er^a and Er^b, requires a journey into their historical development. By exploring their origins, we can gain valuable insights into the role these high-incidence antigens played in shaping the ER blood group system.

The Er^a Blood

Er^a is a specific blood type within the ER blood group. Daniels et al. elucidated how this blood group type appears to follow a hereditary pattern, passing from one generation to the next.[3,6] In 1988, Hamilton et al.[4] made a noteworthy discovery by identifying a rare antibody known as Er^b. This antibody exhibited reactivity with the RBCs of individuals possessing the Er^a blood type, shedding light on the complexity of blood group systems and the clinical significance of rare antibodies.[10] Er^a and Er^b display a codominant inheritance pattern, indicating that both alleles are regularly inherited as codominant traits within specific populations. This pattern contributes to the prevalence of Er^a individuals in certain groups.[11] While Er^a is primarily observed in individuals of European descent, isolated instances of Er^a have surfaced in other populations, exemplified by the identification of a Mexican family with this blood type, signifying its presence in diverse populations.[12]

The Er^b Type

The Er^b group typically refers to a family of genes and proteins that play a crucial role in regulating various physiological processes, particularly in the context of cellular growth and development.[13] One well-known member of this group is the ER, which exists in two major types, ERα and ERβ. These receptors are primarily associated with responding to the hormone estrogen and are found in various tissues throughout the body. They function as transcription factors, influencing the expression of specific genes that control functions like cell proliferation, differentiation, and apoptosis. ERβ, in particular, has gained increasing attention for its role in modulating estrogen signaling and influencing a range of health outcomes, including those related to cancer, cardiovascular health, and neurological conditions. The Er^b group, as a whole, represents a fascinating area of research, shedding light on how hormonal signaling impacts diverse aspects of human physiology and disease.

Er3 Blood Type

Er3, a notable antigen within the ER blood group system, holds significance alongside other antigens like Er^a Er^b, Er4, and Er5. Its identification through serological analysis of red blood cells has made it a focal point in blood group classification and transfusion medicine research. Studies suggest that Er3 antibodies can interact with red blood cells expressing the Er(a-) phenotype, potentially causing mild hemolysis following the transfusion of incompatible red cells.[6] While the direct clinical impact of Er3 may be limited, comprehending its role within the intricate ER blood group system is crucial for precise blood typing and ensuring transfusion safety.

The discovery of the Er3 antigen gains additional significance in the context of peculiar blood group cases. Instances such as the identification of an Er(a-b-) phenotype in unrelated individuals and the occurrence of an Er(a+b-) daughter with an Er(a-b+) mother hint at the existence of a third, uncommon gene.[4] This complexity becomes more evident in a specific case where a closely related couple gave birth to a child with Er(a-b-) blood type. This individual, producing an antibody known as anti-Er3, displayed reactivity with all tested RBCs, including those with Er(a-), indicating a potential complete absence of the Er antigen—a rare occurrence. The anti-Er3 also exhibited reactions with RBCs from another Er(a-b-) individual, suggesting a shared absence of the Er antigen.[6] This intricate scenario highlights the intricate nature of blood group genetics, showcasing how different genes can influence the manifestation of antigens and, consequently, our blood types.

Er4 and Er5

Er4 and Er5 are found at a high frequency in the general population. The clinical significance of antibodies against Er4 and Er5 is poorly understood due to a lack of data, but two cases of severe hemolytic disease of the fetus and newborn have been reported in women with these antibodies.[14] The presence of alloantibodies can cause problems during transfusion if there is a mismatch between donor and recipient, as well as triggering attacks on the immune system during pregnancy.[15]

■ MOLECULAR BASIS OF THE ER BLOOD GROUP

Various studies have shown that the *PIEZO1* gene, located on chromosome 16, encodes a mechanically activated cation channel that plays a pivotal role in mechanosensation.[15] This gene is expressed in various tissues, including RBCs, where it modulates cell volume and deformability.[14]

The molecular structure of PIEZO1 is intriguing and pivotal to its function. It is characterized by a three-bladed propeller-like structure with multiple transmembrane domains. This unique architecture allows PIEZO1 to respond to mechanical stimuli by undergoing conformational changes that lead to the opening of ion channels, enabling the flow of ions such as calcium (Ca^{2+}) and sodium (Na^+).[16]

In terms of its functions, PIEZO1 is a versatile mechanosensor with implications in multiple physiological systems. Notably, in the context of the circulatory system, PIEZO1 plays a vital role in regulating blood cell volume and deformability. When RBCs traverse through capillaries or experience changes in pressure, PIEZO1 activation helps them adapt to these mechanical challenges. This function is crucial for the efficient circulation of RBCs in the body and the maintenance of proper blood pressure.

Mutations in the *PIEZO1* gene have been linked to various physiological conditions, including hereditary xerocytosis, a disorder characterized by the abnormal hydration and shape of RBCs.[16]

The genetic variations that govern Er^a and Er^b antigens are closely intertwined with the *PIEZO1* gene. Specific missense mutations within PIEZO1 lead to amino acid substitutions in the extracellular domain of the Piezo1 mechanosensor ion channel. These mutations are responsible for the distinct antigenic properties of Er^a and Er^b. Understanding these genetic nuances is not only essential for blood group classification but also sheds light on the broader role of mechanosensation in RBC biology.[16]

■ MECHANISMS OF ER ANTIGEN EXPRESSION

These mechanisms are fundamental in ensuring precise blood matching for safe and effective transfusions. The expression of Er^a and Er^b antigens is intricately regulated at the molecular level. These antigens belong to a broader family of blood group antigens, and their genetic basis is rooted in the *PIEZO1* gene, as discussed in the previous section. The *PIEZO1* gene encodes a mechanosensor protein that senses changes in cell volume and shape. The mechanosensitivity of this protein allows it to respond to mechanical forces acting on the cell membrane.

Recent studies have shed light on the exact mechanisms by which PIEZO1 influences ER antigen expression. The mechanosensor function of PIEZO1 enables it to detect changes in cell shape that occur during blood flow in the circulatory system. When mechanical forces are exerted on RBCs, PIEZO1 is activated, leading to changes in the conformation of the extracellular domain of the protein. This, in turn, affects the exposure and availability of Er^a and Er^b antigens on the cell surface.[8,16]

Understanding these molecular mechanisms is pivotal for improving blood typing techniques and ensuring accurate and safe blood transfusions. In practice, this knowledge can lead to the development of more precise and reliable blood typing assays that take into account the mechanosensitive nature of ER antigen expression.

Piezo1's mechanosensitive properties have far-reaching implications, contributing significantly to pulmonary function, blood pressure regulation, and fluid balance within the renal system. These insights underscore the vital role of mechanosensation in maintaining organ functionality and hold promise for innovative treatments in pulmonary medicine and nephrology.

■ CLINICAL SIGNIFICANCE OF ER BLOOD GROUP

Blood typing and compatibility testing: Blood typing involves the identification of specific blood group antigens, including Er^a and Er^b, using serological methods.[3] The compatibility testing ensures that donor blood is a suitable match for the recipient, preventing adverse reactions during transfusions.[4]

Er^a and Er^b antibodies in transfusion reactions: Er^a and Er^b antibodies, once developed, can lead to immune responses during transfusions, causing hemolytic reactions.[3] This highlights the necessity of accurate blood typing to anticipate and mitigate potential complications associated with ER blood group antigens.

Clinical implications beyond transfusions: Anti-Era antibodies, falling under the IgG class, may not result in observable hemolysis but can impact laboratory tests, particularly in the context of DAT.[4] The clinical significance of these antibodies varies, emphasizing the need for a nuanced understanding of their implications in different clinical scenarios.

Significance in pregnancy and hemolytic disease: The ER blood group's significance in pregnancy lies in the potential development of Era antibodies in ER-negative pregnant women carrying an ER-positive fetus. This scenario underscores the importance of early and accurate blood typing during antenatal care to proactively manage and mitigate risks associated with ER antibodies during pregnancy.[12,13]

Evaluating Clinical Significance

Additional assessments, including monocyte phagocytosis assays and in vivo red cell survival studies, have been conducted to assess the clinical significance of Er^a antibodies. These investigations collectively suggest that Er^a antibodies typically do not have a clinically significant impact.[3,4,7] Conversely, anti-Er3 antibodies have demonstrated potential clinical significance.[12,13]

■ ER ANTIGENS IN BLOOD TRANSFUSIONS: SAFE PRACTICES

Ensuring Transfusion Safety: Managing Anti-Er Antibodies

In the realm of transfusion medicine, the significance of anti-Er antibodies cannot be overstated. Individuals producing anti-Er^a antibodies, often stemming from a history of blood transfusions or pregnancies, exhibit a distinct immunoglobulin profile falling under the IgG class, which notably does not activate the complement system. In contrast, patients with anti-Er^a antibodies, upon testing their red blood cells (RBCs) with Er^a(+) cells post-transfusion, displayed positive results in direct antiglobulin tests (DAT) without observable hemolysis.[10] Another facet emerges with anti-Er3 antibodies, reacting with Er^a(−) red cells, leading to mild hemolysis after incompatible red cell transfusion.[17]

Significance of Anti-Er Antibodies in Transfusion Medicine

This section underscores the paramount importance of precise blood matching to avert transfusion reactions attributed to Er^a and Er^b antibodies. Rigorous protocols and best practices are imperative to ensure the safe and effective transfusion of blood, considering the potential consequences associated with these antibodies. State-of-the-art technology and serologic testing methods employed by blood banks and transfusion services play a pivotal role in accurately determining a patient's ER blood group. Screening for Er^a and Er^b antigens and assessing donor blood compatibility with the recipient's blood group are integral components of these meticulous procedures.

In cases where patients have a documented history of Er^a and Er^b antibodies or previous transfusion reactions linked to ER antigens, blood banks implement special precautions. These may involve selecting donors negative for the corresponding antigen and conducting crossmatch procedures to affirm compatibility. The entire transfusion process, from blood collection and typing to product administration, demands meticulous attention to detail. Health professionals are adeptly trained to recognize clinical signs of transfusion reactions and respond promptly to mitigate their impact.

Advancements in blood banking technology, including extended blood typing and antigen matching, have significantly enhanced the safety of blood transfusions. These advancements facilitate the selection of donor units closely aligned with the recipient's antigen profile, thereby reducing the risk of adverse reactions.[18] In summary, the safe practice of blood transfusions, particularly concerning ER antigens, hinges on stringent blood typing, compatibility testing, and the implementation of comprehensive protocols, collectively ensuring patients receive blood products as compatible as possible with their own blood group. This approach is pivotal in enhancing the safety and effectiveness of transfusion medicine in healthcare settings.

HEMOLYTIC DISEASE AND ER BLOOD GROUP

In this section, we undertake a critical examination of the association between Er^a and Er^b antibodies and the development of hemolytic disease in fetuses and newborns.[14] We emphasize the significance of early diagnosis and effective management in the context of neonatal care.

Hemolytic disease of the fetus and newborn (HDFN) is a condition characterized by the destruction of RBCs in the fetus or newborn due to maternal antibodies. The most well-known example of HDFN is Rh hemolytic disease, where maternal antibodies against the RhD antigen cause hemolysis in RhD-positive fetuses.

The relationship between the ER blood group and HDFN is an intriguing and less-studied aspect of this condition. When an ER-negative mother carries an ER-positive fetus, there is a risk of developing Er^a antibodies. These antibodies can cross the placental barrier and attack the fetal RBCs, leading to hemolysis and potential complications for the newborn.

Early diagnosis and effective management of HDFN associated with ER antigens are crucial for ensuring the well-being of the newborn. This typically involves close monitoring of maternal antibody titers, fetal blood sampling, and, in severe cases, intrauterine transfusions to support the affected fetus.

Moreover, advances in medical technology have enabled noninvasive prenatal testing (NIPT), allowing healthcare providers to assess the risk of HDFN and other conditions from maternal blood samples. The ability to detect Er^a and Er^b antibodies in maternal blood is a critical advancement in the diagnosis and management of ER-related HDFN.

In neonatal care, it is essential to provide supportive care for newborns affected by HDFN. This may involve phototherapy to manage jaundice resulting from hemolysis and, in severe cases, blood transfusions to replenish the infant's RBC supply.

Ultimately, understanding the association between Er^a and Er^b antibodies and HDFN emphasizes the importance of early and accurate diagnosis and the implementation of effective management strategies to ensure the well-being of affected newborns.[16]

■ BROADER IMPLICATIONS AND FUTURE HORIZONS

In this concluding section of our chapter, we take a step back to reflect on the broader implications of Er^a, Er^b, and Piezo1 beyond the realm of blood biology. We discuss potential applications in fields such as neurobiology, regenerative medicine, and cardiovascular health and suggest areas for future research to uncover the complexities of these systems fully.

Er^a and Er^b antigens, closely associated with the *PIEZO1* gene, offer intriguing insights into the broader field of mechanosensation. While their clinical significance in blood group classification is evident, their implications extend beyond the laboratory. These antigens serve as a window into the world of mechanosensation, a fundamental cellular process with implications in various biological contexts.[4]

One area of potential application is in neurobiology. The ability of PIEZO1 to sense mechanical forces has sparked interest in its role in the nervous system. Research suggests that PIEZO1 channels may be involved in the mechanosensation of neurons and other cells in the nervous system. Understanding these mechanisms could open new avenues for studying the perception of mechanical stimuli in neurons and the potential for therapeutic interventions in conditions like neuropathic pain.

In regenerative medicine, the mechanosensitivity of PIEZO1 presents intriguing possibilities. Researchers are exploring how mechanical cues can influence stem cell behavior and differentiation. Manipulating PIEZO1 activation in stem cells may hold the key to directing their development and tissue repair, opening new prospects for regenerative therapies.

In cardiovascular health, the role of PIEZO1 in blood pressure regulation has implications for hypertension management. Developing interventions that modulate PIEZO1 activity could offer novel approaches to blood pressure control, potentially reducing the reliance on pharmaceutical agents.

As we look to the future, there are exciting avenues for research. Further exploration of the mechanosensitive properties of PIEZO1 and its role in diverse biological processes remains a fertile ground for scientific inquiry. We anticipate studies investigating the nuances of Er^a and Er^b antigens, their interactions with PIEZO1, and their relevance in health and disease.

In conclusion, the ER blood group, Er^a and Er^b antigens, and the *PIEZO1* gene represent a captivating intersection of genetics, biology, and clinical medicine. Their implications extend beyond their established roles in blood biology, reaching into neurobiology, regenerative medicine, and cardiovascular health. As we chart the course for future research, we are poised to unlock the full potential of these intricate systems, offering new insights into human biology and medical science.

CONCLUSION

This chapter has offered a comprehensive overview of the ER blood group, Er^a and Er^b antigens, and the *PIEZO1* gene. It has emphasized their clinical and scientific importance and highlighted their relevance in diverse fields. Our journey through the history, clinical implications, molecular mechanisms, and broader applications of these components underscores their intricate nature and their potential for future advancements in understanding human biology and medical science.

REFERENCES

1. Reid ME, Lomas-Francis C, Olsson ML. The blood group antigen factsbook. Academic press; 2012.
2. International Society of Blood Transfusion. Red cell immunogenetics and blood group terminology. Dostupno na http://www. isbtweb. org/working-parties/red-cell-immunogenetics-and-blood-group-terminology/. Pristupljeno 2.8 (2021).
3. Daniels GL, Judd WJ, Moore BP, et al. A 'new' high frequency antigen Era. Transfusion. 1982;22(3):189-93
4. Hamilton JR, Beattie KM, Walker RH, Hartrick MB. Erb, an allele to Era, and evidence for a third allele, Er. Transfusion. 1988;28(3):268-71.
5. Thompson HW, Skradski KJ, Thoreson JR, Polesky HF. Survival of Er(a+) red cells in a patient with allo-anti-Era. Transfusion. 1985;25:140-1.
6. Arriaga F, Mueller A, Rodberg K, Ciesielski D, Poole J, Banks J, et al. A new antigen of the Er collection. Vox Sang 2003;84:137-9.

7. Wang S, Wang B, Shi Y, Möller T, Stegmeyer Rl, Strilic B, et al. Mechanosensation by endothelial PIEZO1 is required for leukocyte diapedesis. Blood, The Journal of the American Society of Hematology. 2022;140(3):171-83.
8. Zarychanski R, Schulz VP, Houston BL, M Yelena, SH Donald, S Brian et al. Mutations in the mechanotransduction protein PIEZO1 are associated with hereditary xerocytosis. Blood. 2012;120(9):1908-15.
9. Coste B, Mathur J, Schmidt M, JE Taryn, R Sanjeev, MJ Petrus et al. Piezo1 and Piezo2 are essential components of distinct mechanically activated cation channels. Science. 2010;330(6000):55-60.
10. Naoki K, Okuma S, Uchiyama E, Nishizaki T, Okubo Y, Daniels G et al. Er(a-) red cell phenotype in Japan. Transfusion 1991;31:572-3.
11. Rowe GP. On the inheritance of Er and the frequency of Era. Transfusion 1988;28:87-88.
12. Long W, Steinmetz CL, Aranda Ll, et al. The first reported example of anti-Era in a patient of Mexican descent. Vox Sang 2010;99(Suppl. 1):333-4.
13. Poole J, Cordoba R, Marais I, et al. The second example of anti-Erb and its clinical significance in pregnancy. Vox Sang 2010;99(Suppl. 1):340 [Abstract].
14. Karamatic Crew, Vanja, AT Louise, JS Timothyl, AA Samahi, J Benjamin, AS Frances, et al. Missense mutations in PIEZO1, which encodes the Piezo1 mechanosensor protein, define Er red blood cell antigens. Blood. 2023;141(2):135-46.
15. Zupan V, Dornase A, Fairbanks VF, Kim HC. Hemolytic disease of the newborn due to anti-Erb, anti-Wrb, and anti-Wra. Vox Sanguinis. 1990;58(1):35-7.
16. Glogowska E, RS Eve, M Yelena, PS Vincent, LG Kimberly, W John et al. Novel mechanisms of PIEZO1 dysfunction in hereditary xerocytosis. Blood. 2017;130(16):1845-56.
17. Denomme GA. Laboratory identification of IgG antibodies to high-frequency blood group antigens. Transfus Med Rev. 2007;21(3):239-48.
18. Bolton-Maggs, Paula H, Cohen H. Serious Hazards of T ransfusion (SHOT) haemovigilance and progress is improving transfusion safety. British journal of haematology. 2013;163(3):303

CHAPTER 2

Precursor Myeloid Neoplasms: Recent Insights

Jyotsna Suri

■ INTRODUCTION

Precursor myeloid neoplasms (PMNs) refer to hematological disorders that exhibit abnormal proliferation and differentiation of myeloid precursor cells in the bone marrow. These conditions are in certain cases risk factors and precursors for acute myeloid leukemia (AML) and other related diseases.[1]

The World Health Organization (WHO) classification of tumors of various organ systems provides a unified system of tumor classification. It is regularly updated to incorporate advancements in our understanding of diseases, based on ongoing research conducted by various researchers and physicians. This classification serves as a globally accepted standard for diagnosing tumors, conducting research, registering cancer cases, and monitoring public health-related to cancer.

The classification and diagnosis of these disorders have evolved with the integration of newer technologies and molecular profiling. Improved understanding of genetic and epigenetic alterations has contributed to a more precise and personalized approach to diagnose and prognosticate these neoplasms. Tailored therapeutic approaches and precision of risk assessments have been made possible by the identification of specific genetic variants, such as mutations in the genes *DNMT3A*, *TET2*, and *ASXL1*. Furthermore, emerging insights into the clonal architecture and clonal evolution of PMNs have shed light on disease progression and treatment response. Ongoing research continues to unravel the complex biology and heterogeneity of PMNs, paving the way for the development of novel diagnostic and therapeutic approaches. These efforts aim to improve patient outcomes by tailoring treatment strategies based on individual risk profiles, molecular characteristics, and response to therapy.

For the WHO classification of hematolymphoid tumors, 4th edition was released in 2008 and revised in 2017. The recent 5th edition of the Hematopoietic Neoplasms classified according to the proposed WHO 5th edition and the International Consensus Classification (ICC) 5th edition (hence referred to as WHO 2022 and ICC 2022 classification, respectively) is based on lineage, dominant clinical attribute, and dominant biological attribute and has been released online and in print form in 2023.

In the latest edition, numerous changes and updates have lead to complete rewriting of revised hierarchical classification structure, revisions of terminology, nomenclature, diagnostic criteria, updates of pathogenesis, and clinical and genetic attributes. Also, there is inclusion of some nonhematolymphoid tumors and non-neoplastic lesions for the first time. The recent classification is based on integration of data compiled based on morphologic (cytology and histology), immunophenotypic, molecular, and cytogenetic details.[2]

It is widely recognized that hematolymphoid tumors are primarily divided into two major categories: Myeloid and lymphoid. These categories are subsequently refined based on factors such as histomorphologic features, clinical data, maturation stage, phenotypic characteristics, and cytogenetic molecular genetic findings.[2]

In the updated classification of hematolymphoid tumors, a significant change has occurred within the myeloid neoplasia group. For the first time, precursor lesions have been incorporated as distinct entities. This comprises clonal hematopoiesis (CH), with a focus on clonal cytopenias of undetermined significance (CCUS) and clonal hematopoiesis of indeterminate potential (CHIP). With this adjustment, a uniform global definition has been developed, improving the comparability of findings in subsequent investigations.

It encompasses various precursor disease states, which can, over a period of time, lead to the development of myeloid malignancy like myelodysplastic syndrome (MDS) or AML. Clonal hematopoiesis is the first discernible stage in this cycle **(Table 1)**.

Clonal hematopoiesis is the term used to describe a cell population originating from a mutant multipotent stem cell with a selective growth advantage but no inexplicable cytopenias, hematological malignancies, or

TABLE 1: Differences between various precursor myeloid conditions.

	CHIP	ICUS	CCUS
Somatic mutations	+	−	+
Cytopenias	−	+	+
Risk of transformation to MDS/AML	Low	Low	Low to high
Dysplasia	Absent	Absent	Absent
Increased blast percentage	−	−	−

(AML: acute myeloid leukemia; CCUS: clonal cytopenias of undetermined significance; CHIP: clonal hematopoiesis of indeterminate potential; ICUS: idiopathic cytopenia of uncertain significance; MDS: myelodysplastic syndrome)
Source: With permission from Osman (2021).[6]

other clonal diseases. CH is more common as people age. Following the identification and acknowledgement of precursor myeloid lesions (PMLs), significant advancements have already been made, in recognizing the association of these entities with progression to myeloid malignancies and their link to increased mortality, predominantly related to cardiovascular causes. The higher risk is generally attributable to a theory that involves abnormal macrophage gene transcription, increased expression of inflammatory pathways, and encouragement of atherogenesis.[3,4]

Clonal hematopoiesis of indeterminate potential is the term used to describe the earliest discernible phases of the formation of PMNs. When a hematopoietic stem cell (HSC) develops a somatic mutation in a gene linked to myeloid malignancies, the process is known as clonal hematopoiesis. This mutation leads to the expansion of the mutated cell population compared with other stem cells. In individuals without diagnosed hematologic disorders or unexplained cytopenias, this expansion is characterized by a variant allele fraction (VAF) of 2% or more.

All mature blood cells throughout life are produced by HSCs. A single lineage of HSCs makes a disproportionately large contribution to the population of mature blood cells during CH. It is interesting to note that age-related CH does not result from a straightforward depletion in HSCs. In fact, older people have more abundant HSCs in their bone marrow than younger people.

There are standardized criteria for CCUS, MDS, and MDS/myeloproliferative neoplasms (MPNs) that can be used to characterize cytopenia, a frequent characteristic of CH. These criteria include absolute neutrophil counts $< 1.8 \times 10^9$/L for leukopenia, platelet counts $< 150 \times 10^9$/L for thrombocytopenia, and hemoglobin (Hb) values < 13 g/dL in males and <12 g/dL in females for anemia.[5,6]

Clonal hematopoiesis of indeterminate potential is characterized by the presence of somatic mutations linked to hematologic malignancies in people without cytopenias or signs of an underlying hematologic malignancy. Among the many distinctive gene mutations, *DNMT3A*, *TET2*, and *ASXL1* are often occurring ones. An increased (>10-fold) risk of developing a hematopoietic malignancy is related to CHIP, which is generally frequent in the aging population.[1]

The number of mutations present in an individual affects the likelihood of progression to CHIP. The presence of several driving mutations points to clonal evolution, whereby the blood cells pick up additional mutations along the way to become fully malignant cells.

Blood counts in CHIP are within normal range; however, a larger red cell distribution width (RDW) is linked to a higher risk of progression. Red blood cell size variation is quantified by the RDW. A greater RDW may indicate ineffective hematopoiesis (the production of blood cells), which is thought to be the underlying cause of declining counts and the progression to malignant conditions.

Clonal cytopenias of undetermined significance is characterized by the development of low blood cell counts in one or morel lineages. The development of a myeloid malignancy is being sped up by this situation. Comparatively, CCUS is linked to the presence of clones and ineffective blood cell formation, which results in low blood cell counts in one or more blood cell lineages. Although having low blood cell counts in one or more blood cell lineages, idiopathic cytopenia of uncertain significance (ICUS) does not match the requirements for MDS. The lack of somatic driver mutations distinguishes ICUS from CCUS, which is unrelated to clonal processes. This distinction is essential as CCUS is linked to a noticeably worse prognosis. CHIP has a very low probability of developing myeloid malignancies, whereas CCUS significantly raises this risk. The predisposing genetic alterations observed in CCUS are not present in idiopathic cytopenia of undetermined significance (IDUS), which has a varied illness trajectory.[3,5,7]

■ MANAGEMENT OF MYELOID PRECURSOR CONDITIONS

Since PML is a newly recognized and introduced subcategory in the classification of hematolymphoid neoplasms, much prospective studies are still not available on this topic. Hence, this entity currently requires management and follow-up of patients based on experience and opinion of experts in this field.

There is ongoing relevant discussion regarding the investigations to be done in incidentally discovered cases of PMLs as these lesions have high prevalence in older population and are uncertain in progression and clinical course.

Establishing follow-up clinics (with a multidisciplinary team of professionals) for counseling, monitoring, and regular follow-up of patients of PMLs can be done and has already been started by some institutions. Patients should be advised to undergo regular complete blood count every 3-6 months and a bone marrow aspiration/trephine biopsy in case of cytopenias. Also keeping increased mortality because of cardiovascular risk associated with CHIP/CCUS in mind, such patients should be evaluated regularly and managed accordingly.[8,9]

Studies are needed to determine optimal treatment approaches, including the use of targeted therapies and HSC transplantation for high-risk patients of PMLs.

In addition, more research is needed to identify predictive biomarkers and risk stratification tools that can help guide treatment decisions for high-risk individuals with PMLs. This will not only aid in selecting appropriate therapeutic interventions but also help in monitoring treatment response and disease progression.[8,10]

Collaborative efforts across multiple institutions and countries will be essential to collect sufficient data and conduct large-scale clinical trials. This will enable the development of evidence-based guidelines for the management of high-risk PMLs and improve patient outcomes.

> **BOX 1** | **Recommended management and follow-up of cases of PMLs.**
>
> - *ICUS*:
>   - CBC with differential, history, and physical annually or semiannually
> - *CCUS*:
>   - CBC with differential every 3–6 months
>   - History and physical annually or semiannually
>   - Repeat bone marrow biopsy if counts worsen
>   - Assess cardiovascular risk
> - *CHIP*:
>   - Routine health maintenance
>   - Consider annual CBC with differential
>   - Assess cardiovascular risk
>
> (CBC: complete blood count; CCUS: clonal cytopenias of undetermined significance; CHIP: clonal hematopoiesis of indeterminate potential; ICUS: idiopathic cytopenia of uncertain significance; PMLs: precursor myeloid lesions)

Moreover, it is crucial to establish a standardized reporting system for PMLs to facilitate data collection and comparison across different studies. This will help in identifying common patterns and trends, ultimately leading to a better understanding of the disease and improved treatment strategies.

Overall, the establishment of specific therapeutic interventions for high-risk PMLs is an ongoing research area. Further studies, collaboration, and the development of evidence-based guidelines are necessary to optimize patient care and improve outcomes in this population **(Box 1)**.

CONCLUSION

Since precursor myeloid neoplasms is a newly recognized entity in latest classification of hematolymphoid neoplasms; there is lot of scope of research in this field. Consistent monitoring; follow-up along with reassurance, education and counseling of patients and attendants plays a critical role in effectively managing these conditions.

REFERENCES

1. Arber D, Orazi A, Hasserjian RP, Borowitz MJ, Calvo KR, Kvasnicka HM, et al. International consensus classification of myeloid neoplasms and acute leukemias: Integrating morphologic, clinical, and genomic data. Blood. 2022;140(11):1200-28.
2. Alaggio R, Amador C, Anagnostopoulos I, Attygalle AD, Araujo IBO, Berti E, et al. The 5th edition of the World Health Organization Classification of haematolymphoid tumours: Lymphoid neoplasms. Leukemia. 2022;36(7):1720-48.
3. Zink F, Stacey SN, Norddahl GL, Frigge ML, Magnusson OT, Jonsdottir I, et al. Clonal hematopoiesis, with and without candidate driver mutations, is common in the elderly. Blood. 2017;130:742-52.

4. Jaiswal S, Natarajan P, Silver AJ, Gibson CJ, Bick AG, Shvartz E, et al. Clonal hematopoiesis and risk of atherosclerotic cardiovascular disease. N Engl J Med. 2017;377:111-21.
5. Malcovati L, Gallì A, Travaglino E, Ambaglio I, Rizzo E, Molteni E, et al. Clinical significance of somatic mutation in unexplained blood cytopenia. Blood. 2017;129:3371-8.
6. Osman AEWG. When are idiopathic and clonal cytopenias of unknown significance (ICUS or CCUS)? Hematol Am Soc Hematol Educ Program. 2021;2021:399-404.
7. Jaiswal S, Fontanillas P, Flannick J, Manning A, Grauman PV, Mar BG, et al. Age-related clonal hematopoiesis associated with adverse outcomes. N Engl J Med. 2014;371: 2488-98.
8. Gondek LP, DeZern AE. Assessing clonal haematopoiesis: Clinical burdens and benefits of diagnosing myelodysplastic syndrome precursor states. Lancet Haematol. 2020;7:e73-e81.
9. Steensma DP, Bolton KL. What to tell your patient with clonal hematopoiesis and why: Insights from 2 specialized clinics. Blood. 2020;136:1623-31.
10. Xie Z, Nanaa A, Saliba An, He R, Viswanatha D, Nguyen P, et al. Treatment outcome of clonal cytopenias of undetermined significance: A single-institution retrospective study. Blood Cancer J. 2021;11:43.

CHAPTER 3

Gene Therapy in Hematological Diseases

Summyia Farooq, Nuzhat Samoon

■ INTRODUCTION

Gene therapy involves the therapeutic intervention in a patient's genetic disorder by the introduction of specific genetic material that modifies cellular functions.[1] This method effectively modifies an individual's genetic composition, aiming to restore the functionality of essential proteins.[1] Proteins serve as the cellular workhorses and form the structural foundation of the body's tissues.[1] Gene therapy offers compensation for genetic alterations through various methods. One such approach is gene transfer therapy, which involves the introduction of new genetic material into cells. If a mutated gene leads to a defective or absent protein crucial for normal cellular function, gene transfer therapy can insert a healthy copy of the gene to restore the protein's functionality. Alternatively, even in the presence of a genetic alteration, gene therapy can introduce an alternative gene that encodes instructions for a protein essential for enabling proper cellular function. This approach aims to compensate for genetic deficiencies and promote normal cellular activities. Genome editing represents a relatively new technique with potential applications in gene therapy. Instead of adding new genetic material, genome editing employs gene-editing tools to modify the existing DNA within a cell. This technology allows for precise additions, removals, or alterations of genetic material at specific locations in the genome. One well-known genome editing method is CRISPR-Cas9.

In gene therapy, the use of vectors is a critical step for delivering genetic material to the target tissues or cells. Vectors are engineered to transport and deliver genetic material. There are two primary types of vectors: viral and non-viral. Viral vector-based gene therapy involves the in vivo introduction of therapeutic genes into a patient using these vectors. These vectors are derived from retroviruses, adenoviruses (Ads), or adeno-associated viruses (AAVs) **(Figs. 1 and 2)**. Alternatively, a therapeutic transgene can be delivered ex vivo, where a patient's cells are extracted, cultured outside of the patient's body, genetically modified, and subsequently reintroduced into the patient after the therapeutic transgene therapy.

CHAPTER 3: Gene Therapy in Hematological Diseases   17

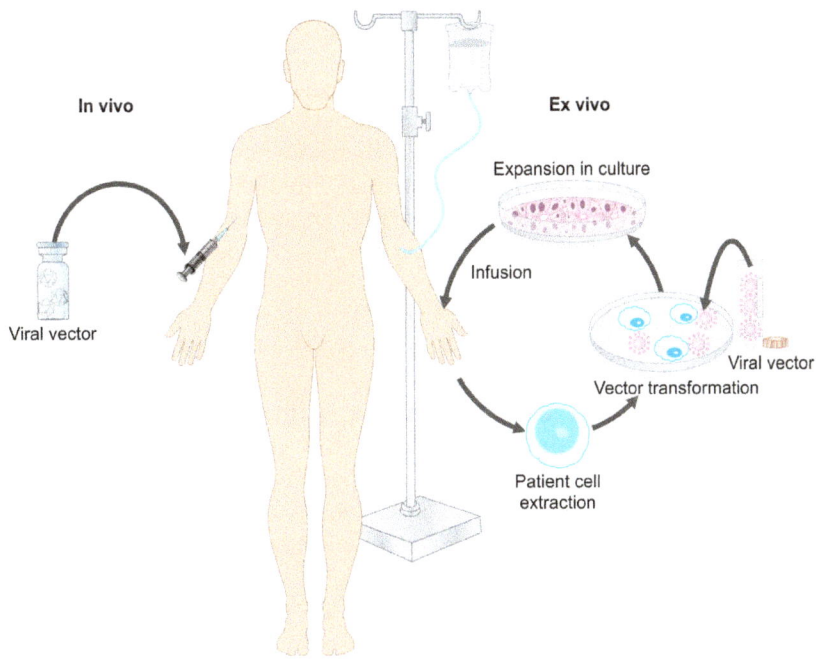

FIG. 1: Illustration of two primary methods of gene therapy.

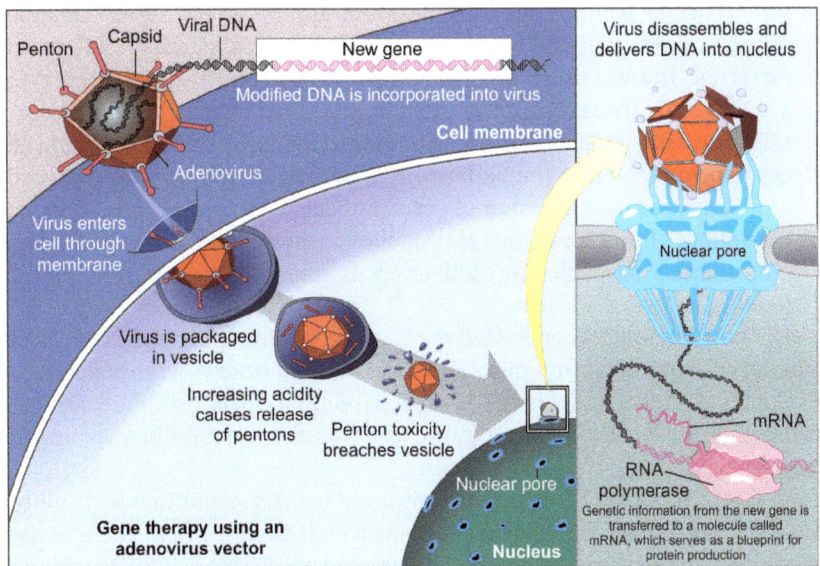

FIG. 2: The diagram illustrates the direct insertion of a new gene into a cell. To facilitate this process, a carrier known as a vector is genetically engineered to transport and deliver the gene. An adenovirus is employed to introduce the DNA into the nucleus of the cell. It is important to emphasize that the introduced DNA does not become integrated into a chromosome within the cell. Instead, it remains separate from the host cell's chromosomal DNA. This method ensures that the newly introduced gene functions independently without permanent integration into the cell's genomic DNA.

There are four fundamental gene therapy approaches, each serving a distinct purpose:
1. *Gene replacement*: This approach involves the substitution of a malfunctioning gene with a fully functional one. The non-working gene is replaced by a functional counterpart to restore normal cellular function.
2. *Gene silencing*: In this method, a toxic mutated gene is intentionally deactivated or "silenced." This silencing prevents the expression of the harmful gene, thereby mitigating its detrimental effects.
3. *Gene addition*: Gene addition entails the introduction of an exogenous gene in excess to influence cellular function positively. This approach involves augmenting the genetic makeup with additional genetic material to enhance cellular processes.
4. *Gene editing*: Gene editing allows for permanent manipulation of a patient's genome. This approach involves precise alterations to the patient's genetic code, enabling the modification of specific genes to correct or modify their function permanently.

These four gene therapy approaches offer diverse strategies for addressing genetic diseases and disorders.[2]

- *In vivo gene therapy*: In this approach, a vector carrying a therapeutic transgene is directly administered into the patient. The therapeutic genetic material is introduced into the patient's body to address the specific genetic condition.
- *Ex vivo gene therapy*: Ex vivo gene therapy involves a more complex process. First, patient's cells or cells from an allogeneic source are extracted. These cells are then genetically modified using a vector carrying a therapeutic transgene. After genetic modification, the cells undergo a selection and expansion process in culture. Finally, the engineered cells are reintroduced into the patient. This method allows for precise genetic modification and expansion of corrected cells before reintroduction into the patient's body. These two approaches, in vivo and ex vivo gene therapy, offer distinct strategies for delivering therapeutic genetic material and treating genetic disorders.

Dr Stanfield Rogers conducted the initial gene therapy trial on two sisters afflicted with hyperargininemia.[3] His approach was based on the observation that patients infected with the Shope papilloma virus exhibited reduced serum arginine levels. Regrettably, the trial was unsuccessful in reversing the disease.

In 1980, Dr Martin Cline made an attempt to insert recombinant β-globin into the bone marrow cells of two patients with β-thalassemia.[4] The transfected cells were then reintroduced into the patients. While groundbreaking at the time, this pioneering ex vivo gene therapy attempt also ended in failure.

It was not until the early 1990s that viral vector gene therapies achieved clinical success. A trial led by French Anderson, Michael Blaese, and Steven Rosenberg employed an ex vivo strategy to treat a patient named DeSilva, who suffered from adenosine deaminase deficiency severe combined immunodeficiency disease (ADA-SCID). Several infusions of T cells transformed with a recombinant retrovirus carrying the *ADA* gene were administered, marking the first successful gene therapy in humans.[5,6]

Viral vector systems for gene therapy typically consist of several essential components, each with distinct functions:
- *Protein capsid and/or envelope*: The protein capsid and/or envelope of the viral vector encapsulate the genetic payload (transgene) and play a crucial role in determining the vector's tissue or cell tropism, that is, the specific types of cells it can infect. They also contribute to antigen recognition, which may trigger an immune response.
- *Transgene*: The transgene is the gene of interest that is introduced into the target cells. This transgene serves to confer a desired therapeutic effect when expressed in the affected cells.
- *Regulatory cassette*: The regulatory cassette includes a combined enhancer/promoter region that can function as an episome or integrate into the host cell's chromosomes. It controls the stable or transient somatic expression of the transgene, regulating when and how the gene of interest is expressed.

The majority of gene therapy vectors are based on three primary viral strategies: Ads, AAVs, and lentiviruses (retroviruses). These viruses are commonly used as vector platforms for gene delivery **(Fig. 3)**. These platforms hold significant promise for future applications as commercialized drugs and in ongoing clinical trials within the field of gene therapy.

Adenovirus vectors are known for their large payload capacities, making them suitable for transient targeted gene delivery. These vectors are derived from a large and complex non-enveloped virus that primarily causes infections of the upper respiratory tract.

The structure of Ad is characterized by an icosahedral protein capsid, which serves as a protective shell for its genetic material. Within this capsid, Ad can accommodate a linear, double-stranded DNA genome ranging from 26 to 45 kilobases in length. The Ad genome features hairpin-like inverted terminal repeats (ITRs).[7,8] These ITRs play a crucial role in promoting primase-independent DNA replication, facilitating the replication of the Ad genome.

The Ad genome encodes five "early-phase" genes, namely *E1A, E1B, E2, E3,* and *E4*.[7] These early-phase genes are transcribed before the initiation of viral DNA replication. Among these, the "immediate-early" *E1A* gene is essential for the transcription of other viral genes (e.g., *E1B, E2, E3,* and *E4*) responsible for viral DNA synthesis. E1B, in particular, plays a critical role in counteracting the host cell's activation of apoptosis by binding to and inactivating p53, thereby permitting viral replication to proceed.[9] These characteristics make Ad vectors valuable tools for gene therapy applications.

The "late-phase" genes (L1–L5) play a crucial role in various aspects of the Ad lifecycle, including virus assembly, release, and the lysis of the host cell.[10] These late-phase gene products are derived from the five late transcriptional

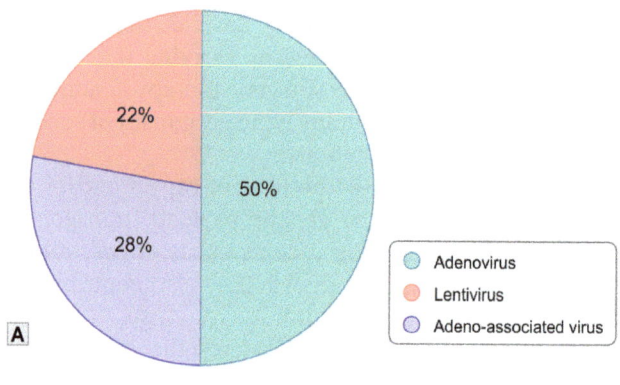

Vectors	Number of clinical trials
Adenovirus	575
Adeno-associated virus	250
Lentivirus	315
Total	1,140

FIGS. 3A AND B: Illustration of a summary of viral vectors that have been utilized in clinical trials for gene therapy. (A) A pie chart provides a visual representation of the percentage distribution of viral vectors used in these clinical trials, categorizing them into adenovirus, adeno-associated virus, or lentivirus vectors. (B) A table displays the current number of clinical trials associated with each type of viral vector, offering specific data on the utilization of adenovirus, adeno-associated virus, and lentivirus vectors. The data source for this information is the Wiley database on gene therapy trials worldwide. This figure serves as a valuable reference for understanding the prevalence and distribution of viral vectors in the context of gene therapy clinical trials.

units. These units are generated through alternative splicing and polyadenylation of the major late messenger RNAs, as depicted in **Figure 4**.[11] This orchestrated process ensures the production of key components necessary for the final stages of the viral lifecycle, ultimately leading to the release of new viral particles and the destruction of the host cell. The Ad viral capsid has a diameter ranging from 90 to 100 nanometers (nm) and is constructed from various structural proteins. These proteins include hexon (capsid protein II), penton base (capsid protein III), fiber (capsid protein IV), capsid protein precursors, such as pIIIa, pVI, and pVIII, and capsid protein IX. Additionally, the virion core contains proteins denoted as V, VII, and X.[12]

Hexons are the most abundant structural components, and they form the majority of the capsid. At the apex of the icosahedral vertices, there are 12 penton proteins, which give rise to the protruding fibers. These fibers are essential for the virus's attachment to host cells.

CHAPTER 3: Gene Therapy in Hematological Diseases

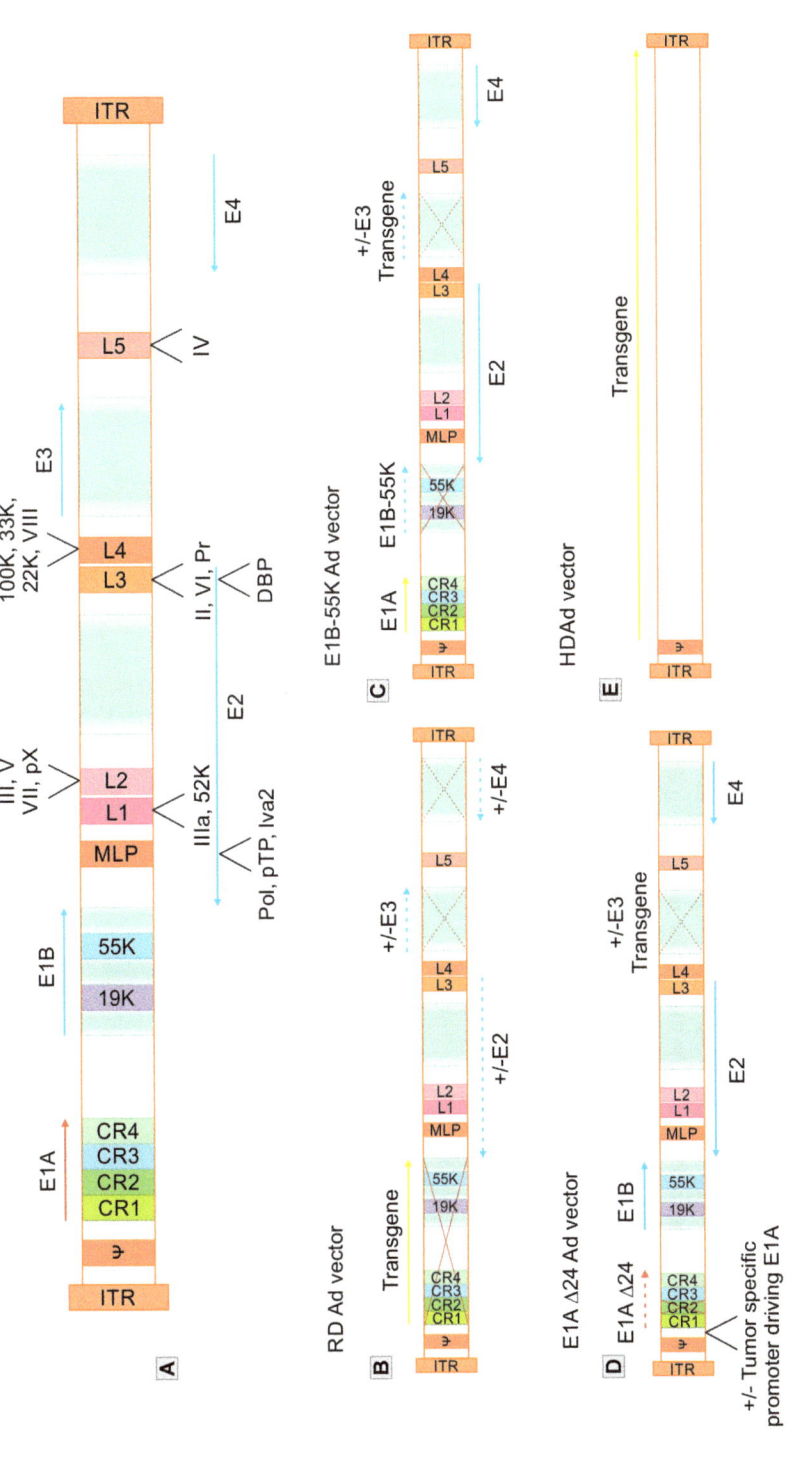

FIGS. 4A TO E: A schematic representation of the wild-type adenovirus type 5 (Ad5) genome and common genetic modifications made in Ad5-based vectors. *Continued...*

FIGS. 4A TO E: *Continued...* (A) The top section displays the structure of the wild-type Ad5 genome. It consists of a 36-kilobase (kb) genome featuring four early transcription elements (E1, E2, E3, and E4), five late expression genes (L1–L5), cis-packaging elements (ψ), and two inverted terminal repeat sequences (ITR). Various genes in the genome are labeled, such as E1A, E1B, E2, E3, and E4, each with specific functions. (B) The replication-defective (RD) vector is depicted, where the E1A and E1B regions are deleted and replaced with an expression cassette containing an exogenous promoter and a transgene of interest. Deletion of E3 and E4 regions may also occur to accommodate larger insertions and eliminate leaky expression of other viral genes. (C) The E1B-55K replication-competent vector is shown, with the E1B-55K region being deleted. In some vectors, the E3 region is deleted and replaced with an expression cassette. (D) The E1A-Δ24 (Δ24) replication-competent vector is illustrated. In this vector, the CR2 region in E1A is deleted, and the E1A promoter can be replaced with various tumor-specific promoters to drive the expression of the CR2-deleted *E1A* gene. Similar to other designs, the E3 region can be deleted and replaced with an expression cassette. (E) Helper-dependent Ad vectors (HDAds) are shown at the bottom. In these vectors, most or all of the Ad genomic elements are replaced with a therapeutic expression cassette. However, cis-packaging sequences (ψ) and ITRs are retained. HDAds are propagated in the presence of an Ad helper vector (yellow arrow) (Reference not provided). These genetic modifications allow Ad5-based vectors to be tailored for specific gene therapy applications.

The V, VII, and X proteins primarily associate with the viral genome and play crucial roles in processes such as genome replication, condensation, and other assembly processes.[13] These structural and core proteins collectively contribute to the formation and functionality of the Ad capsid.

The IIIa proteins are located on the inner surface of the capsid and play a pivotal role in driving the assembly of the packaged genome. They achieve this by binding to L1 52/55K and stabilizing the vertex regions through interactions with the penton base, hexon, and VI proteins.[14]

The VI proteins serve dual functions. They link the viral core to the inner icosahedral shell, contributing to the structural integrity of the virus. Additionally, they act as lytic factors during endosomal disruption, facilitating the release of the viral genome into the host cell's cytoplasm.[15]

The VIII proteins are responsible for binding to the peripentonal hexons, thereby contributing to the stabilization of the viral capsid.[16]

The terminal protein (pTP) plays a crucial role in gene replication. It covalently attaches to the 5-ends of the Ad genome, enhancing the replication process.[17] These various proteins and their functions collectively enable the Ad to carry out its infectious cycle.

Adenovirus vectors play a significant role in gene therapy, primarily due to their unique advantages and attributes:

- *High transduction efficiency*: Ad vectors are known for their ability to efficiently transduce both quiescent (non-dividing) and dividing cells. This characteristic is particularly advantageous in delivering therapeutic genes to various cell types, making them versatile tools in gene therapy applications.
- *Epichromosomal determination*: Ad vectors exhibit epichromosomal determination in host cells. This means that the genetic material introduced by the vector remains separate from the host cell's chromosomal DNA. This is beneficial as it prevents integration of the therapeutic gene into the host genome, reducing the risk of unintended genetic disruptions.
- Broad *tissue tropism*: Ad vectors possess a wide range of tropism, allowing them to target and infect various types of tissues effectively. This versatility is essential for addressing a broad spectrum of genetic diseases and disorders affecting different tissues and organs.
- *Scalable production systems*: Ad vectors offer the attainability of expandable production systems. This scalability is critical for producing the large quantities of vectors needed for clinical applications, ensuring that gene therapy treatments are readily available.[18]

Despite these advantages, it is important to note that Ad vectors are derived from human serotypes HAd2 and HAd5. One of the primary challenges in Ad vector development is overcoming the pre-existing viral immunity that exists in a significant portion of the general population.[19] This issue necessitates strategies for vector modifications and immunomodulation to enhance the safety and efficacy of Ad-based gene therapy.

The development of Ad vectors has progressed through various generations, each with distinct characteristics and improvements. The first generation of Ad vectors is characterized as follows:

First generation: In this early stage, Ad vectors were engineered using transgene cassettes of up to 4.5 kilobases (kb) in length. These vectors were created by replacing the E1A/E1B region of the Ad genome with the transgene of interest. Notably, the removal of the *E1A* gene renders the recombinant Ad (rAd) unable to replicate within the host cell.[20]

To overcome this limitation and facilitate the production of first-generation Ad vectors, complementary cell lines such as HEK293 were designed. These cell lines were engineered to express the *E1A* and *E1B* genes, which are essential for Ad replication. Therefore, the introduction of E1A and E1B into these cells enabled the production of first-generation Ad vectors.[21] These vectors served as early tools in the field of gene therapy but had limitations related to the potential for host immune responses and restricted transgene capacity. Subsequent generations of Ad vectors aimed to address these limitations and improve vector performance.

The second generation of Ad vectors indeed made significant improvements, but it continued to face some notable challenges:

- *Host immune response*: Despite the enhancements in the second-generation Ad vectors, the de novo expression of Ad proteins within the transduced cells could still activate the host immune response. This immune response remained a concern, potentially leading to the clearance of vector-transduced cells and thereby limiting the efficacy of the therapy.[22]
- *Potential for replication-competent adenovirus (RCA) generation*: The risk of generating RCA persisted due to the potential for spontaneous homologous recombination between the vector and the E1 region from HEK293 during genome amplification. The generation of RCA raised safety concerns and had the potential to affect the reliability of Ad vector production (reference not provided).

In the second generation of Ad vectors, efforts were made to address these issues by deleting additional early gene regions such as E2a, E2b, or E4, allowing for larger transgene cassettes. New vector forms, including temperature-sensitive rAd vectors, were developed by making specific genetic modifications. These modifications aimed to reduce late gene expression and lower the cytotoxic T-lymphocyte response.[23-27] To compensate for the deleted genes, engineered production cell lines were used. However, the deletion of *E2* and/or *E4* genes resulted in reduced vector titers, which could negatively impact the process of viral vector amplification.[28] Despite these challenges, the second-generation Ad vectors represented an improvement in terms of immune responses and transgene capacity.

The third generation of Ad vectors, often referred to as "gutless" or "helper-dependent" Ad vectors, represent a significant advancement in gene therapy:
- These vectors, also known as "high-capacity" adenoviral vectors (HCAds), are characterized by the deletion of nearly all viral sequences from the Ad genome, except for the packaging signal and ITRs. As a result, HCAds can accommodate much larger transgenes, with a capacity of approximately 36 kb.[29]
- The HCAd genome is transfected into HEK293 producer cells that express Cre recombinase. In the presence of Cre recombinase, the HCAd genome is processed and activated for replication. Replication and packaging are permitted by the viral proteins provided by the helper genome.[30] This helper-dependent system enhances the safety and efficiency of HCAds.
- HCAds offer several advantages over previous generations of Ad vectors. They have reduced immunogenicity, which decreases the likelihood of provoking immune responses in the host. HCAds also enable prolonged transduction within the host cell, leading to sustained therapeutic effects. Moreover, their significantly larger cargo capacity allows for the accommodation of multiple transgene cassettes or therapeutic genes. These genes can be driven by their larger native promoters and enhancers, enabling the mimicry of physiological levels of gene expression, which can be crucial for certain therapeutic applications (reference not provided).

The development of third-generation HCAds represents a substantial step forward in gene therapy, with the potential to overcome many of the limitations associated with earlier Ad vector generations.

Adeno-associated virus vectors are an essential tool in gene therapy, and they have a unique structure and genome. Here are some key characteristics of AAV vectors:
- *Discovery*: AAV vectors were discovered by Bob Atchison in 1965.[31] These vectors are known as dependoparvoviruses because they rely on other viruses, such as Ad, to provide essential functions for their life cycle.
- *Dependence on Helper viruses*: AAV is classified as a dependoparvovirus because it lacks the necessary genes for replication and expression of its own genome. Instead, it relies on helper functions provided by other viruses, including the *Ad E1, E2a, E4*, and *VA RNA* genes.[32,33] This dependence on helper viruses is a critical aspect of AAV biology.
- *Genome*: The AAV genome is a single-stranded DNA. It contains four known open reading frames (ORFs). The first ORF encodes several Rep proteins, including Rep40, Rep52, and Rep68, as well as three viral capsid proteins: VP1, VP2, and VP3.[34] These proteins play essential roles in AAV replication and capsid formation.
- *Sub-genomic mRNAs*: AAV also utilizes nested sub-genomic mRNAs. One of these is the assembly-activating protein (AAP), which is involved in shuttling capsid monomers to the nucleolus, where capsid assembly occurs.[35] Another recently discovered sub-genomic mRNA is the

membrane-associated accessory protein (MAAP),[36] which likely plays a role in AAV biology, although its functions are still being elucidated.

○ Adeno-associated virus vectors have become a prominent choice in gene therapy due to their safety profile, versatility, and ability to deliver therapeutic genes to target cells effectively. Their dependence on helper viruses, such as Ad, is harnessed in the laboratory to create recombinant AAV vectors for gene therapy applications **(Fig. 5)**.

Adeno-associated virus has become a valuable vector for gene therapy due to its unique characteristics and versatility. Here are some key points regarding AAV as a vector for gene therapy:

- *Vector genome cloning*: The AAV genome was first successfully cloned by researchers, including Samulski et al.[37] This breakthrough allowed for the manipulation and engineering of recombinant AAV (rAAV) vectors for various applications.
- *Gutted genome for transgene packaging*: A significant advancement in AAV vector technology was the realization that the vector's genome could be "gutted," meaning nearly all viral genes could be removed, leaving only the essential ITR elements. The gutted genome could then be replaced with a promoter of choice and the gene of interest. This innovation opened the door to using AAV vectors to deliver specific genes for therapeutic purposes.
- *Human trials*: In 1995, the first demonstration of an AAV vector used in humans occurred when researchers delivered the cystic fibrosis transmembrane regulator (*CFTR*) gene, packaged with the AAV2 capsid (rAAV2-CFTR), into a cystic fibrosis patient.[38] This marked a significant milestone in the development of AAV-based gene therapy.

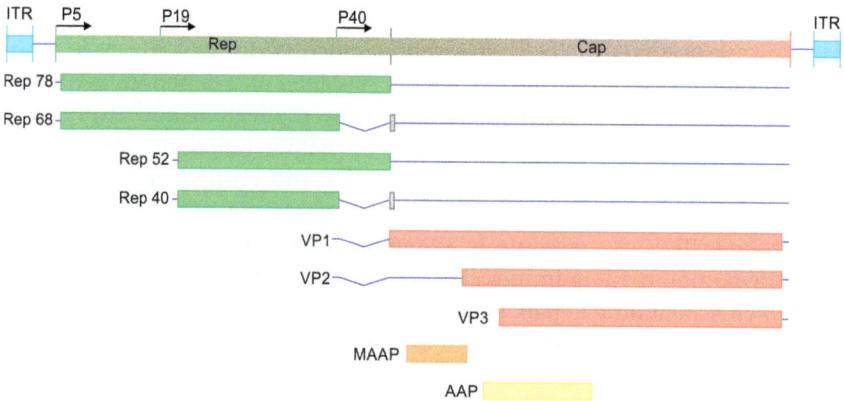

FIG. 5: Schematic of the AAV genome and sites used for PCR screening. The AAV genome comprised four known open reading frames, rep (green), cap (salmon), MAAP (orange), and AAP (yellow). The rep and cap ORFs encode four and three isoforms, respectively. Transcription is driven by the viral P5, P19, and P40 promoters (arrows). The genome is flanked by inverted terminal repeat (ITR, cyan) sequences.

- *Vector size limitation*: A key consideration in AAV vector design is that the wild-type AAV genome is approximately 4.7 kb in size. Consequently, AAV vectors are limited to a capacity of approximately 5 kb. This size constraint can be a limitation when attempting to package larger or multiple transgenes.
- *Strategies for expanding vector size*: To overcome the size limitation, researchers have developed various strategies, such as using ITR-mediated recombination to create dual-vector systems that can express "oversized" transgenes.[39-41] Other approaches for expanding vector size include homology-based methods,[42] RNA trans-splicing,[43] or protein "trans-splicing" through split intein designs.[44,45]

These advancements in AAV vector design and engineering have expanded the utility of AAV vectors in gene therapy, making them a valuable tool for delivering therapeutic genes to treat a wide range of genetic diseases and disorders.

Lentivirus vectors, which belong to the retroviridae family, are essential tools in gene therapy. Here are some key details about their structure and genome:

- *Retroviruses*: Lentiviruses are a genus within the retroviridae family. Retroviruses are spherical, enveloped viruses with single-stranded RNA genomes. They have a diameter of approximately 100 nanometers.[46,47]
- *RNA genome*: Lentiviral particles encapsulate two sense-strand RNA molecules that are bound by nucleocapsid proteins. The viral genome contains long terminal repeats (LTRs) that have unique sequences (U5 and U3) at the 5′ and 3′ termini, respectively. The R sequence is common to both ends. A cis-acting sequence, known as psi, is located just outside of the LTR and is crucial for signaling viral genome encapsulation.[48,49]
- *Core protein genes*: Retroviruses, including lentiviruses, have essential core protein genes. These genes include gag, pol, and env. The gag gene encodes information for transmembrane and envelope glycoproteins that determine the virus's cellular tropism.[50] Tat supports transcriptional activation and RNA polymerase II elongation by binding adjacently to the LTR.[51] Rev orchestrates nuclear export of spliced and unspliced viral RNA by binding to a motif in the env gene region.[52]
- *Auxiliary genes*: Lentiviruses, such as HIV-1, have an additional set of auxiliary genes, including vif, vpr, vpu, and nef. These auxiliary genes play roles in increasing the viral titer and enhancing the pathogenicity of the virus.[53,54]
- *Lentiviral vectors in gene therapy*: Lentiviruses are used as vectors in gene therapy due to their ability to effectively deliver genes into target cells. They have a relatively large packaging capacity, capable of accommodating up to 9 kb of genetic material.[55] This makes them suitable for transferring larger or multiple genes for therapeutic purposes.

Lentivirus vectors have proven valuable in gene therapy applications due to their efficient gene delivery and capacity to carry relatively large transgenes. They are commonly used to treat genetic diseases and disorders by introducing therapeutic genes into patients' cells.

Lentiviral vectors offer distinct advantages in gene therapy, particularly when high-level expression of multiple genes is necessary to achieve therapeutic outcomes for specific diseases. Here are some key advantages and considerations:

- *Multigene expression*: Lentiviral vectors have demonstrated the capability to express multiple genes from a single vector.[56-58] This feature is crucial for addressing diseases or conditions that require the coordinated expression of several genes to achieve therapeutic effects.
- *Transduction of postmitotic and quiescent cells*: Lentiviral vectors can transduce postmitotic and quiescent cells effectively. In contrast, other retrovirus-based platforms, such as gamma-retroviral vectors, typically require active cell division for successful infection. Quiescent cells, which are not actively dividing, are often resistant to viral infection due in part to the innate immune response. Stimulation of mitotic entry can facilitate viral transduction in these cells.[59-63]
- *Immune responses*: Depending on the specific design of the lentiviral vector, they can elicit relatively weak immune responses.[64-66] This is advantageous because a robust immune response can limit the effectiveness of gene therapy. Lentiviral vectors are engineered to minimize immunogenicity, allowing for more successful and sustained gene expression.

These characteristics make lentiviral vectors a preferred choice in gene therapy when multiple gene expression and the transduction of non-dividing cells are critical requirements. Their ability to achieve high-level expression in a variety of cell types, along with their relatively low immunogenicity, positions them as valuable tools for addressing a wide range of genetic diseases and disorders.

Recent medical advances in gene therapy and molecular studies have had a significant impact on the development of safer and better-tolerated therapies for patients with hematologic cancers. These clinically functional "gene therapies" are now showing promising roles in hematological disorders. Here are some key points regarding these advances:

- *Improved delivery systems*: Advances in delivery systems have contributed to more efficient treatments and better clinical outcomes for patients with hereditary diseases in hematology. These improvements have led to decreased genotoxicity, making gene therapy safer and more effective.
- *Gene editing technologies*: One of the notable recent advances in the field is the application of gene-editing technologies for the treatment of human diseases. Technologies such as zinc-finger nucleases, CRISPR/Cas, and TALENs can be used to edit target genes, allowing for gene knockdown or repair. These technologies offer the potential to "correct" or "repair" mutant genes, bringing them back to normal without causing genotoxicity in other genes.

These advancements represent significant progress in the development of gene therapies for hematological disorders. They offer hope for improved treatment options and potentially curative approaches for patients with genetic blood disorders and hematologic cancers. Gene-editing technologies, in particular, hold great promise for the precise correction of genetic mutations, leading to better patient outcomes and reduced side effects. Achieving the correction of 100% of malignant cells, especially in actively proliferating cells, can be challenging. Even if the initial disease-inducing mutation is normalized, it may not necessarily lead to the elimination of all malignant cells. In response to this challenge, treatment strategies have been designed to specifically target and eliminate malignant cells. One notable recent advancement in this regard is CAR-T-cell therapy, particularly in its application to B-cell malignancies. CAR-T-cell therapy represents a significant breakthrough in the field of cancer treatment and offers a promising approach for precisely targeting and eradicating malignant cells. Immuno-gene therapy, exemplified by approaches like GVAX and granulocyte macrophage colony-stimulating factor (GM-CSF) producing whole tumor cell vaccines, has demonstrated promising results in the treatment of hematological malignancies. These therapies harness the power of the immune system to target and combat cancer cells.

Additionally, the use of RNA interference and suicide gene-based strategies for regulating graft-versus-host disease (GVHD)[67] has been actively researched in the context of hematological malignancies. These techniques aim to enhance the safety and efficacy of therapies, particularly in the context of stem cell transplantation and allogeneic therapies.

Second-generation chimeric antigen receptors (CARs) represent important tools in immuno-gene therapy. They enable the redirection of antigen-specific T cells independently of the HLA-restriction, allowing[68] for a more targeted and effective immune response against cancer cells. These advancements in immuno-gene therapy hold significant promise for improving the outcomes of patients with hematological malignancies.

Chimeric antigen receptors are innovative immune cell receptors designed to enhance the targeting of specific antigens on the surface of cancer cells. These CARs are hybrid receptors that consist of several components:
- *Ligand for cell surface molecule*: The CAR includes a ligand that binds to a specific cell surface molecule or antigen expressed on the target cancer cell. This ligand is often a single-chain variable fragment (scFv) derived from a monoclonal antibody or an antigen-binding fragment (Fab).
- *Signaling domains*: The CAR is equipped with signaling domains that are crucial for initiating and regulating T-cell functions. These signaling domains are typically derived from the CD3ζ chain and other co-stimulatory molecules, such as CD28 or 4-1BB.

The CAR is designed to redirect T-cell function toward cancer cells expressing the targeted antigen. This means that CAR-T cells express both their endogenous T-cell receptor (TCR) and the transduced CAR. This dual-receptor system allows CAR-T cells to specifically recognize and attack cancer cells that express the target antigen, providing a highly precise and effective immunotherapy approach for certain hematological malignancies and solid tumors.[69,70]

The production of CAR-T cells for clinical purposes is a carefully controlled process that involves several key steps:

- *T-cell collection*: The process begins with the collection of T cells from the patient's blood, which is typically accomplished through leukapheresis. During this procedure, a blood sample is taken, and the T cells are separated from the rest of the blood components.
- *T-cell isolation and activation*: The isolated T cells are then subjected to activation using antibodies specific for CD3 and/or CD28. This activation step stimulates the T cells and promotes their proliferation, which is essential for generating a sufficient number of CAR-T cells.
- *Transduction*: The T cells are transduced with the *CAR* gene. This genetic modification equips the T cells with the ability to recognize and target-specific antigens on cancer cells.
- *Cell expansion*: The transduced T cells are cultured and expanded in a controlled environment until the desired dose of CAR-T cells is achieved. This step is crucial to generate a sufficient quantity of therapeutic cells for treatment.
- *Quality control and assurance*: The CAR-T cells undergo a series of pre-defined quality control and assurance assays. These tests confirm the functionality and sterility of the CAR-T-cell product. Quality control measures ensure that the CAR-T cells meet the required standards for safety and efficacy.
- *Product release*: Once the CAR-T-cell product successfully passes quality control and assurance assessments, it is released for clinical use. This means that the CAR-T cells are deemed safe, functional, and ready for infusion into the patient.

The production of CAR-T cells is a highly regulated and precise process, with strict quality control measures in place to ensure the safety and effectiveness of the therapy.[71]

Studies that have evaluated CD19-targeted T cells in patients with B-cell malignancies have demonstrated the potency of CAR-engineered T cells. The clinical outcome of CAR-based approaches is influenced by several key parameters:

- *CAR design*: The design of the CAR is a critical factor. Different generations of CARs have been developed, with second-generation CARs being particularly effective. These CARs incorporate both activating and co-stimulatory signaling domains, leading to improved T-cell activation, cytokine secretion, expansion, and persistence.
- *T-cell production methods*: The methods used to produce CAR-T cells play a significant role in determining their function and clinical outcomes.

The isolation, activation, transduction, and expansion of T cells must be carefully optimized to generate high-quality therapeutic cells.
- *Conditioning chemotherapy*: The conditioning chemotherapy regimen used in conjunction with CAR-T-cell therapy can impact its effectiveness. Appropriate conditioning can help prepare the patient's immune system to receive and respond to CAR-T-cell treatment.
- *Patient selection*: Selecting the right patients for CAR-T-cell therapy is crucial. Factors, such as disease type and stage, overall health, and previous treatments can influence the outcomes of CAR-based approaches.

CARs have been developed to target various cell surface molecules, including CD19, HER2, GD2, prostate-specific membrane antigen (PSMA), and mesothelin. Among these, CAR-modified T-cells targeting CD19 have shown some of the most promising clinical outcomes. These therapies have demonstrated significant efficacy in treating patients with B-cell malignancies, offering a potential breakthrough in the management of these diseases.[72-75]

CD19 is a cell surface molecule that is primarily expressed by most B-cell leukemias and lymphomas. Importantly, it is not expressed in the tissues of normal B lineage cells. This unique expression pattern makes CD19 an ideal target for immunotherapies, such as CAR-T-cell therapy, aimed at treating B-cell malignancies.[76]

Patients with chronic lymphocytic leukemia (CLL) who undergo infusion of autologous CD19-targeted T cells may experience certain side effects or toxicities. Some common toxicities associated with this treatment approach include fever, hypotension (low blood pressure), lymphopenia (a decrease in the number of lymphocytes), and delayed tumor lysis syndrome. These side effects are important to monitor and manage during the course of treatment to ensure the safety and well-being of the patients.[74,75,77,78]

Bi-specific CARs represent an intriguing advancement in the field of CAR-T-cell therapy. These bi-specific CARs are designed to enhance the safety and efficacy of the approach by equipping T cells with the ability to recognize and target two distinct tumor antigens. There are two main approaches to achieve this:

1. *Dual CARs (CAR1 and CAR2)*: In this approach, T cells are genetically modified to express two fully autonomous CARs. Each CAR is specific for a unique tumor antigen. This means that a single T cell can effectively target and attack cancer cells expressing either of these two antigens. This approach increases the versatility of CAR-T cells and broadens their effectiveness against a wider range of cancer cells.[79,80]
2. *Co-expression of CAR and CCR*: In another approach aimed at reducing tumor activity, T cells are engineered to co-express a CAR and a chimeric cytokine receptor (CCR). The CCR is designed to interact with specific cytokines, which can affect the immune response. This combination can help modulate the T-cell response to the tumor, potentially reducing tumor activity.[79,80]

Both of these strategies represent innovative approaches to enhance the safety and efficacy of CAR-T-cell therapy by expanding the range of tumor antigens that can be targeted and by modulating the T-cell response to improve therapeutic outcomes.

Suicide gene therapy is an approach used to prevent GVHD in stem cell or organ transplant recipients. In this strategy, donor T cells are genetically modified ex vivo (outside the body) before being infused into the patients. These genetically modified T cells carry a suicide gene that can be activated to eliminate the T cells if they cause adverse effects, such as GVHD. Two methods have been tested in clinical trials:

1. *Thymidine kinase gene and ganciclovir*: In one approach, a vector is used to introduce the thymidine kinase gene into the donor T cells. After infusion, if these modified T cells cause GVHD or other complications, the drug ganciclovir can be administered. Thymidine kinase-expressing T cells will phosphorylate ganciclovir, leading to the death of these T cells, thus helping to control the adverse immune response.[81]
2. *Caspase-9*: Another system involves the incorporation of caspase-9 into T cells. Caspase-9 is a protein that can be triggered to initiate a self-destructive process in the T cells. To activate caspase-9, a dimerizing drug called AP1903 is administered. This drug induces the dimerization of caspase-9, leading to the selective elimination of the modified T cells. This approach offers a way to control GVHD by eliminating problematic T cells.[82]

Suicide gene therapy has shown promise as a means to regulate and manage GVHD, making it a potentially valuable strategy to improve the safety of stem cell or organ transplant procedures.

RNA interference (RNAi) and gene silencing are powerful techniques for targeting specific genes, and they have shown promise in various medical applications:

- *Double-stranded RNA (dsRNA)*: Double-stranded RNA is an effective way to target-specific genes. It can induce RNA interference by triggering the degradation of messenger RNA (mRNA) molecules that carry the genetic information for the target gene. This approach has been widely used in research and therapeutic applications.[83]
- *MicroRNAs (miRNA)*: Endogenous regulatory microRNAs, which are approximately 22 nucleotides long, play a role in gene regulation by binding to specific mRNA sequences and promoting their degradation or inhibiting their translation. These small RNAs are generated from longer primary transcripts (pri-miRNAs) and can be involved in the regulation of various genes and cellular processes.
- *Short interfering RNA (siRNA)*: Exogenous delivery of short-interfering RNA (siRNA) is another method to induce RNA interference. SiRNAs are synthetic molecules that can specifically target and silence the expression of a particular gene. They can be used to bypass the need for cellular transduction and nuclear processing. However, siRNAs are susceptible

to rapid degradation by ribonucleases, which can limit their systemic therapy applications.
- *Immunomodulatory approaches*: RNAi-based approaches have been explored in the treatment of various conditions, including cancer and inflammatory diseases like rheumatoid arthritis. By silencing the genes associated with inflammation, such as TNF, IL1, IL6, and IL18, these approaches aim to improve the pathological changes associated with the diseases.[84]
- *RNAi-mediated silencing of specific genes*: In specific medical contexts, RNAi has been used to target and silence the expression of particular genes associated with diseases. For example, silencing the MLL fusion gene (*MLL-AF9*) in precursor B-cell acute lymphoblastic leukemia (B-ALL) can lead to the arrest of cell maturation and halt the malignant behavior of these cells.[85]
- Hematopoietic stem cell (HSC) transplantation is an essential treatment option for various malignant and non-malignant disorders of the blood and immune systems. HSCs are multipotent stem cells that express the CD34 antigen and are primarily located in the bone marrow. Traditionally, HSCs have been harvested directly from the bone marrow, often obtained via the iliac crest.
- An alternative method for obtaining HSCs is from peripheral blood following treatment with hematopoietic growth factors, such as granulocyte-colony-stimulating factor (G-CSF), which is also known as Neupogen or Filgrastim. The G-CSF treatment is administered to donors twice daily over a period of 4–5 days to mobilize HSCs into the peripheral blood circulation.
- After G-CSF mobilization, the collection of HSCs is typically performed via leukapheresis. During leukapheresis, a specialized machine is used to separate the white blood cells from other blood components, including plasma and red blood cells, based on density centrifugation. This process results in a collection of white blood cells, which includes the CD34$^+$ HSC population. Additionally, the collected white blood cell compartment contains lymphocytes, granulocytes, and monocytes.
- For successful HSC transplantation and gene therapy applications, it is crucial to obtain a sufficient number of CD34$^+$ cells. This often involves collecting over 6 million CD34$^+$ cells per kilogram (kg) of the patient's body weight to ensure that a minimum of 3–5 million gene-modified cells per kg can be reintroduced to the patient.
- While G-CSF mobilization is effective in many cases, it may not be equally successful in all patients, particularly in those with conditions such as sickle-cell disease.[86] In such cases, alternative strategies and agents may be considered to enhance the collection of CD34$^+$ HSCs for transplantation.
- In cases where HSCs mobilize poorly with G-CSF, leading to an insufficient number of collected CD34$^+$ cells, alternative strategies have been

explored. Plerixafor, which is an inhibitor of C-X-C chemokine receptor type 4 (CXCR4), a receptor responsible for the homing of HSCs to the bone marrow, has been used to enhance HSC mobilization. Plerixafor can be used in conjunction with G-CSF mobilization or on its own, resulting in a substantial increase in the collection of CD34⁺ stem cells.[87] However, even with these advancements, in some cases, such as Fanconi anemia, it remains challenging to obtain adequate numbers of CD34⁺ cells.[88]

- HSC transplantation (HSCT) is a well-established and effective treatment for various malignant and non-malignant disorders of the blood and immune systems, including leukemia, lymphoma, and myeloma.[89] The primary goal of HSCT is to replenish the bone marrow and reconstitute the immune system with functional hematopoietic lineages.
- Allogeneic HSCT, which involves the transplantation of HSCs harvested from a healthy donor, is a crucial therapeutic option for the cure of rare inherited diseases of the blood and immune systems. These inherited disorders encompass a wide range of conditions, including primary immune deficiencies, hemoglobinopathies, lysosomal storage and metabolic diseases, and bone marrow failure syndromes.[90]
- While allogeneic HSCT can provide curative benefits, it has its limitations, including the requirement for a genetically matched donor, which may not be available for up to 70% of cases. Additional challenges associated with allogeneic HSCT include graft rejection, delayed immune reconstitution, GVHD, and a significant risk of mortality. This approach is also applicable when a gene modification correction is needed to treat specific genetic disorders.
- The treatment of primary immune deficiencies has also seen significant advancements with the use of gene-modified HSCs.[73] Conditions like adenosine deaminase deficiency (ADA), X-linked severe combined immunodeficiency (X-SCID), Wiskott–Aldrich syndrome (WAS), and chronic granulomatosis disease (CGD) can be treated with autologous transplantation of the patient's own HSCs, which have been genetically modified to correct the underlying genetic cause of the disease. This approach offers a preferred treatment option for these patients.
- A breakthrough in stem cell biology has been the development of induced pluripotent stem cells (iPSCs), which are derived from a patient's mature cells.[88] These autologous stem cells have the potential to differentiate into various mature cell types and can be expanded in culture. Genetic modification of HSCs for therapeutic applications has been approved by the European Medicines Agency for two drugs.
- The first approved drug, Strimvelis (developed by GlaxoSmithKline, UK), is indicated for the treatment of a rare primary immune disorder known as ADA-SCID.[91] Strimvelis involves the transplantation of autologous gene-modified HSCs that express functional ADA. Clinical data have shown a 100% survival rate over a median follow-up of 7 years for 18 study participants.[92]

- The second treatment, Zynteglo (developed by Bluebird Bio, USA), is designed to replace functional beta-hemoglobin in HSCs from patients with transfusion-dependent beta-thalassemia. Clinical development data have demonstrated that patients treated with Zynteglo achieved either complete transfusion independence or a near two-thirds reduction in the annual number and volume of blood transfusions.[93] These therapeutic developments represent significant progress in the treatment of these challenging genetic disorders.
- Indeed, successful *HSC* gene therapy is a complex process with various critical aspects that need careful consideration. These aspects include:
  - Collection of high numbers of HSCs: Ensuring that a sufficient quantity of HSCs is collected is essential. This may involve strategies such as mobilization with growth factors like G-CSF or the use of agents like plerixafor to enhance HSC harvests. In some cases, as with Fanconi anemia, collecting adequate numbers of CD34$^+$ cells can be particularly challenging.
  - Safe and efficient cell processing: Processing the collected HSCs and introducing the desired genetic modifications must be done safely and efficiently to avoid potential complications. This involves gene transfer techniques, culture conditions, and quality control measures to ensure the integrity and functionality of the modified cells.
  - Optimal transplantation protocols: Determining the best transplantation protocols, including conditioning chemotherapy and the timing of HSC infusion, is crucial for the success of the therapy. The goal is to achieve effective engraftment of gene-modified HSCs that will persist in the long term and express therapeutic genes in all blood lineages.
- These considerations are essential for ensuring the effectiveness and safety of *HSC* gene therapy in the treatment of various blood and immune system disorders.

VIRAL VECTOR DELIVERY

Viral vectors have played a pivotal role in the field of gene-modified cell therapies. These vectors are derived from natural viruses and have been genetically engineered to efficiently transduce target cells and deliver genetic material. Different types of viral vectors are available, and they serve various purposes in gene therapy. In the 1980s, the concept of utilizing retroviral vectors for direct genomic integration emerged.[94] Due to their procedural accessibility and ease of manipulation, hematopoietic cells became prime candidates for gene therapy applications.[95] Here, we will discuss adenoviral and adeno-associated viral vectors (rAAVs):
- *Adenoviral vectors*: Adenovirus-based vectors are known for their substantial transgene carrying capacity, which allows them to accommodate extensive or multiple gene expression cassettes within the

vector genome.[96,97] While these vectors may not be the primary choice for treating blood disorders, they have shown effectiveness in generating virus-specific T-cell populations.[98]

- *Adeno-associated viral vectors*: Adeno-associated viral vectors are another important class of viral vectors. They are known for their versatility and safety in gene therapy applications. These vectors can deliver genetic material for transient genetic effects, making them suitable for a wide range of applications. They are particularly valuable for delivering therapeutic genes to target cells.

These viral vectors, including adenoviral and adeno-associated viral vectors, have opened up new possibilities in the field of gene therapy by enabling the efficient and precise delivery of therapeutic genes to target cells, offering hope for the treatment of various genetic and acquired disorders.

Adeno-associated viral vectors have several advantages and characteristics that make them valuable tools in gene therapy:

- *Low immunogenicity*: rAAVs have a lower tendency to provoke an immune response compared with adenoviral vectors. This reduced immunogenicity is a significant advantage, as it can help prevent the immune system from clearing the vector-transduced cells.[99,100]
- *Efficient packaging*: rAAVs are efficiently packaged to yield high vector titers, making them suitable for delivering therapeutic genes to target cells.
- *Preexisting immunity*: In general, preexisting immunity to rAAVs is low, particularly for specific serotypes like serotypes 8 and 9. This lower preexisting immunity can improve the effectiveness of rAAV-based gene therapy.
- *Limited transgene size*: One limitation of rAAVs is their constraint in accommodating larger transgenes. The AAV genome is single-stranded, and rAAV preparations consist of a mixture of particles, each carrying one of the two viral strands. This can result in a delay in gene expression following transduction. Therefore, rAAVs are better suited for smaller transgenes of up to 4,700 nucleotides.

Despite these limitations, rAAVs are valuable tools in gene therapy due to their safety, efficiency, and reduced immunogenicity, offering hope for the treatment of various genetic and acquired disorders.

Gamma-retroviral and lentiviral vectors are widely used for gene therapy in the hematopoietic system. These vectors are designed for stable integration of therapeutic genes into the DNA of hematopoietic cells. However, there are some concerns associated with the use of viral vectors, particularly the risk of insertional mutagenesis.

Here is an overview of these vectors and the concerns related to insertional mutagenesis:

- *Integration process*: After transduction of patient cells, viral RNA is converted to DNA by the reverse transcriptase enzyme present in the viral vector. This newly synthesized DNA is then integrated into the cellular

genome, and the process is mediated by the integrase enzyme provided by the viral vector.
- *Risk of insertional mutagenesis*: One of the significant concerns with viral vectors, particularly gamma-retroviral vectors, is the risk of insertional mutagenesis. This refers to the possibility of the integrated DNA disrupting or activating nearby genes, potentially leading to unwanted side effects, including malignant transformation of the genetically modified cells.
- *Clinical studies*: Initial clinical studies using gamma-retroviral vectors showed promise in the treatment of primary immune deficiency patients, achieving a cure in the majority of cases. However, later cases revealed treatment-related hematological malignancies in some patients.
- *Insertion near proto-oncogenes*: Gamma-retroviral vectors tend to insert their DNA near proto-oncogenes, which are genes that can promote cell growth and division. When the viral vector integrates near a proto-oncogene and activates it, it can lead to malignant transformation of the modified cells.
- *ADA-SCID exception*: Interestingly, no malignancies have been reported in ADA-SCID patients who received gene therapy with gamma-retroviral vectors even after treating a significant number of patients. The reasons for this observation are not entirely understood and it remains a subject of study.

While these vectors have shown great promise in gene therapy, the risk of insertional mutagenesis remains a key concern, and ongoing research aims to better understand and mitigate these risks to ensure the safety and efficacy of gene therapy approaches.

Lentiviral vectors offer several advantages in the context of gene therapy, particularly in the hematopoietic system as compared with gamma-retroviral vectors. Here are some key points regarding lentiviral vectors:
- *Limited immunogenicity*: Lentiviral vectors are known for their limited immunogenicity, which means they are less likely to provoke an immune response when introduced into the patient.
- *Nonspecific integration*: Lentiviral vectors tend to integrate into the host genome in a more nonspecific manner. This characteristic eliminates the risk of integration near proto-oncogenes, which can reduce the potential for malignant transformation.
- *Safety record*: Remarkably, despite the numerous instances of HIV infection, which is caused by a lentivirus, no hematological malignancies have been associated with lentiviruses. This suggests that lentiviral vectors have a relatively good safety record.
- *Target cell range*: Lentiviral vectors are capable of infecting a wide range of target cells, including non-dividing cells. This broader target cell range is advantageous in gene therapy applications.
- *Transduction rates*: While lentiviral vectors offer many advantages, they may have lower transduction rates in certain types of cells. For example,

the transduction rate in CD34⁺ cells can be as low as 10%, compared with over 90% in T cells when using equivalent vector-to-target cell ratios.
- *Alternative vectors*: Researchers have explored alternative viral vectors in gene therapy. For example, foamy viruses, which are non-pathogenic retroviruses not known to infect humans, exhibit a diffuse pattern of genomic integration. This pattern avoids integration into genes or regulatory elements, which can reduce the risk of unwanted side effects.[101] Alpha-retroviral vectors, which exhibit a more uniform pattern of genomic integration, particularly within intergenic regions, are also being considered for therapeutic gene transfer.[102,103]
- *Functional validation*: The therapeutic potential of these alternative vectors has been validated in various ways, such as through the functional correction of conditions like CGD in cell lines and transduced human cells that successfully engraft in animal models.

Overall, lentiviral vectors have shown promise in gene therapy applications, particularly for their safety profile, broad target cell range, and ability to avoid integration near proto-oncogenes. Researchers continue to explore and develop alternative viral vectors to improve the safety and efficacy of gene therapy.

■ THE GVAX APPROACH

The GVax approach in the context of chronic myelogenous leukemia (CML) involves several key components:
- *Engineering HLA-negative CML cells*: In this approach, CML cells that lack the human leukocyte antigen (HLA) markers are genetically engineered. These cells are manipulated to express GM-CSF.
- *Mixing with patient-derived cml cells*: The GM-CSF-expressing CML cells are then mixed with irradiated patient-derived CML cells. These patient-derived cells contain antigens that are recognized by the immune system.
- *Intradermal vaccine*: The combination of engineered CML cells expressing GM-CSF and patient-derived CML cells is administered as an intradermal vaccine. This means that the vaccine is injected into the skin.[104]
- *Maintaining deep remission*: The primary goal of this approach is to maintain deep remission in CML patients. Deep remission refers to a state in which minimal or no detectable disease is present.

Toll-like receptors (TLRs) are also integrated into this approach to activate innate immune responses.[105] TLRs are receptors that can recognize specific molecular patterns associated with invading microorganisms.[106] They trigger gene expression programs that activate various components of the innate immune system, including neutrophils, mast cells, and natural killer (NK) cells.[107-109]

The combination of GM-CSF-expressing autologous tumor cell vaccination with TLR activation has shown promise in the treatment of CML patients. It has led to complete molecular remissions and deep responses, indicating effective control of the disease.

However, further development and refinement of the GVax approach are necessary to fully harness its potential as an in situ and whole-cell tumor vaccination strategy. This research is crucial for improving the treatment outcomes and quality of life for patients with CML and potentially for other cancer types as well.

■ GENE EDITING AND TRANSPOSON-BASED SYSTEMS

In contrast to older genome modification methods, modern gene-editing tools aim to precisely target-specific sites in the human genome using site-specific nucleases. There are four classes of these nucleases which include:
1. Engineered meganucleases
2. Zinc-finger nucleases (ZFNs)
3. Transcription activator-like effector nucleases (TALENs)
4. CRISPR-Cas9

These nucleases share a common mechanism, which involves creating a double-strand break (DSB) in the DNA at the targeted locus. Once the DSB is created, the cell's natural DNA repair mechanisms come into play. There are two main methods of repair:
1. *Nonhomologous end joining (NHEJ)*: This method often results in occasional nucleotide deletions or insertions at the site of the DSB. It can be used to disrupt a specific gene.
2. *Homology-directed repair (HDR)*: HDR utilizes homologous DNA as a template to precisely repair the DSB. This method enables the introduction, deletion, or modification of nucleotides when coupled with an exogenous piece of DNA that is homologous to the target genomic region.

These site-specific nucleases have revolutionized genetic research, offering promising applications in gene therapy and the treatment of genetic diseases.[110] The choice of which nuclease to use may depend on factors, such as specificity, efficiency, and ease of design for a particular application.

Gene-editing techniques, while highly promising for gene therapy, do indeed come with certain challenges and concerns:
- *Off-target effects (OTE)*: One significant concern in the application of gene-editing techniques is the possibility of off-target effects. OTE refer to unintended changes at genomic sites other than the intended target. These off-target changes can lead to adverse outcomes, such as the activation of oncogenes (genes that can promote cancer) or the inactivation of tumor suppressor genes (genes that normally inhibit cancer). Minimizing OTE is a critical consideration in the development of safe and effective gene-editing therapies.
- *Cytotoxicity*: Engineered nucleases, including CRISPR-Cas9, can be cytotoxic when they are expressed for extended periods or at high levels. Prolonged expression of nucleases may harm the cells being edited, leading to undesirable outcomes. Therefore, controlling the expression

of these nucleases and ensuring they are active only during the editing process is essential.
- *Efficiency*: When applied to modifying HSCs for therapeutic purposes, gene-editing techniques can be less efficient compared with using viral vectors. Achieving high efficiency in gene editing is crucial to ensure that a sufficient number of cells receive the desired genetic modifications.
- *Safety Validation*: The use of gene-editing techniques in clinical applications, particularly in the context of modifying HSCs, requires rigorous safety validation. Ensuring that the edited cells do not pose risks, such as tumorigenesis or immune reactions, is essential before these techniques can be widely adopted for clinical use.

Addressing these concerns and optimizing the precision and safety of gene-editing techniques is an ongoing focus of research and development in the field of gene therapy

Transposon-based systems represent another class of non-viral gene modification approaches. Transposons are naturally occurring DNA elements capable of changing their positions within the genome. They contain a recognition domain for transposase, the enzyme responsible for the "cut and paste" function. After excision by transposase, the transposon is inserted in a semi-random manner into the patient's cell genome.[90] Three transposon-based systems have been developed for therapeutic purposes: Sleeping beauty, PiggyBac, and Tol2. Notably, transposon-based systems are being successfully applied in the development of CAR-T cells, with clinical trials in progress.[111,112]

■ GENE THERAPY EX VIVO

The approach you are describing is known as ex vivo gene therapy, which involves modifying cells outside the patient's body and then reinfusing them into the patient. This approach is often used in HSCT and gene therapy for blood-related disorders.

Advantages
- *Cell selection*: Ex vivo gene therapy allows for the selection and enrichment of the modified cells, ensuring that the desired therapeutic effect is achieved.
- *Immune avoidance*: It helps avoid potential immune responses against the modified cells since the cells can be tested and manipulated outside the patient's body.
- *Precise modification*: Researchers can carefully edit or modify the cells to ensure that they function as intended.
- *Suitable for various disorders*: It can be applied to various genetic disorders and diseases, especially those related to hematopoietic (blood-forming) cells.

Challenges and Concerns

- *Preparation and conditioning*: As you mentioned, the process often requires intense conditioning regimens, which can lead to short-term side effects like low blood cell counts, mouth sores, and a higher risk of infections.
- *Long-term risks*: There are concerns about potential long-term side effects, such as infertility, organ damage, and the development of secondary cancers due to the high-dose treatments used in conditioning.
- *Complexity*: Ex vivo gene therapy is a complex and resource-intensive process that requires specialized facilities and expertise.

It is important for clinicians and researchers to carefully weigh the potential benefits against the risks and closely monitor patients undergoing these therapies. As the field of gene therapy continues to advance, ongoing research is essential to better understand and mitigate the potential risks associated with ex vivo gene therapies.

To make this process safer, some researchers are working on new ways to prepare the bone marrow. These approaches include using special toxins and antibodies that target-specific markers on the cells we want to modify, such as c-Kit, CD47, and CD45.[113-115]

CONCLUSION

In conclusion gene therapy has important role in following hematological disorders.

Hemoglobinopathies like sickle-cell disease and β-thalassemia, X-SCID, and ADA-SCID.

Lysosomal storage disorders, leukemia, lymphomas, and multiple myelomas. In many non-hematological disorders, such as genetic disorders, muscular dystrophies, spinal muscular atrophy, many infectious diseases, autoimmune diseases, HIV, and malignancies. It is also used in development of certain vaccines.

REFERENCES

1. Kim YK. RNA Therapy: current status and future potential. Chonnam Med J. 2020;56(2):87-93.
2. Bulcha JT, Wang Yi, Ma Hong, Tai PWL, Gao G. Viral vector platforms within the gene therapy landscape. Signal Transduct Target Ther. 2021;6(1):53.
3. Terheggen HG, Lowenthal A, Lavinha F, Colombo JP, Rogers S. Unsuccessful trial of gene replacement in arginase deficiency. Z Kinderheilkd. 1975;119(1):1-3.
4. Cline MJ. Perspectives for gene therapy: inserting new genetic information into mammalian cells by physical techniques and viral vectors. Pharm Ther. 1985;29(1):69-92.
5. Anderson WF. Human gene therapy. Science. 1992;256:808-13.
6. Kohn DB, Mitsuya H, Ballow M, Selegue JE, Barankiewicz J, Cohen A, et al. Establishment and characterization of adenosine deaminase deficient human T cell lines. J Immunol. 1989;142(11):3971-7.

7. Arrand JR, Roberts RJ. The nucleotide sequences at the termini of adenovirus-2 DNA. J Mol Biol. 1979;128(4):577-94.
8. Shinagawa M, Padmanabhan RV, Padmanabhan R. The nucleotide sequence of the right-hand terminal Smal-K fragment of adenovirus type 2 DNA. Gene. 1980;9(1-2):99-114.
9. Yang ZR, Wang HF, Zhao J, Peng YY, Wang J, Guinn BA, et al. Recent developments in the use of adenoviruses and immunotoxins in cancer gene therapy. Cancer Gene Ther. 2007;14(7):599-615.
10. Tooze J, Acheson NH, Broker TR, Flint SJ. DNA Tumor Viruses. New York: Cold Spring Harbor Laboratory, 1981.
11. Fields BN, Knipe DM, Howley PM. Fields' fundamental virology. Philadelphia, PA; London: Lippincott Williams & Wilkins; 2007.
12. Russell WC. Adenoviruses: update on structure and function. J Gen Virol. 2009;90(Pt 1): 1-20.
13. Saban SD, Silvestry M, Nemerow GR, Stewart PL. Visualization of alpha-helices in a 6-angstrom resolution cryoelectron microscopy structure of adenovirus allows refinement of capsid protein assignments. J Virol. 2006;80(24):12049-59.
14. San Martín C, Glasgow JN, Borovjagin A, Beatty MS, Kashentseva EA, Curiel DT, et al. Localization of the N-terminus of minor coat protein IIIa in the adenovirus capsid. J Mol Biol. 2008;383(4):923-34.
15. Wodrich H, Henaff D, Jammart B, Segura-Morales C, Seelmeir S, Coux O, et al. A capsid-encoded PPxY-motif facilitates adenovirus entry. PLoS Pathog. 2010;6(3):e1000808.
16. Fabry CM, Rosa-Calatrava M, Conway JF, Zubieta C, Cusack S, Ruigrok RW, et al. A quasi-atomic model of human adenovirus type 5 capsid. EMBO J. 2005;24(9):1645-54.
17. Liu H, Naismith JH, Hay RT. Adenoviruses: Model and Vectors in Virus-Host Interactions: Virion-Structure, Viral Replication and Host-Cell Interactions. In: Doerfler W, Bohm P, (Eds). USA: Springer: 2003. pp. 131-64.
18. Lee CS, Bishop ES, Zhang R, Yu X, Farina EM, Yan S, et al. Adenovirus-mediated gene delivery: potential applications for gene and cell-based therapies in the new era of personalized medicine. Genes Dis. 2017;4(2):43-63.
19. Singh S, Kumar R, Agrawal B. Adenoviral Vector-based Vaccines and Gene Therapies: Current Status and Future Prospects. In: Desheva YA (Ed). Adenoviruses. Intech Open Publishers: London, United Kingdom; 2018. Vol. 1. pp. 1-39.
20. McGrory WJ, Bautista DS, Graham FL. A simple technique for the rescue of early region I mutations into infectious human adenovirus type 5. Virology. 1988;163(2):614-7.
21. Akusjärvi, G. Proteins with transcription regulatory properties encoded by human adenoviruses. Trends Microbiol. 1993;1(5):163-70.
22. Yang Y, Nunes FA, Berencsi K, Furth EE, Gönczöl E, Wilson JM. Cellular immunity to viral antigens limits E1-deleted adenoviruses for gene therapy. Proc Natl Acad Sci USA. 1994;91(10):4407-11.
23. Gorziglia MI, Kadan MJ, Yei S, Lim J, Lee GM, Luthra R, et al. Elimination of both E1 and E2 from adenovirus vectors further improves prospects for in vivo human gene therapy. J Virol. 1996;70(6):4173-8.
24. Engelhardt JF, Ye X, Doranz B, Wilson JM. Ablation of E2A in recombinant adenoviruses improves transgene persistence and decreases inflammatory response in mouse liver. Proc Natl Acad Sci USA. 1994;91(13):6196-200.
25. Amalfitano A, Hauser MA, Hu H, Serra D, Begy CR, Chamberlain JS. Production and characterization of improved adenovirus vectors with the E1, E2b, and E3 genes deleted. J Virol. 1998;72(2):926-33.
26. Osada T, Yang XY, Hartman ZC, Glass O, Hodges BL, Niedzwiecki D, et al. Optimization of vaccine responses with an E1, E2b and E3-deleted Ad5 vector circumvents pre-existing anti-vector immunity. Cancer Gene Ther. 2009;16(9):673-82.

27. Gao GP, Yang Y, Wilson JM. Biology of adenovirus vectors with E1 and E4 deletions for liver-directed gene therapy. J Virol. 1996;70(12):8934-43.
28. Lusky M, Christ M, Rittner K, Dieterle A, Dreyer D, Mourot B, et al. In vitro and in vivo biology of recombinant adenovirus vectors with E1, E1/E2A, or E1/E4 deleted. J Virol. 1998;72(3):2022-32.
29. Wang Q, Finer MH. Second-generation adenovirus vectors. Nat Med. 1996;2(6):714-6.
30. Alba R, Bosch A, Chillon M. Gutless adenovirus: last-generation adenovirus for gene therapy. Gene Ther. 2005;12 Suppl 1:S18-27.
31. Hartigan-O'Connor D, Amalfitano A, Chamberlain JS. Improved production of gutted adenovirus in cells expressing adenovirus preterminal protein and DNA polymerase. J Virol. 1999;73(9):7835-41.
32. Atchison RW, Casto BC, Hammon WM. Adenovirus-associated defective virus particles. Science 1965;149(3685):754-6.
33. Matsushita T, Elliger S, Elliger C, Podsakoff G, Villarreal L, Kurtzman GJ, et al. Adeno-associated virus vectors can be efficiently produced without helper virus. Gene Ther. 1998;5(7):938-45.
34. Xiao X, Li J, Samulski RJ. Production of high-titer recombinant adeno-associated virus vectors in the absence of helper adenovirus. J Virol. 1998;72(3):2224-32.
35. Linden RM, Berns KI. Molecular biology of adeno-associated viruses. Contrib Microbiol. 2000;4:68-84.
36. Sonntag F, Schmidt K, Kleinschmidt JA. A viral assembly factor promotes AAV2 capsid formation in the nucleolus. Proc Natl Acad Sci USA. 2010;107(22):10220-5.
37. Ogden PJ, Kelsic ED, Sinai S, Church GM. Comprehensive AAV capsid fitness landscape reveals a viral gene and enables machine-guided design. Science. 2019;366(6469):1139-43.
38. Samulski RJ, Berns KI, Tan M, Muzyczka N. Cloning of adeno-associated virus into pBR322: rescue of intact virus from the recombinant plasmid in human cells. Proc Natl Acad Sci USA. 1982;79(6):2077-81.
39. Flotte T, Carter B, Conrad C, Guggino W, Reynolds T, Rosenstein B, et al. A phase I study of an adeno-associated virus-CFTR gene vector in adult CF patients with mild lung disease. Hum Gene Ther. 1996;7(9):1145-59.
40. Duan D, Yue Y, Yan Z, Engelhardt JF. A new dual-vector approach to enhance recombinant adeno-associated virus-mediated gene expression through intermolecular cis activation. Nat Med. 2000;6(5):595-8.
41. Nakai H, Storm TA, Kay MA. Increasing the size of rAAV-mediated expression cassettes in vivo by intermolecular joining of two complementary vectors. Nat Biotechnol. 2000;18(5):527-32.
42. Sun L, Li J, Xiao X. Overcoming adeno-associated virus vector size limitation through viral DNA heterodimerization. Nat Med. 2000;6(5):599-602.
43. Ghosh A, Yue Y, Lai Y, Duan D. A hybrid vector system expands adeno-associated viral vector packaging capacity in a transgene-independent manner. Mol Ther. 2008;16(1):124-30.
44. Lai Y, Yue Y, Liu M, Ghosh A, Engelhardt JF, Chamberlain JS, et al. Efficient in vivo gene expression by trans-splicing adeno-associated viral vectors. Nat Biotechnol. 2005;23(11):1435-9.
45. Chew WL, Tabebordbar M, Cheng JK, Mali P, Wu EY, Ng AH, et al. A multifunctional AAV-CRISPR-Cas9 and its host response. Nat Methods. 2016;13(10):868-74.
46. Li J, Sun W, Wang B, Xiao X, Liu XQ. Protein trans-splicing as a means for viral vector-mediated in vivo gene therapy. Hum Gene Ther. 2008;19(9):958-64.
47. Campbell S, Vogt VM. In vitro assembly of virus-like particles with Rous sarcoma virus Gag deletion mutants: identification of the p10 domain as a morphological determinant in the formation of spherical particles. J Virol. 1997;71(6):4425-35.

48. Vogt VM. Retroviruses. In: Coffin JM, Hughes SH, Varmus HE, (Eds). Cold Spring Harbor; 1997.
49. Beasley BE, Hu WS. cis-Acting elements important for retroviral RNA packaging specificity. J Virol. 2002;76(10):4950-60.
50. Watanabe S, Temin HM. Encapsidation sequences for spleen necrosis virus, an avian retrovirus, are between the 5' long terminal repeat and the start of the gag gene. Proc Natl Acad Sci USA. 1982;79(19):5986-90.
51. Hanawa H, Kelly PF, Nathwani AC, Persons DA, Vandergriff JA, Hargrove P, et al. Comparison of various envelope proteins for their ability to pseudotype lentiviral vectors and transduce primitive hematopoietic cells from human blood. Mol Ther. 2002;5(3):242-51.
52. Bieniasz PD, Grdina TA, Bogerd HP, Cullen BR. Recruitment of cyclin T1/P-TEFb to an HIV type 1 long terminal repeat promoter proximal RNA target is both necessary and sufficient for full activation of transcription. Proc Natl Acad Sci USA. 1999;96(14):7791-6.
53. Neville M, Stutz F, Lee L, Davis LI, Rosbash M. The importin-beta family member Crm1p bridges the interaction between Rev and the nuclear pore complex during nuclear export. Curr Biol. 1997;7(10):767-75.
54. Basmaciogullari S, Pizzato M. The activity of Nef on HIV-1 infectivity. Front Microbiol. 2014;5:232.
55. Seissler T, Marquet R, Paillart JC. Hijacking of the Ubiquitin/Proteasome Pathway by the HIV Auxiliary Proteins. Viruses. 2017;9(11):322.
56. Naldini L, Blömer U, Gallay P, Ory D, Mulligan R, Gage FH, et al. In vivo gene delivery and stable transduction of nondividing cells by a lentiviral vector. Science. 1996 12;272(5259):263-7.
57. Zhu Y, Feuer G, Day SL, Wrzesinski S, Planelles V. Multigene lentiviral vectors based on differential splicing and translational control. Mol Ther. 2001;4(4):375-82.
58. Yu X, Zhan X, D'Costa J, Tanavde VM, Ye Z, Peng T, et al. Lentiviral vectors with two independent internal promoters transfer high-level expression of multiple transgenes to human hematopoietic stem-progenitor cells. Mol Ther. 2003;7(6):827-38.
59. Tian J, Andreadis ST. Independent and high-level dual-gene expression in adult stem-progenitor cells from a single lentiviral vector. Gene Ther. 2009;16(7):874-84.
60. Rausell A, Muñoz M, Martinez R, Roger T, Telenti A, Ciuffi A. Innate immune defects in HIV permissive cell lines. Retrovirology. 2016;13(1):43.
61. Bukrinsky MI, Stanwick TL, Dempsey MP, Stevenson M. Quiescent T lymphocytes as an inducible virus reservoir in HIV-1 infection. Science. 1991;254(5030):423-7.
62. Ohashi K, Park F, Kay MA. Role of hepatocyte direct hyperplasia in lentivirus-mediated liver transduction in vivo. Hum Gene Ther. 2002;13(5):653-63.
63. Park F, Ohashi K, Chiu W, Naldini L, Kay MA. Efficient lentiviral transduction of liver requires cell cycling in vivo. Nat Genet. 2000;24(1):49-52.
64. Stevenson M, Stanwick TL, Dempsey MP, Lamonica CA. HIV-1 replication is controlled at the level of T cell activation and proviral integration. EMBO J. 1990;9(5):1551-60.
65. Abordo-Adesida E, Follenzi A, Barcia C, Sciascia S, Castro MG, Naldini L, et al. Stability of lentiviral vector-mediated transgene expression in the brain in the presence of systemic antivector immune responses. Hum Gene Ther. 2005;16(6):741-51.
66. Baekelandt V, Eggermont K, Michiels M, Nuttin B, Debyser Z. Optimized lentiviral vector production and purification procedure prevents immune response after transduction of mouse brain. Gene Ther. 2003;10(23):1933-40.
67. Nikolova D. Current trends in the gene therapy of hematologic disorders. Acta Medica Bulgarica. 2021;XLVIII:4.
68. Sadelain M, Rivière I, Brentjens R. Targeting tumours with genetically enhanced T lymphocytes. Nat Rev Cancer. 2003;3(1):35-45.

69. Sadelain M, Brentjens R, Rivière I. The promise and potential pitfalls of chimeric antigen receptors. Curr Opin Immunol. 2009;21(2):215-23.
70. Davila ML, Sadelain M. Biology and clinical application of CAR T cells for B cell malignancies. Int J Hematol. 2016;104(1):6-17.
71. Wang X, Rivière I. Manufacture of tumor- and virus-specific T lymphocytes for adoptive cell therapies. Cancer Gene Ther. 2015;22(2):85-94.
72. Davila ML, Brentjens R, Wang X, Rivière I, Sadelain M. How do CARs work?: Early insights from recent clinical studies targeting CD19. Oncoimmunology. 2012;1(9):1577-83.
73. Maher J, Brentjens RJ, Gunset G, Rivière I, Sadelain M. Human T-lymphocyte cytotoxicity and proliferation directed by a single chimeric TCRzeta /CD28 receptor. Nat Biotechnol. 2002;20(1):70-5.
74. Kochenderfer JN, Wilson WH, Janik JE, Dudley ME, Stetler-Stevenson M, Feldman SA, et al. Eradication of B-lineage cells and regression of lymphoma in a patient treated with autologous T cells genetically engineered to recognize CD19. Blood. 2010;116(20):4099-102.
75. Kochenderfer JN, Dudley ME, Feldman SA, Wilson WH, Spaner DE, Maric I, et al. B-cell depletion and remissions of malignancy along with cytokine-associated toxicity in a clinical trial of anti-CD19 chimeric-antigen-receptor-transduced T cells. Blood. 2012;119(12):2709-20.
76. Li YS, Wasserman R, Hayakawa K, Hardy RR. Identification of the earliest B lineage stage in mouse bone marrow. Immunity. 1996;5(6):527-35.
77. Jensen MC, Popplewell L, Cooper LJ, DiGiusto D, Kalos M, Ostberg JR, et al. Antitransgene rejection responses contribute to attenuated persistence of adoptively transferred CD20/CD19-specific chimeric antigen receptor redirected T cells in humans. Biol Blood Marrow Transplant. 2010;16(9):1245-56.
78. Savoldo B, Ramos CA, Liu E, Mims MP, Keating MJ, Carrum G, et al. CD28 costimulation improves expansion and persistence of chimeric antigen receptor-modified T cells in lymphoma patients. J Clin Invest. 2011;121(5):1822-6.
79. Kloss CC, Condomines M, Cartellieri M, Bachmann M, Sadelain M. Combinatorial antigen recognition with balanced signaling promotes selective tumor eradication by engineered T cells. Nat Biotechnol. 2013;31(1):71-5.
80. Lanitis E, Poussin M, Klattenhoff AW, Song D, Sandaltzopoulos R, June CH, et al. Chimeric antigen receptor T Cells with dissociated signaling domains exhibit focused antitumor activity with reduced potential for toxicity in vivo. Cancer Immunol Res. 2013;1(1):43-53.
81. Lupo-Stanghellini MT, Provasi E, Bondanza A, Ciceri F, Bordignon C, Bonini C. Clinical impact of suicide gene therapy in allogeneic hematopoietic stem cell transplantation. Hum Gene Ther. 2010;21(3):241-50.
82. Di Stasi A, Tey SK, Dotti G, Fujita Y, Kennedy-Nasser A, Martinez C, et al. Inducible apoptosis as a safety switch for adoptive cell therapy. N Engl J Med. 2011;365(18):1673-83.
83. Fire A, Xu S, Montgomery MK, Kostas SA, Driver SE, Mello CC. Potent and specific genetic interference by double-stranded RNA in Caenorhabditis elegans. Nature. 1998;391(6669):806-11.
84. Khoury M, Louis-Plence P, Escriou V, Noel D, Largeau C, Cantos C, et al. Efficient new cationic liposome formulation for systemic delivery of small interfering RNA silencing tumor necrosis factor alpha in experimental arthritis. Arthritis Rheum. 2006;54(6):1867-77.
85. Fleischmann KK, Pagel P, Schmid I, Roscher AA. RNAi-mediated silencing of MLL-AF9 reveals leukemia-associated downstream targets and processes. Mol Cancer. 2014;13:27.
86. Lagresle-Peyrou C, Lefrère F, Magrin E, Ribeil JA, Romano O, Weber L, et al. Plerixafor enables safe, rapid, efficient mobilization of hematopoietic stem cells in sickle cell disease patients after exchange transfusion. Haematologica. 2018;103(5):778-86.

87. Pantin J, Purev E, Tian X, Cook L, Donohue-Jerussi T, Cho E, et al. Effect of high-dose plerixafor on CD34+ cell mobilization in healthy stem cell donors: results of a randomized crossover trial. Haematologica. 2017;102(3):600-9.
88. Adair JE, Sevilla J, Heredia CD, Becker PS, Kiem HP, Bueren J. Lessons learned from two decades of clinical trial experience in gene therapy for Fanconi anemia. Curr Gene Ther. 2017;16(5):338-48.
89. Passweg JR, Baldomero H, Bader P, Basak GW, Bonini C, Duarte R, et al. Is the use of unrelated donor transplantation leveling off in Europe? The 2016 European Society for Blood and Marrow Transplant activity survey report. Bone Marrow Transplant. 2018;53(9):1139-48.
90. Booth C, Gaspar HB, Thrasher AJ. Treating Immunodeficiency through HSC Gene Therapy. Trends Mol Med. 2016;22(4):317-27.
91. Aiuti A, Roncarolo MG, Naldini L. Gene therapy for ADA-SCID, the first marketing approval of an ex vivo gene therapy in Europe: paving the road for the next generation of advanced therapy medicinal products. EMBO Mol Med. 2017;9(6):737-40.
92. Cicalese MP, Ferrua F, Castagnaro L, Pajno R, Barzaghi F, Giannelli S, et al. Update on the safety and efficacy of retroviral gene therapy for immunodeficiency due to adenosine deaminase deficiency. Blood. 2016;128(1):45-54.
93. Thompson AA, Walters MC, Kwiatkowski J, Rasko JEJ, Ribeil JA, Hongeng S, et al. Gene Therapy in Patients with Transfusion-Dependent β-Thalassemia. N Engl J Med. 2018 19;378(16):1479-93.
94. Gorman CM, Lane DP, Rigby PW. High efficiency gene transfer into mammalian cells. Philos Trans R Soc Lond B Biol Sci. 1984;307(1132):343-6.
95. Bregni M, Magni M, Siena S, Di Nicola M, Bonadonna G, Gianni AM. Human peripheral blood hematopoietic progenitors are optimal targets of retroviral-mediated gene transfer. Blood. 1992;80(6):1418-22.
96. Beatty MS, Curiel DT. Chapter two--Adenovirus strategies for tissue-specific targeting. Adv Cancer Res. 2012;115:39-67.
97. Puntel M, Ghulam Muhammad AKM, Farrokhi C, Vanderveen N, Paran C, Appelhans A, et al. Safety profile, efficacy, and biodistribution of a bicistronic high-capacity adenovirus vector encoding a combined immunostimulation and cytotoxic gene therapy as a prelude to a phase I clinical trial for glioblastoma. Toxicol Appl Pharmacol. 2013;268(3):318-30.
98. Nienhuis AW. Development of gene therapy for blood disorders: an update. Blood. 2013;122(9):1556-64.
99. Xiao PJ, Lentz TB, Samulski RJ. Recombinant adeno-associated virus: clinical application and development as a gene-therapy vector. Ther Deliv. 2012;3(7):835-56.
100. Nathwani AC, Rosales C, McIntosh J, Rastegarlari G, Nathwani D, Raj D, et al. Long-term safety and efficacy following systemic administration of a self-complementary AAV vector encoding human FIX pseudotyped with serotype 5 and 8 capsid proteins. Mol Ther. 2011;19(5):876-85.
101. Erlwein O, McClure MO. Progress and prospects: foamy virus vectors enter a new age. Gene Ther. 2010;17(12):1423-9.
102. Kaufmann KB, Brendel C, Suerth JD, Mueller-Kuller U, Chen-Wichmann L, Schwäble J, et al. Alpharetroviral vector-mediated gene therapy for X-CGD: functional correction and lack of aberrant splicing. Mol Ther. 2013;21(3):648-61.
103. Corrigan-Curay J, Cohen-Haguenauer O, O'Reilly M, Ross SR, Fan H, Rosenberg N, et al. Challenges in vector and trial design using retroviral vectors for long-term gene correction in hematopoietic stem cell gene therapy. Mol Ther. 2012;20(6):1084-94.
104. Smith BD, Kasamon YL, Kowalski J, Gocke C, Murphy K, Miller CB, et al. K562/GM-CSF immunotherapy reduces tumor burden in chronic myeloid leukemia patients with residual disease on imatinib mesylate. Clin Cancer Res. 2010;16(1):338-47.

105. Uematsu S, Akira S. Innate immune recognition of viral infection. Uirusu. 2006;56(1):1-8.
106. Iwasaki A, Medzhitov R. Toll-like receptor control of the adaptive immune responses. Nat Immunol. 2004;5(10):987-95.
107. Hayashi F, Means TK, Luster AD. Toll-like receptors stimulate human neutrophil function. Blood. 2003;102(7):2660-9.
108. Supajatura V, Ushio H, Nakao A, Akira S, Okumura K, Ra C, et al. Differential responses of mast cell Toll-like receptors 2 and 4 in allergy and innate immunity. J Clin Invest. 2002;109(10):1351-9.
109. Brackett CM, Kojouharov B, Veith J, Greene KF, Burdelya LG, Gollnick SO, et al. Toll-like receptor-5 agonist, entolimod, suppresses metastasis and induces immunity by stimulating an NK-dendritic-CD8+ T-cell axis. Proc Natl Acad Sci USA. 2016;113(7):E874-83.
110. Gupta RM, Musunuru K. Expanding the genetic editing tool kit: ZFNs, TALENs, and CRISPR-Cas9. J Clin Invest. 2014;124(10):4154-61.
111. Kebriaei P, Izsvák Z, Narayanavari SA, Singh H, Ivics Z. Gene Therapy with the Sleeping Beauty Transposon System. Trends Genet. 2017;33(11):852-70.
112. Kebriaei P, Singh H, Huls MH, Figliola MJ, Bassett R, Olivares S, et al. Phase I trials using Sleeping Beauty to generate CD19-specific CAR T cells. J Clin Invest. 2016;126(9):3363-76.
113. Czechowicz A, Kraft D, Weissman IL, Bhattacharya D. Efficient transplantation via antibody-based clearance of hematopoietic stem cell niches. Science. 2007;318(5854):1296-9.
114. Chhabra A, Ring AM, Weiskopf K, Schnorr PJ, Gordon S, Le AC, et al. Hematopoietic stem cell transplantation in immunocompetent hosts without radiation or chemotherapy. Sci Transl Med. 2016;8(351):351ra105.
115. Palchaudhuri R, Saez B, Hoggatt J, Schajnovitz A, Sykes DB, Tate TA, et al. Non-genotoxic conditioning for hematopoietic stem cell transplantation using a hematopoietic-cell-specific internalizing immunotoxin. Nat Biotechnol. 2016;34(7):738-45.

CHAPTER 4

Role of Flow Cytometry in Transfusion Medicine

Aparna Bhardwaj, Gaurav Raturi, Sanjay Kaushik, Saqib Ahmed

■ INTRODUCTION

Flow cytometry (FCM) is a newer technology that has been useful in many places, including modern laboratories and research centers. This technology dates back to the early 1970s when antibodies were initially tagged with fluorescent labels with cell sorting and fluorescence microscopy, to build the first fluorescence-activated cell sorter. Shortly thereafter, a commercial flow cytometer was introduced by Becton Dickinson and the use of FCM blossomed as scientists embraced the technique to sort and isolate individual cells. This technique employs the principle of sorting and counting cells or particles while passing in a single file against a single or multiple laser sources in a buffered solution. Fluorescently labeled cell components when passed through a laser source excite the flourochrome and emit light that has a longer wavelength than the light source. Several detectors are carefully placed around the stream, at the point where the fluid passes the light stream. The detector which is in line with the light beam measures forward scatter (FSC) and the other one which is placed perpendicular to the light beam measures side scatter (SSC). This is then detected by different detectors known as photomultiplier tubes (PMTs) that pick up a combination of scattered and fluorescent light and convert it to a digital pulse. The data are then analyzed by a computer attached to a flow cytometer using special software. The digital signal's intensity is saved in a computer and presented as a relative scale called a channel. These results are then displayed as dot plots or histograms. Usually, FSC can identify the cell volume, while SSC detects the inner complexity of particles, such as nuclear structure or cytoplasmic granule content. Therefore, the light scattering method separates and distinguishes cells of varying sizes and granularity.[1-3]

Flow cytometry is a versatile testing technique used for evaluating a wide range of materials, such as DNA and bacteria. It is commonly employed for cell phenotypic characterization, counting, sorting, and cycle analysis. Additionally, FCM is utilized in cancer biology, measuring apoptosis markers, virology, and infectious disease screening. Owing to its expanding range of applications, FCM is now considered an essential diagnostic tool in medical laboratories. FCM is a versatile testing technique used for evaluating a wide range of materials, such as DNA and bacteria. It is commonly employed for cell phenotypic characterization, counting, sorting, and cycle analysis. Additionally, FCM is utilized in cancer biology, measuring apoptosis markers, virology, and infectious disease screening. Owing to its expanding range of applications, FCM is now considered an essential diagnostic tool in medical laboratories. FCM has been extensively used for red blood cell (RBC) characterization, leucocyte subpopulation analysis in leukemia/lymphoma diagnosis, and cell enumeration in stem cell grafts.[1,2] Owing to the numerous current and potential applications of FCM in transfusion medicine, it has been recognized as a separate entity with vast applications in modern blood banking. FCM can accurately identify individual cell populations and cell epitopes through a technique that is both sensitive and reproducible.[3]

The main utilization of FCM in modern blood banking is for:
- Quality control of blood/blood components
  - Quantification of residual white blood cells (rWBCs) in leucodepleted cellular blood products (platelets, red cell concentrate) and plasma
  - To rule out contamination of blood components
  - Determination of RBC or other cell component survival in vivo/in vitro
- Immunohematology
  - Red blood cell immunology
    - Semiquantification of red cell antigen
    - Red cell phenotyping to resolve ABO discrepancy and detection of chimerism
    - Detecting fetal erythrocytes in fetomaternal hemorrhage and estimation of red cell survival
    - Diagnose genetic disorders of erythrocytes [paroxysmal nocturnal hemoglobinuria (PNH)]
    - Diagnosis and characterization of red cell autoantibody in autoimmune hemolytic anemia (AIHA) (direct coomb's negative or positive)
    - Quantification of D antigen
  - Platelet immunology
    - Detecting platelet antibodies (allo or autoantibody)
    - Platelet crossmatching
    - Verifying platelet functionality in platelet units
  - Assessment of the integrity and functionality of granulocyte and monocyte
- Hematopoietic stem cell transplantation (HSCT)
  - Enumeration of CD34$^+$ stem cells
  - Human leukocyte antigen (HLA) crossmatching

■ QUALITY CONTROL OF BLOOD COMPONENTS

Quantification of Residual White Blood Cells in Leucodepleted Cellular Blood Products (Platelets, Red Cell Concentrate) and Plasma

Blood product transfusion therapy has advanced significantly in the last few years. In modern blood banking, component therapy is emphasized over whole blood transfusion, as it makes the process more effective. Blood is donated as whole blood, which can be separated into components by differential centrifugation. These components include red cell concentrate, fresh frozen plasma (FFP), cryoprecipitate, and random donor platelets (RDPs). This approach allows for optimal survival of each component and reduces the risk of transfusion to a minimum, as only the specific component required is transfused to the patient. Additionally, component therapy avoids the use of unnecessary components that may be contraindicated in a patient. Transfusion centers now emphasize the administration of leukodepleted blood products, which decreases the potential risk of cell-mediated adverse events such as nonhemolytic febrile transfusion reaction (NHFTR), transfusion-related immunomodulation (TRIM), alloimmunization to HLAs, or graft-versus-host disease (GVHD).[4,5] It is estimated that the average number of white blood cells in one unit of whole blood is around 10^9. To ensure that there are no cell-mediated adverse events after the transfusion of blood components, it is essential to quantify the rWBCs in leucodepleted cellular blood products such as platelets, red cell concentrate, and plasma to ensure robust quality control. It is essential for transfusion medicine services to accurately enumerate rWBCs in cellular components following leucodepletion, to ensure their quality. Accurately counting low levels of residual leukocytes in various blood components is challenging. According to the guidelines of the European Committee on blood transfusion, RBC units should not contain more than 1×10^6 leukocytes per unit in 90% of blood components. In India and the USA, the acceptable limit of rWBCs is 5×10^6 leukocytes per unit, as per quality control criteria.[6] Enumeration in whole blood samples can be done using automated cell counters. However, the enumeration of rWBC by automation in various blood components is a limiting factor. This is because the cell concentration of rWBC is far below the range of linearity of the instruments and the high concentration of platelets (PLTs) or RBCs in the sample to be tested could interfere with the count.[7,8] Flow cytometric bead-based counting is widely accepted as the reference method for enumerating rWBC in leukoreduced blood components. Leukocyte-specific monoclonal antibodies (MoAbs) are also used by FCM analyzers to detect rWBC.

To Rule Out Contamination of Blood Components

Bacterial contamination continues to pose a challenge in the context of blood components. Septic reactions may occur after transfusion of blood components stored under standard conditions due to bacterial proliferation. Bacterial contamination leading to post-transfusion septic reactions has been traditionally associated with platelets due to their storage at room temperature. However, it is important to note that red cell concentrate, FFP, and stem cell preparations have also been reported to cause septicemia after therapeutic administration. Detecting bacterial contamination in all blood components, particularly in stem cell preparations, is crucial. For this purpose, FCM has become a popular and efficient method for rapid detection of bacteria, achieved through labeling them with fluorescent dyes. This method is applicable to all blood components, including platelet concentrates and stem cell preparations.[8,9]

Determination of RBC or Other Cell Component Survival in vivo/in vitro

Flow cytometry enables the quantitative measurement of viable and nonviable cells within a population by using fluorescent dyes that selectively label either live or dead cells. Viability assessment using FCM is based on various small-molecule dyes with different hydrophobic properties, which can penetrate intact cellular membranes while others cannot. The most commonly used dyes include propidium iodide and 7-amino actinomycin D, which bind to DNA but cannot penetrate intact membranes, rendering dead cells fluorescent. Alternately fluorescent-labeled annexin V can be combined with viability dyes to differentiate viable cells (annexin V-negative) from apoptotic cells (annexin V-positive). Another method known as the annexin V/PI assay is widely used to differentiate between apoptotic and necrotic cells in which cells are simultaneously labeled with annexin V and propidium iodide.[10,11]

■ IMMUNOHEMATOLOGY

Red Blood Cell Immunology

Semiquantification of Red Cell Antigen

Flow cytometry is an important technique used to determine antigen expression on erythrocytes and to identify any aberrant antigen expression. This methodology involves the use of different antibodies, either in combination or alone, to detect specific epitopes. It enables the verification of new variants of blood group antigens, thus leading to the identification of new blood group systems.[11,12] Thus the use of FCM in determining ABO antigen expression can be enumerated as:

- Determining whether an individual is homozygous or heterozygous for alleles that produce normal amounts of ABH antigens[3]
- Determining alterations in ABH antigens during blood bank storage[11,12]
- Analyze the decrease of ABH antigen levels in patients with hemato-lymphoid malignancies where the loss of A and B antigens along with a decrease in H antigen levels occurred[12,13]

Red Cell Phenotyping to Resolve ABO Discrepancy and Detection of Chimerism

ABO discrepancies are frequently encountered and can endanger patients through transfusion of incompatible blood products. The ABO discrepancies are classified into four groups based on unexpected reactions in forward or reverse grouping, as well as missing reactions in forward cell or reverse typing. FCM, when used in combination with serology and genetic testing, can be extremely helpful in resolving ABO discrepancies. It is particularly useful in resolving discrepancies that arise as a result of weakened expression due to pregnancy or hematological malignancy. Additionally, FCM can also be used to determine and sort discrepancies arising from the Bombay and para-Bombay blood groups.[14]

The phenomenon of chimerism can cause discrepancies in blood groups, which can be either congenital or acquired through blood transfusions.[15] When evaluating such cases, the use of FCM can provide clear evidence of the presence of two distinct populations. It is important to note that ABO discrepancies between the donor and the recipient must be resolved for safe transfusion. Additionally, if chimeric donors are identified, they should refrain from donating blood.

Detecting Fetal Erythrocytes in Fetomaternal Hemorrhage and Estimation of Red Cell Survival

It is crucial to determine the amount of fetomaternal hemorrhage (FMH) in a clinical setting where an RhD-negative woman is carrying an RhD-positive fetus. The Kleihauer-Betke test or the acid elution test is commonly used to detect and estimate the volume of FMH. It is necessary to accurately measure the volume of FMH to determine the appropriate dose of anti-D Ig for sensitized mothers and improve pregnancy outcomes. This test, however, has limitations such as being time-consuming, difficult to perform, and lacking standardization. FCM can be an excellent alternative to traditional methods as it provides faster and more sensitive results. Furthermore, it allows for standardization, ensuring reproducibility, and aiding in determining the correct dosage of anti-D fetomaternal hemorrhage. FMH can be detected through FCM by using indirect or direct immunofluorescence. The indirect immunofluorescence technique involves the labeling of RhD antigen with an anti-D reagent. This is followed by the addition of conjugated IgG antibodies. The direct fluorescence method, on the other hand, uses fluorescein isothiocyanate labeled anti-CD45 MoAb and phycoerythrin (PE) labeled anti-fetal hemoglobin or anti-HbF antibody to detect fetal hemoglobin HbF.[16,17] Although anti-HbF FCM offers the advantage of accurately monitoring FMH levels, it has certain limitations. While the maternal blood group does not interfere with detection, even a small amount of HbF in maternal RBCs can cause errors in distinguishing fetal and maternal cell populations. Additionally, when interpreting FCM results in mothers with hemoglobinopathies, a thorough evaluation is necessary.[17,18]

Genetic Disorders of Erythrocytes (Paroxysmal Nocturnal Hemoglobinuria)

Paroxysmal nocturnal hemoglobinuria is a type of blood disorder that occurs due to mutations in hematopoietic stem cells (HSCs). These mutations affect the *PIGA* gene, which is responsible for producing phosphatidylinositol N-acetylglucosaminyltransferase subunit A. As a result, the gene products like glycosylphosphatidylinositol (GPI) are either defective or absent, leading to a deficiency or absence of GPI-linked proteins, particularly CD55 (decay accelerating factor) and CD59 (glycoprotein). The loss of CD55 and CD59 causes complement-mediated intravascular hemolysis of PNH erythrocytes, which is a defining feature of PNH. The disease is characterized by features such as pancytopenia, intravascular hemolysis, and thrombotic events.[18,19] FCM immunophenotyping is a diagnostic technique that uses MoAbs, namely CD55 and CD59, conjugated with PE to differentiate cell populations. It helps to identify the absence or incomplete expression of one or more GPI-anchored proteins on erythrocytes, leukocytes, and platelets, making it an effective tool in discriminating cell populations and reaching a conclusive diagnosis. As the prevalence of the disease is low in the Indian subcontinent, a high level of suspicion is required to make the correct diagnosis.[19,20]

Diagnosis and Characterization of Red Cell Autoantibody in Autoimmune Hemolytic Anemia (Direct Coomb's Negative or Positive)

Flow cytometry is a useful tool to diagnose AIHA, even if it is Coombs-negative. This is because the direct antiglobulin test (DAT) may miss some cases of Coombs-negative AIHA, while FCM is a more sensitive technique that can detect lower levels of antibodies on RBCs. In fact, FCM can detect as few as 30–40 molecules per RBC, which is much lower than the threshold of approximately 200 molecules required for a positive interpretation of the direct coombs test. Therefore, FCM is a reliable method for detecting and characterizing RBC autoantibodies in cases of DAT-negative AIHA.[21]

Quantification of D Antigen

Unlike ABO antigens, Rh antigens are present only in RBCs. The Rh(D) antigen is highly significant in clinical settings due to its high antigenicity. The genes *RHD* and *RHCE* determine Rh antigenicity, which encodes for the D, C, c, E, and e antigens. Among these, the D antigen is the most immunogenic, followed by c and E. An individual can be designated as Rh positive or Rh negative based on the presence or absence of the D antigen. Additionally, Rh-positive cells with weak expression of D antigen are referred to as weaker variants of D and are termed Du. Based on the quantification of D antigen, various Rh phenotypes have been reported, including normal D positive, weak D, and partial D cases. Weak D in addition may have various variations as genetic weak D, C trans, and

D mosaic, and likewise variable antigen densities may be observed. According to various studies and literature reviews, about 10,000–30,000 D antigens per cell are present on the surface of normal RhD-positive red cells while weak D red cells (Du) have antigen densities between 70 and 4,000 D antigens per cell depending upon the subtype of Du. Even RBCs with <30 D antigen sites can cause alloimmunization in RhD-negative individuals. Therefore, it is beneficial to quantify the D antigen during transfusion. It has been observed that even a small volume of 0.1–1 mL of D-positive red cells can lead to anti-D formation in D-negative recipients, resulting in adverse transfusion reactions. FCM estimation of D antigenic sites on red cells is reliable, sensitive, and less time-consuming, making it suitable for routine use.[22-24]

Platelet Immunology

Detecting Platelet Antibodies (Allo or Autoantibody) and in Platelet Crossmatching

A platelet transfusion may fail due to platelet refractoriness (PR) in the patient. PR occurs when the body fails to respond to platelet transfusions, and it can have immunological or nonimmunological causes. Nonimmunological causes such as fever, sepsis, disseminated intravascular coagulation (DIC), and splenomegaly account for 70–80% of PR cases, while immunological causes, such as alloimmunization against HLAs or human platelet antigens (HPAs), account for only 20% of cases. The majority of PR cases are caused by immunological factors associated with HLA, whereas HPA is responsible for a smaller percentage. FCM is the most reliable method for detecting platelet autoantibodies in patients suspected of having immune thrombocytopenic purpura (ITP). It is highly sensitive, objective, and reproducible, making it the gold standard in HPA detection. FCM can also identify and quantify platelet-specific antibodies, such as PAIgM and PAIgG, which play a crucial role in screening patients for ITP. Apart from platelet crossmatching, FCM can also be used to analyze storage lesions in platelet units through CD62P (P-selectin).[25,26]

Platelet Function in Platelet Units

Flow cytometry is a versatile and sensitive method used for detecting platelet properties and functions. This method employs fluorescently labeled platelets that are passed through one or more laser beams. The signal intensity and light scattering generated during this process indicate cell size and granularity, which enables the precise determination of platelet function and properties. Platelet function can be studied using various platelet agonists to evaluate different aspects of their response. This method is particularly helpful in pediatric patients where sample sizes are limited and in cases of thrombocytopenia where reliable results are independent of the number of cells present.[27,28]

Assessing the Integrity and Functionality of Granulocytes and Monocytes: Analysis of Granulocyte Function

Flow cytometry can be used for the detection of various granulocyte functions including the detection of functional defects in granulocyte reactive oxygen species (ROS) production in human neonates of different gestational age.[29,30]

Analysis of Monocyte Function

Several assays using FCM have been developed to study phagocytes and their interactions with microorganisms. These assays help to study the following: (1) surface receptors and regulatory molecules of phagocytes; (2) membrane potential; (3) phagocytosis of microorganisms, including distinguishing between attachment to the phagocyte surface and actual internalization; (4) phagosomal pH; (5) degranulation and enzymatic activity; (6) intracellular calcium; (7) oxidative metabolism; (8) intracellular killing of microorganisms; (9) degradation of microorganisms; and (10) exocytosis. Additionally, the effect of serum opsonins on phagocyte–microorganism interactions can also be studied.[30]

HEMATOPOIETIC STEM CELL TRANSPLANTATION

Enumeration of CD34$^+$ Stem Cells

Flow cytometry is an important tool in HSCT. It is used to determine the number of CD34$^+$ hematopoietic progenitor cells in stem cell grafts and to measure T-cell content before allogeneic transplantation. To ensure operational and economic efficiency, it is desirable to harvest sufficient peripheral blood (PB) progenitor cells with the least number of collections possible and to accurately predict the optimal timing of leukapheresis. To obtain a yield of more than 1×10^6/kg CD34$^+$ cells in a single apheresis procedure, it is recommended to have a PB-CD34$^+$ cell count of over 20×10^3/µL which can be determined by FCM.[31,32]

Human Leukocyte Antigen Crossmatching

Flow cytometry plays a crucial role in HSCT, including HLA crossmatching. In the pretransplantation phase, it helps evaluate the efficacy of ex vivo T-cell graft depletion by examining HSC graft manipulation. In the post-transplantation phase, it helps determine immune recovery, graft rejection, GVHD, and the graft-versus-leukemia effect.[32,33]

CONCLUSION

With this background it implies that the application of flow cytometery in transfusion medicine is an ingenious technology that may be utilized routinely for effective Quality Control in Blood Bank. Furthermore, it promises to be preferred tool in developing various scientific and research methodologies.

REFERENCES

1. Adan A, Alizada G, Kiraz Y, Baran Y, Nalbant A. Flow cytometry: Basic principles and applications. Crit Rev Biotechnol. 2017;37(2):163-76.
2. McKinnon KM. Flow cytometry: An overview. Curr Protoc Immunol. 2018;120:5.1.1-5.1.11.
3. Chaudhary R, Das SS. Application of flow cytometry in transfusion medicine: The Sanjay Gandhi Post Graduate Institute of Medical Sciences, India experience. Asian J Transfus Sci. 2022;16(2):159-66.
4. Marik PE. Transfusion of blood and blood products. Evidence-Based Critical Care. 2014:585-619.
5. Maličev E, Železnik K, Jazbec K. An evaluation of a volumetric method for the flow cytometric determination of residual leukocytes in blood transfusion units. PLoS One. 2022;17(12):e0279244.
6. European Directorate for the Quality of Medicines & Healthcare. Guide to the Preparation, Use and Quality Assurance of Blood Components: Recommendation Number R (95) 15, 18 edition. Strasbourg: EDQM of the Council of Europe; 2015. pp. 85-95.
7. Saran RK. Transfusion Medicine: Technical Manual. 2. New Delhi: Directorate General of Health Service (DGHS); 2003.
8. Sharma RR, Marwaha N. Leukoreduced blood components: Advantages and strategies for its implementation in developing countries. Asian J Transfus Sci. 2010;4(1):3-8.
9. Hillyer CD, Josephson CD, Blajchman MA, Vostal JG, Epstein JS, Goodman JL. Bacterial contamination of blood components: Risks, strategies, and regulation: Joint ASH and AABB educational session in transfusion medicine. Hematology Am Soc Hematol Educ Program. 2003;2003(1):575-89.
10. Robinson JP, Ostafe R, Iyengar SN, Rajwa B, Fischer R. Flow cytometry: The next revolution. Cells. 2023;12(14):1875.
11. Kummrow A, Frankowski M, Bock N, Werner C, Dziekan T, Neukammer J. Quantitative assessment of cell viability based on flow cytometry and microscopy. Cytometry A. 2013;83(2):197-204.
12. Hult AK. Flow cytometry in transfusion medicine: an overview. VOXS. 2018;13:3-10.
13. Sharon R, Fibach E. Quantitative flow cytometric analysis of ABO red cell antigens. Cytometry. 1991;12(6):545-9.
14. Li HY, Guo K. Blood group testing. Front Med (Lausanne). 2022;9:827619.
15. Leenarets PL, Vandeputte M, Waer M. Determination of mixed chimerism by a simple flow cytometry method. J Immunol Methods. 1990;130(2):163-9.
16. Farias MG, Dal Bó S, Castro SM, da Silva AR, Bonazzoni J, Scotti L, et al. Flow cytometry in detection of fetal red blood cells and maternal F cells to identify fetomaternal hemorrhage. Fetal Pediatr Pathol. 2016;35(6):385-91.
17. Dziegiel MH, Nielsen LK, Berkowicz A. Detecting fetomaternal hemorrhage by flow cytometry. Curr Opin Hematol. 2006;13(6):490-5.
18. Davis BH, Olsen S, Bigelow NC, Chen JC. Detection of fetal red cells in fetomaternal hemorrhage using a fetal hemoglobin monoclonal antibody by flow cytometry. Transfusion. 1998;38(8):749-56.
19. Brodsky RA. Paroxysmal nocturnal hemoglobinuria. Blood. 2014;124(18):2804-11.
20. Brando B, Gatti A, Preijers F. Flow cytometric diagnosis of paroxysmal nocturnal hemoglobinuria: Pearls and pitfalls - A critical review article. EJIFCC. 2019;30(4):355-70.
21. Khungar JM, Prasad Pati HP, Mahapatra M. Diagnosis of auto immune hemolytic anemia by detection of RBC-bound IgG antibodies, using flow-cytometry. Blood. 2012;120(21):5159.

22. Flegel WA. The genetics of the Rhesus blood group system. Blood Transfus. 2007;5(2): 50-7.
23. Jones JW, Lloyd-Evans P, Kumpel BM. Quantitation of Rh D antigen sites on weak D and D variant red cells by flow cytometry. Vox Sang. 1996;71:176-83.
24. Beckers EA, Faas BH, Ligthart P, Overbeeke MA, von dem Borne AE, Schoot CE, et al. Lower antigen site density and weak D immunogenicity cannot be explained by structural genomic abnormalities or regulatory defects of the RHD gene. Transfusion. 1997;37:616-23.
25. Köhler M, Dittmann J, Legler TJ, Lynen R, Humpe A, Riggert J, et al. Flow cytometric detection of platelet-reactive antibodies and application in platelet crossmatching. Transfusion. 1996;36(3):250.
26. Buakaew J, Promwong C. Platelet antibody screening by flow cytometry is more sensitive than solid phase red cell adherence assay and lymphocytotoxicity technique: A comparative study in Thai patients. Asian Pac J Allergy Immunol. 2010;28:177-84.
27. Shen CL, Wu YF. Flow cytometry for evaluating platelet immunophenotyping and function in patients with thrombocytopenia. Tzu Chi Med J. 2022;34(4):381-7.
28. Ramström S, Södergren AL, Tynngård N, Lindahl TL. Platelet function determined by flow cytometry: New perspectives? Semin Thromb Hemost. 2016;42(3):268-81.
29. Wu YC, Huang YF, Lin CH, Shieh CC. Detection of defective granulocyte function with flow cytometry in newborn infants. J MicrobiolImmunol Infect. 2005;38(1):17-24.
30. Lehmann AK, Sornes S, Halstensen A. Phagocytosis: Measurement by flow cytometry. J Immunol Methods. 2000;243(1-2):229-42.
31. Lemos NE, Farias MG, Kubaski F, Scotti L, Onsten TGH, Brondani LA, et al. Quantification of peripheral blood CD34+ cells prior to stem cell harvesting by leukapheresis: A single center experience. Hematol Transfus Cell Ther. 2018;40(3):213-8.
32. Yu H, Yoo J, Hwang JS, Kim M, Bae KH, Jekarl DW, et al. Enumeration of CD34-positive stem cells using the ADAMII image-based fluorescence cell counter. Ann Lab Med. 2019;39:388-95.
33. Maguire O, Tario JD Jr, Shanahan TC, Wallace PK, Minderman H. Flow cytometry and solid organ transplantation: a perfect match. Immunol Invest. 2014;43(8):756-74.

CHAPTER 5

Hematological Changes Associated with COVID-19 Infections

Aarushi Chopra

■ INTRODUCTION

The global onslaught of coronavirus disease 2019 (COVID-19) has not only thrust the medical community into uncharted territories but also explored the intricacies of its impact on various physiological systems. This chapter delves in to nuanced alterations in blood parameters observed in individuals afflicted with COVID-19, seeking to unravel the complex interplay between viral infection and hematopoietic system. The chapter aims to illuminate the evolving landscape of hematological manifestations in COVID-19 shedding light on both the immediate clinical implications and potential long term consequences for affected individuals.

The COVID-19 virus, also called Severe acute respiratory syndrome coronavirus 2 (SARS-CoV-2) upsurge took a heavy toll and precipitated public health disaster throughout the entire planet.

Changes are not mentioned in COVID-19 patients who show no symptoms. Patients with mild signs and symptoms, such as fever, cough, myalgia, and fatigue, only experience minor hematological changes, such as a drop in lymphocyte count (80.4%). Neutrophil, lymphocytopenia, expanded D-dimer, fibrin degradation products (FDPs), extended prothrombin time (PT), and decreased fibrinogen are among the adjustments noted in patients with severe symptoms, including acute breathing problems, acute coronary damage, and neurological signs. These changes serve as indicators of the severity and progression of the illness. These patients are more vulnerable to venous and thrombotic problems.[1]

Multiple systems are affected by the illness known as COVID-19. Prognostic indicators of abnormality in COVID-19 include a decrease in lymphocyte count and an increase in neutrophil count. Other prognostic indicators include hyperferritinemia and raised D-dimer levels along with raised lactate dehydrogenase levels.[2]

Although COVID-19 typically affects either the upper or lower respiratory tract, the virus can also be lost in plasma or serum.[3] Therefore, the possibility that coronaviruses could spread through some blood components is very real. Concerns concerning the safety of blood and the COVID-19 virus have been raised in endemic areas due to the increased detection of subclinical infections in COVID-19 cases.

■ WORLD HEALTH ORGANIZATION'S GUIDELINES FOR MANAGING COVID-19

Moderate
Patients clinically exhibit symptoms like pyrexia, coughing, dyspnea, and fast breathing. However, there was no severe pneumonia (on imaging) along with a SpO_2 of 90% or room air.

Severe
Patients have clinically evident pneumonia symptoms (pyrexia, cough, dyspnea, fast breathing). Additionally, one of the symptoms includes a respiratory rate >30 breaths/min, severe breathing difficulties, or a SpO_2 below 90%.

Critically Ill
These COVID-19 patients either have pulmonary failure requiring artificial ventilation or multiple organ failure requiring monitoring in the critical care unit, or septic shock.

Meaning, acute life-threatening disorder in multiple organs, of septic shock with features of persistent low blood pressure within 1 week of exhibiting medical signs and symptoms, advanced or worsening breathing signs, X-ray chest showing opacities in both lungs not explained by excess in volume, labor or collapse of lung, breathing failure not explained by heart failure or fluid excess, declining oxygenation in adults and children.

According to the computed tomography (CT) severity scores, the degree of the pneumonia was described as follows: Score 0, 1, or 2 (none; 40% parenchymal involvement). According to chest CT severity score (CTSS), COVID pneumonia severity was categorized as mild (score = 7), moderate (score 8–17), and severe (score ≥18).

Analysis of hematological tests such as absolute lymphocyte count and neutrophil count, platelet count, and total white blood cell (WBC) count derived from frequently conducted complete blood picture test counts as a disease progression marker in the control and recognition of high-risk sufferers in time who need critical care services.

■ HEMATOLOGICAL ABNORMALITIES CUTOFF VALUES[4,5]

Male individuals older than 15 years who have hemoglobin levels <13 g/dL have anemia, as do nonpregnant women older than 15 years who have hemoglobin levels <12 g/dL. WBC count overall <3.6 × 10^9/L for leucopenia. Overall platelet count less than 1.5 lac/μL for thrombocytopenia.

Laboratory Findings

Lactic dehydrogenase (LDH): COVID-19 patients had elevated levels of LDH. The liver, lungs, heart, kidneys, brain, striated muscle, and red blood cells (RBCs) all contain LDH. LDH is an illustrative indicator of cellular death in COVID-19.[3]

Erythrocyte sedimentation rate (ESR): COVID-19 has a higher ESR.[6] The effects of the COVID-19 virus include modifications to the properties of RBCs or plasma, which raise ESR.

C-reactive protein (CRP): Tissue damage and elevated inflammatory cytokine levels both contributed to a rise in CRP levels.[7,8]

Changes in liver features may be caused by direct injury to the organ, drugs, congestive or ischemic hepatic disorders, or other factors,[9] and they occasionally lead to an increase in total bilirubin levels.[10] Aspartate aminotransferase (AST) production is up along with alanine aminotransferase (ALT) production with decreased albumin levels.[7]

Patients with COVID-19 have been found to have low levels of albumin, high glutamic-pyruvic transaminase range, and glutamic oxaloacetic transaminase range.[9,10] These results point to the long-term development of liver dysfunction brought on by SARS-CoV-2 and reduced clotting factor synthesis, ultimately leading to coagulation problems. Additionally, the use of antiviral medications such ribavirin, which is linked to liver cell toxicity and reduced synthesis of molecules including coagulation factors, may contribute to coagulation disorder.[11-13] After the COVID-19 sickness has resolved, the ALT, AST, gamma-glutamyl transferase (GGT), and alkaline phosphatase (ALP) levels may still be high for 2-3 months. These altered markers could be the result of the virus directly damaging the liver cells and a systemic inflammatory response brought on by elevated levels of IFN, interleukin (IL)-6, IL-10, and IL-2.[14,15]

■ INJURY FROM ISCHEMIC HYPOXIC REPERFUSION

Ischemic hypoxic reperfusion injury may cause epithelial cells to experience oxidative stress, which lowers nitric oxide production and increases superoxide production. Damage to epithelial cells, exposure of transfer factor on the vascular cell outer membranes and the activation of external coagulation pathways are the effects of this.[12] By directly interacting with ACE2 on the surface of epithelial cells, SARS-CoV-2 may also exacerbate the harm that it causes. When epithelial cells are damaged, transfer factor is expressed more strongly on the cell surface. In addition to losing its anticoagulant capabilities, this harms protein C, tissue factor (TF) pathway inhibitor, and antithrombin 3. Damage to epithelial cells also induces an unbalanced fibrinolytic process which results in coagulation dysfunction.[12]

CHANGES IN KIDNEY FUNCTION

Acute kidney damage causes include (a) SARS-CoV-2 binding to ACE2 receptors first of all leads to direct kidney harm;[16] (b) expanded production of proinflammatory cytokines and chemokines that may cause apoptosis of the renal tubular epithelial cells further leads to direct damage to kidneys; and (c) critical care interventions leads to damage to kidneys. Increased levels of blood urea and creatinine are noticed as a result of damage to kidneys. Complete urine examination shows protein in urine.[17]

Procalcitonin

Calcium regulatory hormone calcitonin's precursor is procalcitonin (PCT). COVID-19 patients show increased levels of PCT which is mediated by expanded range of IL-6 and tumor necrosis factor alpha (TNF-α).[18]

Cardiac Markers

Cardiac troponin I (cTnI), creatine kinase (CK), CK-muscle/brain activity (CK-MB), myoglobin (Mb), alpha-hydroxybutyrate dehydrogenase (α-HBDH), and N-terminal of the prohormone brain natriuretic peptide (NT-proBNP) are all cardiac markers which show marked increase in levels.

Variable Inflammatory Markers

The presence of an inflammation in COVID-19 also leads to increase of cytokines and chemokines such as IL-2, IL-6, IL-7, IL-10, TNF-α, G-CSF, IP-10, MCP-1, and MIP-1α.[19]

HEMATOLOGICAL FINDINGS

Certain variables that act as inflammatory markers in COVID-19 are total leucocyte count, differential neutrophil, monocyte, eosinophils and lymphocyte count, platelet count, and mean platelet volume. Frequently noticeable changes seen in blood profile are anemia, leucocytosis or leucopenia, neutrophilia, low eosinophil count or eosinophilia, thrombocytopenia, and very seldom thrombocytosis is seen.[20]

However, anemia is rarely seen. According to studies, approximately 1.5% patients suffering from COVID-19 needed blood transfusion.[19] Low hemoglobin causes include: (a) RBC membranes are damaged due to presence of angiotensin and ACE2-interacting proteins present on the surface of RBCs, all led by SARS-CoV-2; (b) virus may directly damage heme protein; (c) iron metabolism function is dysregulated; (d) blood loss that took place during the course of renal replacement therapy and gastrointestinal bleeding in patients suffering from COVID-19 with or without use of anticoagulant; (e) cytokine storm leading to auto-immune hemolytic anemia.[21] At the time of admission, red blood cell distribution width (RDW) >14.5% was associated with increase in fatality risk from 11 to 31%.

Lymphopenia that may be seen in 25 to >80% of patients at the time of admission is the most frequently observed laboratory finding in SARS-CoV-2 infection.[7] Causes of lymphopenia include: (a) SARS-CoV-2 infection of lymphocytes as they have ACE2 receptors on their surface that further results in cell lysis;[10] (b) cytokine storm that also causes lymphocyte apoptosis;[22] (c) splenic atrophy associated with cytokine activation that results in a decrease in lymphocytes turnover;[23] severity of COVID-19 increases with lymphopenia. One of the signs for early admission for supportive care in the intensive care unit (ICU) may be a reduced ALC count of around 6,000 cm/L. Patients in the ICU have significant lymphopenia. Direct interaction between the S proteins of SARS-CoV-2 and SARS-CoV to ACE2 receptors expressed on CD34+ hematopoietic stem cells, lymphocytes, monocytes, and macrophages,[24] further initiate infection.[25]

According to reports, SARS-CoV-2 attacks cellular hemoglobin, which may be indicative of aberrant oxygen and carbon dioxide exchange in patients.[26]

A patient's immune system may react to a SARS-CoV-2 infection by producing certain antibodies or immune complexes. HIV-1 glycoprotein 160/120 interacts with antibodies against platelet proteins in thrombocytopenic individuals, increasing the amount of circulating immune complexes.[27,28] Consequently, the reticuloendothelial system detects and eliminates platelets coated with these antibodies or immune complexes. Thus, immune complexes can also harm hematopoietic cells that express related antigens. Therefore, immunological complexes or antibodies can cause cellular damage and indirectly cause apoptosis or prevent hematopoietic stem/progenitor cells from proliferating, which causes hemocytopenia.[29]

THE HEMATOPOIETIC MICROENVIRONMENT IS DESTROYED BY SARS-COV-2

In the bone marrow (BM), the microenvironment plays a crucial part in controlling hematopoiesis. A hematopoietic microenvironment resembling a honeycomb is created by BM stromal cells, endothelial cells (ECs), osteoblasts, macrophages, extracellular matrix, and released cytokines.[30,31] The hematological microenvironment may change as a result of epithelial cell death and malfunction as well as BM mesenchymal stem cells (MSCs).[32-34] SARS-CoV uses the ACE2 receptor, which is also present on the surface of epithelial cells and fibroblasts, to cause cellular death.[35,36] As a result, the virus's ability to connect to the ACE2 receptor may cause harm to epithelial cells. Consequently, it might be inferred that SARS-CoV-2 has an impact on the BM microenvironment. The high expression of ACE2 on the surface of human alveolar tissue can be blamed for the lung damage brought on by SARS-CoV-2.[36] Patients with COVID-19 have diffuse alveolar damage in their lungs, which is accompanied by pulmonary congestion, edema, the development of a hyaline membrane, and fibrosis.[37] Severe alveolar injury inhibits the development and fragmentation of megakaryocytes in the pulmonary microcirculation, leading to thrombocytopenia.[38,39] It also reduces the effective capillary bed of the lung. Additionally, hematopoietic progenitors exterior to the pulmonary arteries may suffer from virus- or inflammation-induced damage that impairs their ability to migrate and differentiate, which can lead to thrombocytopenia.[14] Therefore, thrombocytopenia may result either directly or indirectly from increased platelet consumption and/or decreased platelet synthesis.

In extreme cases, the neutrophil-to-lymphocyte ratio rises. In severe situations, the neutrophil count is also raised.[40] Additionally, the ratios of neutrophil count to albumin and neutrophil to CD4⁺ lymphocytes are rising.[41,42] The ratio of lymphocytes to monocytes can be low, normal, or even higher. Also observed is eosinopenia.[43,44]

Thrombocytopenia may be caused by any of the following: (a) CD13 and CD66a, which function as potential receptors for SARS-CoV-2 internalization, directly damage hematopoietic CD34⁺ stem cells and further reduce platelet production; (b) imperfectly fragmented megakaryocytes, which result in a reduction in platelet production due to damage to the lung and pulmonary capillaries; (c) increased platelet consumption caused by EC damage; (d) decreased thrombopoietin production; (e) anti-platelet autoantibodies also leads to platelet destruction.[45,46]

Very low platelet counts <20,000 or a sudden fall in platelet count >50% over 24-48 hours can occur in preterminal stages of COVID-19.

Increasing values in WBC, ALC, AMC and decreasing LDH is observed in ICU patients as clinical condition improves.

PERIPHERAL BLOOD SMEAR FINDINGS

Blood picture is predominantly normocytic and normochromic. Sometimes the blood image may be dimorphic (microcytic–macrocytic), microcytic hypochromic, or macrocytic. A nucleated RBC (NRBC) and coarse basophilic stippling are present in the RBC series.[47] The most frequent result is lymphopenia with reactive lymphocytes; however, cells occasionally display monocytoid or lymphoplasmacytoid characteristics.[20,48] There are also several big granular lymphocytes with conspicuous azurophilic granules and round to indented nuclei, condensed chromatin, a few with prominent nucleoli, and an abundance of pale blue cytoplasm. These cells are most likely cytotoxic T lymphocytes or natural killer cells. There are other descriptions in the literature of large, unusual-appearing mononuclear cells that are 2-3 times the size of RBCs and have an uneven nuclear membrane, dense chromatin, minimal-to-moderate cytoplasm, and a small number of cytoplasmic granules and vacuoles (also labelled as virocyte).[49] There are cytoplasmic vacuolations in neutrophils, as well as numerous, crowded, dark distinct granulations that resemble poisonous granulations, a basophilic agranular zone in the cytoplasm's periphery, and noticeably condensed chromatin in the nucleus.[20,48] Numerous aberrant nuclear morphologies, such as ring-shaped, pi-shaped, and donut-shaped nuclei, were also seen in neutrophils.[47] These C-shaped, nuclear projection-adorned nuclei, which resemble fetuses, are known as COVID nuclei.[48] Hypogranulations, hypolobation, and pseudo-Pelger–Huët neutrophils are examples of dysmorphic images. Apoptotic cells resembling polymorphs with nuclear fragmentation are found, with liquefied nuclear chromatin and granulated or deep blue cytoplasm. Early phases usually contain immature granulocytes in the form of tiny promyelocytes, myelocytes, or metamyelocytes. There are also occasionally reactive big atypical monocytes with aberrant nuclear structure and cytoplasmic vacuolations.[43,50] Leucoerythroblastic blood images are described infrequently.[51] In COVID-19, platelet morphological abnormalities can be detected in patients with thrombocytosis as well as thrombocytopenia. Giant platelets, typically hyperchromatic, vacuolized, and some displaying pseudopods are among these morphological alterations **(Fig. 1)**.[52]

Cytoplasmic Abnormalities in Neutrophils

- Up to 97% of patients had hypergranular cytoplasm (black, crowded, coarse type), which was frequently described as poisonous[47,49,53-61]
- Cytoplasm with hypogranules.[49,50,54,55,58-63] On the same film, it is not unusual to find both hypergranular/toxic neutrophils and hypogranular neutrophils.
- Existence of small basophilic, agranular cytoplasmic areas, blue areas, or Döhle bodies; these pale blue spots represent endoplasmic reticulum membranes[55,57,59,61,64,65]
- Cytoplasmic vacuoles were discovered in up to 95% of patients[47,49,58,59,61,64,66]
- In severe or fatal cases, lipid-rich lipofuscin from necrotic liver cells is seen as blue-green cytoplasmic inclusions.[53,59]
- Reduced myeloperoxidase (MPO) activity measured by automated blood cell counts in cytochemistry.[67]

Nuclear Abnormalities in Neutrophils

Nuclear hyposegmentation or the absence of nuclear lobes, along with darkly clumped chromatin,[49,50,55,58,60] and atypical nuclear profiles (round, C-shaped, fetus-like, or ring-shaped) are the most frequent findings.[49,65] A comparable morphology is observed in COVID-19 by the majority of authors. The nuclear hyposegmentation with aberrant,[61] hyperdense,[60] or amorphous[55] chromatin is sometimes referred to as a pseudo-Pelger-Huët (PPH) anomaly.[47,55-57,59-62,65,68,69]

Additionally, other reports have mentioned the following nuclear shapes or structural abnormalities:
- Hyper-segmented nuclei[54]
- Detached nuclear fragments[68] are also referred to as inclusions that resemble Howell–Jolly bodies[64]

CHAPTER 5: Hematological Changes Associated with COVID-19 Infections

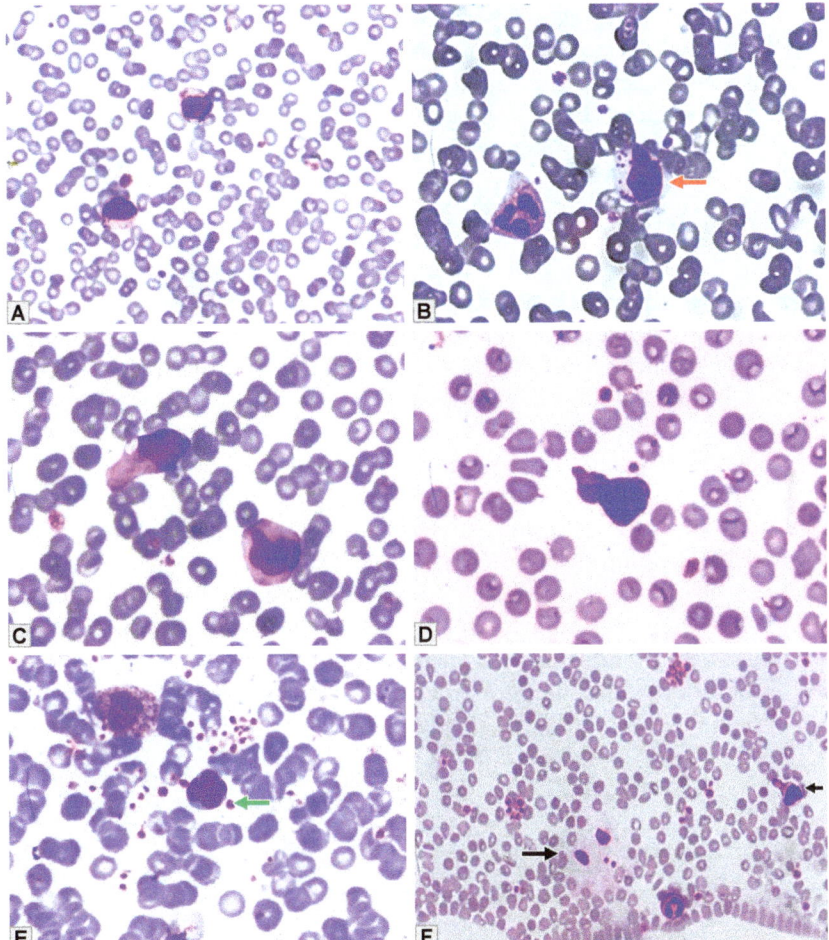

FIGS. 1A TO F: Changes noticed in lymphocytes as shown by peripheral blood smear. (A) Abnormal lymphocytes (virocyte/covicyte) with a characteristic varied azurophilic granule pattern, an open chromatin structure, a conspicuous nucleoli, and an abundance of cytoplasm. (B) Large granular lymphocyte (red arrow). (C and D) Downey cells in (D) display an irregular nucleus and hyperbasophilic cytoplasm with pod development. (E) Lymphocyte that has died (green arrow). (F) Atypical lymphocyte (short black arrow) next to circulating macrophage (wide black arrow). 400–1,000× Leishman.

- Karyorrhexis[49,59,60]
- Karyolysis[59,66]

Abnormality Involving All Neutrophils
- The presence of apoptotic neutrophils in the blood, or pyknosis[55,56,62,66,70,71]
- Smeared or disintegrated neutrophils[60]
- Massive forms[61]

- With an increasing proportion of band forms[55,64] and circulating granulocyte precursors like metamyelocytes, myelocytes, promyelocytes, and even blasts with cytoplasmic granules, myeloid left shift is nearly always present in the body.[47,55,56,63,64] They occasionally form a leucoerythroblastic image with circulating NRBCs.

PLATELETS

When a patient is admitted to the hospital, the platelet count has been reported as normal[20] or decreasing.[7,72,73] The prevalence of low platelet count at admission was 36.2% in one of the earliest clinical presentations from China. Patients with severe or critical conditions may experience a decrease in platelet count, and the count may alter as the disease progresses.[74] In one investigation, a level of $100 \times 10^9/L$ was present in 45.5% of the patients.[72]

In COVID-19, platelets frequently have morphological abnormalities and may exhibit a hyperactive behavior.[75,76] Patients with COVID-19 have been reported to have the following platelet shape characteristics:
- Platelet pleomorphism[67] and anisocytosis[57]
- Large or enormous platelets, even in youngsters.[50,55,56,62,64,66] Platelets in COVID-19 have an increased mean platelet volume in several experiments using automated blood cell counters[47]
- Thrombocytes granulomere which are hyperchromatic[49,59]
- Variable sizes of peripheral clear areas[55]
- Protrusions of pseudopods [55,59]
- Aggregates of platelets[77]

Flowcytometry

Analyzing various populations of peripheral blood cells can be done with the aid of flowcytometric immunophenotyping. ICU patients' CD45+, CD3+, CD4+, CD8+, CD19+, and CD16/56+ levels are significantly reduced. Not all patient groups had an inverted CD4 to CD8 ratio. More frequently, SARS-CoV-2 affects T cells. Patients with COVID-19 had reduced levels of suppressor T cells (CD3+ and CD8+) as well as helper T (Th) cells (CD3+ and CD4+).[78,79] However, CD8 T-cell numbers fell more dramatically. In the B-cell population, COVID-19 patients had lower levels of CD19 expression and higher levels of membrane-bound IgM and IgG, which suggested that B cells undergo plasmacytoid maturation and immunoglobulin switching after viral exposure. Along with greater levels of abnormal and delayed plasma cell maturation, which is also found[80] are the expanded levels of macrophage markers CD80 and CD206.[43] According to some investigators, the amount of HLA-DR present on monocytes correlates with the severity of COVID-19; individuals with severe and critical COVID-19 exhibited decreased levels of HLA-DR. The two primary indicators evaluated in the study by flow cytometry for differentiating between bacterial or other viral infections were CD64 on neutrophils and CD169 on monocytes.[81] The CD4/CD8 ratio was not flipped in ICU patients. Increased concentrations of inflammatory mediators like IL-1B, IL-6, IL-12, IL-18, IL-33, CXCL10, CCL2, and TNF-α cause type 1 helper T cell function to be activated. In contrast to sepsis with DIC, COVID-19 may have a shorter activated partial thromboplastin time (aPTT).

ANTICOAGULANT OF CHOICE

Heparin which is unfractionated, fondaparinux given subcutaneously along with low molecular weight heparin (LMWH) **(Flowchart 1)**.

Bone Marrow Smear

Hematopoiesis, leucopoiesis, and thrombopoiesis are visible in COVID-19's bone marrow, coupled with sporadic myeloid hyperplasia and a shift to the left. Patients with severe COVID-19 exhibit hemophagocytosis and histiocytic proliferation in BM aspirates.[20,83] Through the activation of the IL-1/IL-6 pathway, COVID-19 may increase the risk of hemophagocytic lymphohistiocytosis (HLH). In COVID-19, there is an increase in pleomorphic megakaryocytes, plasma cells, and macrophages.[82]

Coagulation Profile

Coagulopathy is the most frequent cause of death in COVID-19 patients.[84-86] Increases are seen in the FDP, aPTT, D-dimer level, PT, and fibrinogen levels. Additionally elevated are P-selectin, factor VIII, and von Willebrand factor. Additionally elevated in COVID-19 is PAI-1, a plasminogen activator inhibitor. In COVID-19, EC activation and damage brought on by SARS-CoV-2 spike protein binding to receptors and endothelial injury and hypercoagulability brought on by hypoxia are the two main causes of thromboembolism. Blood viscosity is increased; fibrinolysis is reduced in severe COVID-19 cases; complement is activated; prolonged bed rest during illness; dehydration; the presence of other cardiovascular risk factors; and vascular endothelial damage may be brought on by central venous catheterization, mechanical ventilation, and other procedures.[86] When compared with patients with normal or modestly raised D-dimer levels, a high D-dimer value is associated with an increased need for an ICU and a greater fatality rate. Owing to the possibility of venous thrombosis and cytokine storm, a fourfold increase in D-dimer is a sign of high mortality.

Around 91% of those with prolonged aPTT test positive for the lupus anticoagulant. High mortality rate associated with overt DIC.

In COVID-19 without TTP, ADAMTS13 levels of 20–40% were discovered.

Prognosis

In COVID-19, RDW also serves as a complication marker.[78] In COVID-19, lymphopenia appears to be the most important infection severity biomarker. Reduced lymphocyte/leukocyte ratios have been linked to serious illness and/

CHAPTER 5: Hematological Changes Associated with COVID-19 Infections

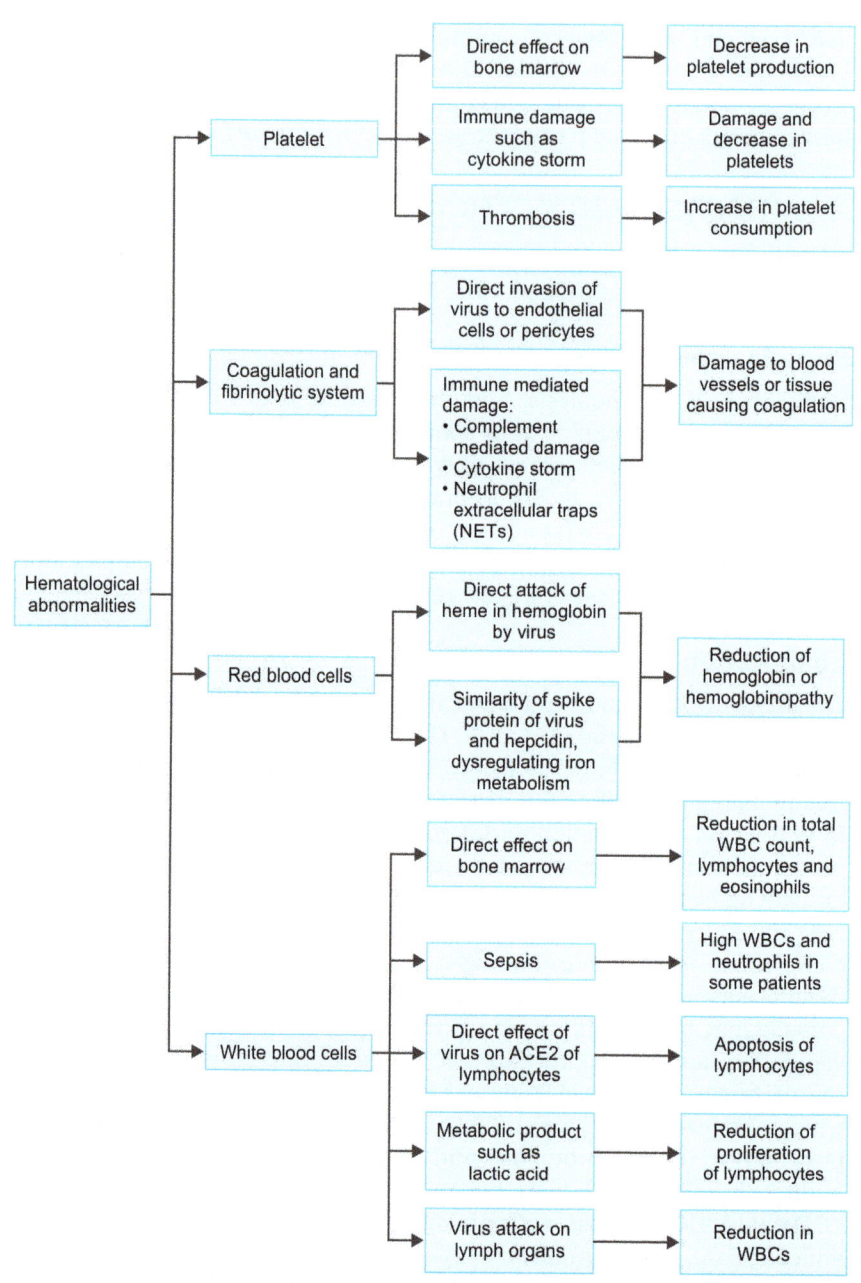

FLOWCHART 1: Chart depicting hematological abnormalities in COVID-19.[82]
(ACE2: angiotensin-converting enzyme 2; WBCs: white blood cells)

or catastrophic consequences.[87] Increased mortality and high neutrophil/lymphocyte and neutrophil/platelet ratios may be signs of myocardial injury.[19,88] The prognostic indicators ESR, CRP, LDH (>250 U/L), and IL-6 are worse. Increased LDH is linked to an increased risk of acute respiratory distress syndrome, death, and multiple organ injury.[3,6,8] The development of ARDS, increased troponin-T levels, cardiac damage, and death are all linked to high CRP levels (>10 mg/L).[74,89,90] The prognosis is poorer when there is hyperferritinemia and elevated bilirubin levels.[10,16] Increased IL-6 and LDH levels have been linked to increased mortality risk.[89] Expanded levels of CD25$^+$ T and CD95$^+$ cells are linked with poor prognosis.

HEMATOLOGICAL CHANGES IN SPECIAL GROUPS

Children have a lower incidence of COVID-19 than do adults. Five percent of the incidents included children under the age of 19 years. The disease appears to progress more slowly in children than in adults. Around 0.3% of cases were severe.

The majority of kids with COVID-19 have normal leukocyte counts. Only 15% of instances were documented to have lymphopenia, and it was not always accompanied by a serious illness.[91-93]

Elevated levels of inflammatory markers such as ferritin [(26% (16–40)], PCT [25% (21–29)], and CRP [19% (16–22)] were found in additional laboratory findings in youngsters.[94] In children with an acute infection, LMWH or unfractionated heparin (UFH) is the anticoagulant of choice. Owing to its consistent pharmacokinetics, pharmacodynamic effects, and longer half-life, it is frequently preferred to UFH.[95] Aside from their anti-inflammatory and immunomodulatory effects, LMWHs may also have an antiviral effect because they interact with the SARS-CoV-2 spike S1 protein receptor-binding domain and prevent the virus from attaching to the receptor.[95] As the illness worsens, higher dosages of LMWH/UFH might be required because of developed heparin resistance and an antithrombin deficit.[95] Less frequently than thrombotic events, bleeding events also have unanswered questions.[77] According to reports, microvascular thrombosis and thrombocytopenia contribute to bleeding events in pediatric patients; the most frequent bleeding event was purpura, which is frequently referred to as chilblains and manifests as petechiae, microhemorrhages in the extremities, erythema, and macular eruptions.[77]

Children with sickle cell disease who were infected with COVID-19 were reported to have asymptomatic (25.5%) or mild-to-moderate symptoms (65.6%), while some also had more severe symptoms (8.2%) in illness-specific hematologic conditions.[96]

Pediatric COVID-19 presentations did not frequently involve severe anemia necessitating transfusion. SARS-CoV-2, however, has the potential to cause autoimmune hemolytic anemia (AIHA) and hemolytic crises in people with congenital hemolytic anemias.[97]

Owing to a genetic defect that affects the red cell membrane's encoding, hereditary spherocytosis is an inherited hemolytic anemia that results in RBCs that are abnormally spherical and less flexible. Hemolysis can be made worse by infections and diseases.

Expecting Mothers

Nearly 80% of pregnant women experience moderate symptoms or are asymptomatic, and they have healthy pregnancies.[7] Around 15% of instances of COVID-19 in pregnant women were classified as severe, and 5% as serious and concomitant.[98] The incidence of mortality was only 0.43%.[99] More recent research has linked placental infection to increased fibrin deposition, which causes fetal discomfort and ultimately results in premature delivery.[100]

The three most prevalent hematological abnormalities are lymphopenia, neutropenia, and thrombocytopenia. There have been reports of hypercoagulability in sick pregnant women.[60] A higher D-dimer (82%), a higher neutrophil count (81%), a higher CRP (69%), and a lower lymphocyte count (59%) are worse prognostic indicators.[101] Along with lower fibrinogen levels, low platelet count, and greater aPTT, with high D-dimer levels. Venous thromboembolism during pregnancy is already recognized to increase the chance of a procoagulant imbalance. Women having C-sections have access to prophylactic anticoagulation to lower the risk of venous thromboembolism.

COVID-19 Infection and Hemoglobinopathies

Infection is one of the main causes of death in people with hemoglobinopathies, such as sickle cell disease and thalassemia. Comorbidities such as inefficient erythropoiesis, chronic hemolytic anemia, iron overload, and hypercoagulability, which render them susceptible to COVID-19 infection sequelae, are the cause of the greater susceptibility.[18,102] When COVID-19 infects a patient who has had a splenectomy, the patient is at risk for developing serious secondary bacterial infections.[18] Despite the fact that the acute chest syndrome (ACS) and the need for critical care support have been linked to the 2009 H1N1 influenza pandemic,[18,19] the majority of COVID-19 chronic hemoglobinopathy patients have a milder version of the disease. The more severe versions are only seen in a small number of people mostly because of hypoxia and VQ mismatch.[18,20]

Other Hematological Conditions and Susceptibility to COVID-19

When compared with the general population, congenital bleeding disorders (such as hemophilia A and von Willebrand disease, vWD) appear to have a low prevalence of COVID-19.[20,22,23] Similarly, even with low dosages of immunosuppressants, patients with ITP do not exhibit elevated infection rates.[22,73] It may be necessary to avoid using larger dosages of steroids and rituximab during the pandemic, and it would be preferable to use IVIG and/or thrombopoietin receptor agonist (TPO) medicines in their place.[73,80]

There is no relationship between the ABO blood group and the severity or fatality of the illness, while people with blood type A may be more vulnerable to contracting COVID-19 while those with blood type O may be less susceptible.[11]

Effect of COVID-19 on Hematologic Cancer Patients' Clinical Results

Patients with hematologic malignancies may experience different results depending on several conditions. However, patients with hematologic malignancies who also have COVID-19 had a greater mortality rate than those who did not.[103]

Patients with hematologic, lung, or metastatic (stage IV) cancer had more severe disease than those who were cancer-free, according to a multicenter study.[104] It has been discovered that mortality is directly correlated with advanced age, disease status, performance status, immunological parameters, and inflammatory levels.[105]

■ BONE MARROW EFFECTS IN COVID-19

Three severely ill COVID-19 patients' bone marrow aspirates revealed hemophagocytosis.[106] Pleomorphic megakaryocytes, plasma cells, macrophages, and hemophagocytosis all increased. Megakaryocytes were discovered in greater numbers in the bone marrow, and their shape suggested that platelet synthesis was active, according to Rapkiewicz et al.[107] Using electron microscopy, rare virions were also found in bone marrow megakaryocytes.

High leukocyte, neutrophil, platelet, and decreased lymphocyte counts in SARS-CoV-2 patients at hospital admission are all connected to COVID-19-related ICU admission.

During hospitalization, low levels of hemoglobin, erythrocytes, and median globular volume were also linked to a higher risk of COVID-19-related ICU admission. Further, elevated LDH levels during hospital admission in SARS-CoV-2 patients are linked to COVID-19-related ICU admission.

Age, gender, lymphocyte/lymphocyte ratio, platelet/neutrophil ratio, erythrocytes, cell hemoglobin concentration mean (CHCM) values, and COVID-19-related mortality risk were all independently associated factors.

■ COVID-19 INFECTION IN MALIGNANCY

Malignancies have the highest frequency of complications among individuals with hematological disorders in the COVID-19 era.[108] The severity of COVID-19 disease, ICU admission, the requirement for mechanical ventilation, and mortality.[108] are some of these problems. This vulnerable subpopulation is experiencing a more aggressive and fatal illness progression cascade. Numerous studies have demonstrated that predictive biomarkers, such as CRP, D-dimer, PT, and serum IL-6 levels, were significantly greater in cancer patients than in noncancer patients, despite the fact that specific pathophysiological changes are still being investigated.[109] More particularly, as this particular subset of patients has a severe and persistent humoral and cellular immune deficit, the coexistence of acute myeloid leukemia in children with COVID-19 provides an unprecedented difficulty.[108,109]

This is demonstrated by the recommendation to postpone acute myeloid leukemia (AML) medication until symptoms subside and the polymerase chain reaction (PCR) results are negative[108] in several nations' cancer institute guidelines. Other research indicates that hematopoietic stem cell transplantation (HSCT; for hematopoietic malignancy and aplasia) or CAR-T therapy have encountered previously unheard-of difficulties due to concern over infection of the donor, recipient, and healthcare personnel.[109] Additionally, leukemoid reactions and overlap syndromes (MDS/MPN) are more likely to occur in individuals with proliferative chronic myelomonocytic leukemia (CMML) because to the higher amount of leukocytes that has been reported in these patients. Therefore, even if they are asymptomatic, they would require a greater type of immunosuppression such as hydroxycarbamide when they are exposed to COVID-19 infection.[110] However, results from smaller cancer centers[111] reported success after a nonmyeloablative conditioning regimen followed by post-transplant cyclophosphamide (PTCy). In these cases, the successful prophylaxis against graft-versus-host disease (GVHD) could also work on the attenuation of COVID-19. Additionally, another single-center study revealed preliminary data showing that organ transplant patient mortality is nearly at prepandemic levels, and they hypothesized that "such patients with an already immune suppressed immune system are not able to produce a cytokine storm and thus do not experience fulminant COVID-19 infection."[112]

Long COVID is defined as persistent symptoms lasting 4–12 weeks; post acute COVID-19 syndrome (PASC) is defined as symptoms lasting more than 12 weeks that cannot be accounted for by a differentiating diagnosis.

Long COVID is also known as persistent symptoms in the absence of a virus, postacute COVID-19 if symptoms last longer than 12 weeks, persistent COVID-19 symptoms with a negative PCR test, or persistent COVID-19 symptoms that appear at least 1 month after the commencement of symptoms.

Age >60 years, obesity, diabetes mellitus, hypertension, ischemic heart disease, chronic obstructive pulmonary disease, asthma, and chronic kidney disease are comorbidities that contribute to long-term illness.

■ HEMATOLOGIC ABNORMALITIES IN LONG COVID

Lymphopenia, Hyperferritinemia, Coagulopathies

Severe acute COVID is related with iron dysregulation, which can cause hyperferritinemia and last for up to 2 months after an acute infection. When there is inflammation, IL-6 is released, which stimulates the production of hepcidin, which then prevents the release of iron from cells, raising ferritin levels and resulting in hyperferritinemia.

Hemophagocytic Lymphohistiocytosis
Long-term COVID leads to HLH leading to multiorgan failure.

Macrophage Activation Syndrome
Excessive cytokines, cytopenia, and hyperferritinemia occurs ultimately leading to septic shock.

Hematological autoimmune diseases associated with COVID-19:
- Autoimmune hemolytic anemia
- *Immune thrombocytopenia (ITP)*: Viral ITP occurs when b lymphocytes produce antibodies that cross react with thrombocytes causing their destruction leading to thrombocytopenia.
- *Abnormal glucose metabolism*: Post-acute COVID-19 patients without a history of diabetes mellitus exhibited a rise in HbA1c.

Blood viscosity, endothelial inflammation, and vascular dysfunction are all further increased by HbA1c.

Every patient with a diagnosis of COVID-19 infection is advised to have baseline measurements of their PT/aPTT, D-dimer, and platelet count. Identifying patients who could require ICU care may be helpful.

CONCLUSION

In conclusion, the exploration of hematological changes in COVID-19 in this chapter unravels a multifaceted landscape of alterations in blood parameters. The identified shifts in hematopoietic elements, coagulation factors and inflammatory markers contribute significantly to our understanding of the virus's impact on the human body. As highlighted in this chapter, the potential implications for diagnosis, prognosis, and therapeutic intervention have been discussed in detail. However, continued research efforts are still required to improve comprehensive healthcare strategies in managing COVID-19 patients.

REFERENCES

1. Agbuduwe C, Basu S. Hematological manifestations of COVID-19: From cytopenia to coagulopathy. Eur J Haematol. 2020;105(5):540-6.
2. Castro RA, Frishman WH. Thrombotic complications of COVID-19 infection: A Review. Cardiol Rev. 2021;29(1):43-7.
3. Henry BM, Aggarwal G, Wong J, Benoit S, Vikse J, Plebani M, et al. Lactate dehydrogenase levels predict coronavirus disease 2019 (COVID-19) severity and mortality: A pooled analysis. Am J Emerg Med. 2020;38:1722-6.
4. WHO. Haemoglobin concentrations for the diagnosis of anemia and assessment of severity: VMNIS vitamin and mineral nutrition information system. Report of a

WHO scientific group. 2011. Available from: http:// www.who.int/vmnis/indica tors/ haemoglobin/en.
5. Tsegaye A, Messele T, Tilahun T, Hailu E, Sahlu T, Doorly R, et al. Immunohematological reference ranges for adult Ethiopians. Clin Diagn Lab Immunol. 1999;6(3):410-4.
6. Ponti G, Maccaferri M, Ruini C, Tomasi A, Ozben T. Biomarkers associated with COVID-19 disease progression. Crit Rev Clin Lab Sci. 2020;57:389-9.
7. Guan WJ, Ni ZY, Hu Y, Liang WH, Ou C-Q, He J-X, et al. China Medical Treatment Expert Group for COVID-19. Clinical characteristics of coronavirus disease 2019 in China. N Engl J Med. 2020;382:1708-20.
8. Liu Y, Yang Y, Zhang C, Huang F, Wang F, Yuan J, et al. Clinical and biochemical indexes from 2019-nCoV infected patients linked to viral loads and lung injury. Sci China Life Sci. 2020;63:364-74.
9. Huang C, Wang Y, Li X, Ren L, Zhao J, Hu Y, et al. Clinical features of patients infected with 2019 novel coronavirus in Wuhan, China. Lancet. 2020;395(10223):497-506.
10. Kumar P, Sharma M, Kulkarni A, Rao PN. Pathogenesis of liver injury in coronavirus disease 2019. J Clin Exp Hepatol. 2020;10(6):641-2.
11. Wang M, Cao R, Zhang L, Yang X, Liu J, Xu M, et al. Remdesivir and chloroquine effectively inhibit the recently emerged novel coronavirus (2019-nCoV) in vitro. Cell Res. 2020;30:269-71.
12. Yan Y, Zou Z, Sun Y, Li X, Xu KF, Wei Y, et al. Anti-malaria drug chloroquine is highly effective in treating avian influenza A H5N1 virus infection in an animal model. Cell Res. 2013;23:300-2.
13. Chaves J, Huen A, Bueso-Ramos C, Vadhan-Raj S. Aerosolized Ribavirin-induced reversible hepatotoxicity in a hematopoietic stem cell transplant recipient with Hodgkin lymphoma. Clin Infect Dis. 2006;42:e72-5.
14. Gameil MA, Marzouk RE, Elsebaie AH, Rozaik SE. Long-term clinical and biochemical residue after COVID-19 recovery. Egypt Liver J. 2021;11:74.
15. Patterson BK, Francisco EB, Yogendra R, Long E, Pise A, Rodrigues H, et al. Persistence of SARS CoV-2 S1 protein in CD16+ monocytes in post-acute sequelae of COVID-19 (PASC) up to 15 months post-infection. Front Immunol. 2022;12:746021.
16. Xiang HX, Fei J, Xiang Y, Xu Z, Zheng L, Li XY, et al. Renal dysfunction and prognosis of COVID-19 patients: A hospital-based retrospective cohort study. BMC Infect Dis. 2021;21:158.
17. Han X, Ye Q. Kidney involvement in COVID-19 and its treatments. J Med Virol. 2021;93:1387-95.
18. Zhou F, Yu T, Du R, Guohui Fan, Ying Liu, Liu Z, et al. Clinical course and risk factors for mortality of adult inpatients with COVID-19 in Wuhan, China: A retrospective cohort study. Lancet. 2020;395:1054-62.
19. Letícia de Oliveira Toledo S, Sousa Nogueira L, das Graças Carvalho M, Rios DRA, de Barros Pinheiro M. COVID-19: Review and hematologic impact. Clin Chim Acta. 2020;510:170-6.
20. Fan BE, Chong VCL, Chan SSW, Lim GH, Lim KGE, Tan GB, et al. Hematologic parameters in patients with COVID-19 infection. Am J Hematol. 2020;95(6):E131-4.
21. Lazarian G, Quinquenel A, Bellal M, Siavellis J, Jacquy C, Re D, et al. Autoimmune haemolytic anaemia associated with COVID-19 infection. Br J Haematol. 2020;190: 29-31.
22. Liao YC, Liang WG, Chen FW, Hsu JH, Yang JJ, Chang MS. IL-19 induces production of IL-6 and TNF-alpha and results in cell apoptosis through TNF-alpha. J Immunol. 2002;169:4288-97.
23. Chan JF, Zhang AJ, Yuan S, Poon VK, Chan CC, Lee AC. Simulation of the clinical and pathological manifestations of coronavirus disease 2019 (COVID-19) in golden Syrian

hamster model: implications for disease pathogenesis and transmissibility. Clin Infect Dis. 2020;71:2428-46.
24. Chan JF, Kok KH, Zhu Z, Chu H, To KK, Yuan S, et al. Genomic characterization of the 2019 novel human-pathogenic coronavirus isolated from a patient with atypical pneumonia after visiting Wuhan. Emerg Microbes Infect. 2020;9:221-36.
25. Xu H, Zhong L, Deng J, Peng J, Dan H, Zeng X, et al. High expression of ACE2 receptor of 2019-nCoV on the epithelial cells of oral mucosa. Int J Oral Sci. 12:82020.
26. Liu W, Li H. COVID-19: Attacks the 1-beta chain of hemoglobin and captures the porphyrin to inhibit human heme metabolism. ChemRxiv. 2020.
27. Scaradavou A. HIV-related thrombocytopenia. Blood Rev. 2002;16:73-6.
28. Nardi M, Tomlinson S, Greco MA, Karpatkin S. Complement-independent, peroxide-induced antibody lysis of platelets in HIV-1-related immune thrombocytopenia. Cell. 2001;106(5):551-61.
29. Yang M, Li CK, Li K, Hon KLE, Ng MHL, Chan PKS, et al. Hematological findings in SARS patients and possible mechanisms (review). Int J Mol Med. 2004;14:311-5.
30. Taichman RS. Blood and bone: Two tissues whose fates are intertwined to create the hematopoietic stem-cell niche. Blood. 2005;105:2631-9.
31. Ru YX, Dong SX, Zhao SX, Li Y, Liang HY, Zhang MMF, et al. One cell one niche: Hematopoietic microenvironments constructed by bone marrow stromal cells with fibroblastic and histiocytic features. Ultrastruct Pathol. 2019;43:117-25.
32. Lord BI. The architecture of bone marrow cell populations. Int J Cell Cloning. 1990;331:317-31.
33. Kiel MJ, Yilmaz ÖH, Iwashita T, Yilmaz OH, Terhorst C, Morrison SJ. SLAM family receptors distinguish hematopoietic stem and progenitor cells and reveal endothelial niches for stem cells. Cell. 2005;121:1109-21.
34. Sugiyama T, Kohara H, Noda M, Nagasawa T. Maintenance of the hematopoietic stem cell pool by CXCL12-CXCR4 chemokine signaling in bone marrow stromal cell niches. Immunity. 2006;25:977-88.
35. Hamming I, Timens W, Bulthuis ML, Lely AT, Navis GJ, van Goor H. Tissue distribution of ACE2 protein, the functional receptor for SARS coronavirus. A first step in understanding SARS pathogenesis. J Pathol. 2004;203:631-7.
36. Ye J, Zhang B, Xu J, Chang Q, McNutt MA, Korteweg C, et al. Molecular pathology in the lungs of severe acute respiratory syndrome patients. Am J Pathol. 2007;170:538-45.
37. Xu Z, Shi L, Wang Y, Zhang J, Huang L, Zhang C, et al. Pathological findings of COVID-19 associated with acute respiratory distress syndrome. Lancet Respir Med. 2020;8:420-2.
38. Niinikoski J, Goldstein R, Linsey M, Hunt TK. Effect of oxygen-induced lung damage on tissue oxygen supply. Acta Chir Scand. 1973;139:591-5.
39. Yang M, Ng MH, Li CK. Thrombocytopenia in patients with severe acute respiratory syndrome (review). Hematology. 2005;10:101-5.
40. Cavalcante-Silva LHA, Carvalho DCM, Lima ÉA, Galvão JGFM, de França da Silva JS, de Sales-Neto JM, et al. Neutrophils and COVID-19: The road so far. Int Immunopharmacol. 2021;90:107233.
41. Wang H, Zhang Y, Mo P, Liu J, Wang H, Fan Wang F, et al. Neutrophil to CD4+ lymphocyte ratio as a potential biomarker in predicting virus negative conversion time in COVID-19. Int Immunopharmacol. 2020;85:106683.
42. Varim C, Yaylaci S, Demirci T, Kaya T, Nalbant A, Dheir H, et al. Neutrophil count to albumin ratio as a new predictor of mortality in patients with COVID-19 infection. Rev Assoc Med Bras (1992). 2020;662(Suppl 2):77-81.
43. Zhang D, Guo R, Lei L, Liu H, Wang Y, Wang Y, et al. Frontline science: COVID-19 infection induces readily detectable morphologic and inflammation-related phenotypic changes in peripheral blood monocytes. J Leukoc Biol. 2021;109:13-22.

44. Du Y, Tu L, Zhu P, Mu M, Wang R, Yang P, et al. Clinical features of 85 fatal cases of COVID-19 from Wuhan: A retrospective observational study. Am J Respir Crit Care Med. 2020;201:1372-9.
45. Pavord S, Thachil J, Hunt BJ, Murphy M, Lowe G, Laffan M, et al. Practical guidance for the management of adults with immune thrombocytopenia during the COVID-19 pandemic. Br J Haematol. 2020;189:1038-43.
46. Aggarwal M, Dass J, Mahapatra M. Hemostatic abnormalities in COVID-19: An update. Indian J Hematol Blood Transfus. 2020;36:1-11.
47. Kaur G, Sandeep F, Olayinka O, Gupta G. Morphologic changes in circulating blood cells of COVID-19 patients. Cureus. 2021;13:e13416.
48. Singh A, Sood N, Narang V, Goyal A. Morphology of COVID-19-affected cells in peripheral blood film. BMJ Case Rep. 2020;13:e236117.
49. Nath D, Madan U, Singh S, Tiwari N. CBC parameters and morphological alterations in peripheral blood cells in COVID-19 patients: Their significance and correlation with clinical course. Int J Health Clin Res. 2020;3:95-108.
50. Ahnach M, Ousti F, Nejjari S, Houssaini MS, Dini N. Peripheral blood smear findings in COVID-19. Turk J Haematol. 2020;37:310-2.
51. Mitra A, Dwyre DM, Schivo M, Thompson GR, Cohen SH, Ku N, et al. Leukoerythroblastic reaction in a patient with COVID-19 infection. Am J Hematol. 2020;95:999-1000.
52. Zini G, Bellesi S, Ramundo F, d'Onofrio G. Morphological anomalies of circulating blood cells in COVID-19. Am J Hematol. 2020;95:870-2.
53. Cantu MD, Towne WS, Emmons FN, Mostyka M, Borczuk A, Salvatore SP, et al. Clinical significance of blue-green neutrophil and monocyte cytoplasmic inclusions in SARS-CoV-2 positive critically ill patients. Br J Haematol. 2020;190:e89-92.
54. Salib C, Teruya-Feldstein J. Hypersegmented granulocytes and COVID-19 infection. Blood. 2020;135:2196.
55. Zini G, Bellesi S, Ramundo F, d'Onofrio G. Morphological anomalies of circulating blood cells in COVID-19. Am J Hematol. 2020;95:870-2.
56. Lüke F, Orsó E, Kirsten J, Poeck H, Grube M, Wolff D, et al. Coronavirus disease 2019 induces multi-lineage, morphologic changes in peripheral blood cells. EJHaem. 2020;1:376-83.
57. Nazarullah A, Liang C, Villarreal A, Higgins RA, Mais DD. Peripheral blood examination findings in SARS-CoV-2 infection. Am J Clin Pathol. 2020;154:319-29.
58. Singh S, Madan J, Nath D, Tiwari N. Peripheral blood smear morphology - A red flag in COVID-19. Int J Trop Dis Health. 2020;2020(41):54-8.
59. Berber I, Cagasar O, Sarici A, Berber NK, Aydogdu I, Ulutas O, et al. Peripheral blood smear findings of COVID-19 patients provide İnformation about the severity of the disease and the duration of hospital stay. Mediterr J Hematol Infect Dis. 2021;13:e2021009.
60. Gabr H, Bastawy S, Abdel Aal AA, Khalil NM, Fateen M. Changes in peripheral blood cellular morphology as diagnostic markers for COVID-19 infection. Int J Lab Hematol. 2022;44:454-60.
61. Horiuchi Y, Hayashi F, Iwasaki Y, Matsuzaki A, Nishibe K, Kaniyu K, et al. Peripheral granular lymphocytopenia and dysmorphic leukocytosis as simple prognostic markers in COVID-19. Int J Lab Hematol. 2021;43:1309-18.
62. Schapkaitz E, De Jager T, Levy B. The characteristic peripheral blood morphological features of hospitalized patients infected with COVID-19. Int J Lab Hematol. 2021;43(3):e130-4.
63. Alnor A, Sandberg MB, Toftanes BE, Vinholt PJ. Platelet parameters and leukocyte morphology is altered in COVID-19 patients compared to non-COVID-19 patients with similar symptomatology. Scand J Clin Lab Invest. 2021;81:213-7.
64. Pezeshki A, Vaezi A, Nematollahi P. Blood cell morphology and COVID-19 clinical course, severity, and outcome. J Hematop. 2021;14:221-8.

65. Jain S, Meena R, Kumar V, Kaur R, Tiwari U. Comparison of hematologic abnormalities between hospitalized coronavirus disease 2019 positive and negative patients with correlation to disease severity and outcome. J Med Virol. 2022;94:3757-67.
66. Singh A, Verma SP, Kushwaha R, Ali W, Reddy HD, Singh US. Hematological changes in the second wave of SARS-CoV-2 in North India. Cureus. 2022;14:e23495.
67. Zini G, Arcuri P, Ladiana R, Tanzarella ES, Pascale GD, Onofrio GD. Vaccination does not affect leukocyte morphologic abnormalities of severe COVID-19. Am J Hematol. 2022;97(8):E310-11.
68. Singh A, Sood N, Narang V, Goyal A. Morphology of COVID-19-affected cells in peripheral blood film. BMJ Case Rep. 2020;13:e236117.
69. Akçabelen YM, Gürlek Gökçebay D, Yaralı N. Dysplastic changes of peripheral blood cells in COVID-19 infection. Turk J Haematol. 2021;38:72-3.
70. Gérard D, Henry S, Thomas B. SARS-CoV-2: A new aetiology for atypical lymphocytes. Br J Haematol. 2020;189:845.
71. Frater JL, Zini G, d'Onofrio G, Rogers HJ. COVID-19 and the clinical hematology laboratory. Int J Lab Hematol. 2020;42(Suppl 1):11-8.
72. Rohlfing AK, Rath D, Geisler T, Gawaz M. Platelets and COVID-19. Hamostaseologie. 2021;41:379-5.
73. Fischer K, Hoffmann P, Voelkl S, Meidenbauer N, Ammer J, Edinger M, et al. Inhibitory effect of tumor cell-derived lactic acid on human T cells. Blood. 2007;109:3812-9.
74. Lippi G, Plebani M, Henry BM. Thrombocytopenia is associated with severe coronavirus disease 2019 (COVID-19) infections: A meta-analysis. Clin Chim Acta. 2020;506:145-8.
75. Comer SP, Cullivan S, Szklanna PB, Weiss L, Cullen S, Kelliher S, et al. COCOON study investigators. COVID-19 induces a hyperactive phenotype in circulating platelets. PLoS Biol. 2021;19:e3001109.
76. Hottz ED, Azevedo-Quintanilha IG, Palhinha L, Palhinha L, Teixeira L, Barreto EA, et al. Platelet activation and platelet-monocyte aggregate formation trigger tissue factor expression in patients with severe COVID-19. Blood. 2020;136:1330-41.
77. McDaniel CG, Commander SJ, DeLaura I, Cantrell S, Leraas HJ, Moore CB, et al. Coagulation abnormalities and clinical complications in children with SARS-CoV-2: A systematic review of 48,322 patients. J Pediatr Hematol Oncol. 2022;44(6):323-35.
78. Erdinc B, Sahni S, Gotlieb V. Hematological manifestations and complications of COVID-19. Adv Clin Exp Med. 2021;30:101-7
79. Moratto D, Chiarini M, Giustini V, Serana F, Magro P, Roccaro AM, et al. Flow cytometry identifies risk factors and dynamic changes in patients with COVID-19. J Clin Immunol. 2020;40:970-3.
80. Rendeiro AF, Casano J, Vorkas CK, Singh H, Morales A, DeSimone RA, et al. Profiling of immune dysfunction in COVID-19 patients allows early prediction of disease progression. Life Sci Alliance. 2020;4:e202000955.
81. Bourgoin P, Soliveres T, Barbaresi A, Loundou A, Belkacem IA, Arnoux I, et al. CD169 and CD64 could help differentiate bacterial from COVID-19 or other viral infections in the emergency department. Cytometry A. 2021;99:435-45.
82. Rahman A, Niloofa R, Jayarajah U, Mel SD, Abeysuriya V, Seneviratne SL. Hematological abnormalities in COVID-19: A narrative review. Am J Trop Med Hyg. 2021;104:1188-201.
83. Harris CK, Hung YP, Nielsen GP, Stone JR, Ferry JA. Bone marrow and peripheral blood findings in patients infected by SARS-CoV-2. Am J Clin Pathol. 2021;155:627-37.
84. Wool GD, Miller JL. The impact of COVID-19 disease on platelets and coagulation. Pathobiology. 2021;88:15-27.
85. Tang N, Li D, Wang X, Sun Z. Abnormal coagulation parameters are associated with poor prognosis in patients with novel coronavirus pneumonia. J Thromb Haemost. 2020;18:844-7.

86. Al-Samkari H, Karp Leaf RS, Dzik WH, Carlson JCT, Fogerty AE, Waheed A, et al. COVID-19 and coagulation: Bleeding and thrombotic manifestations of SARS-CoV-2 infection. Blood. 2020;136:489-500.
87. Deng Y, Liu W, Liu K, Fang YY, Shang J, Zhou L, et al. Clinical characteristics of fatal and recovered cases of coronavirus disease 2019 in Wuhan, China: A retrospective study. Chin Med J (Engl). 2020;133:1261-7.
88. Guo T, Fan Y, Chen M, Wu X, Zhang L, He T, et al. Cardiovascular implications of fatal outcomes of patients with coronavirus disease 2019 (COVID-19). JAMA Cardiol. 2020;5:811-8
89. Wu C, Chen X, Cai Y, Xia J, Zhou X, Xu S, et al. Risk factors associated with acute respiratory distress syndrome and death in patients with coronavirus disease 2019 pneumonia in Wuhan, China. JAMA Intern Med. 2020;180:934-3.
90. Terpos E, Ntanasis-Stathopoulos I, Elalamy I, Kastritis E, Sergentanis TN, Politou M, et al. Hematological findings and complications of COVID-19. Am J Hematol. 2020;95: 834-47.
91. Henry BM, Lippi G, Plebani M. Laboratory abnormalities in children with novel coronavirus disease. Clin Chem Lab Med. 2019;2020(58):1135-8.
92. Patel NA. Pediatric COVID-19: systematic review of the literature. Am J Otolaryngol. 2020;41:102573.
93. Meena J, Yadav J, Saini L, Yadav A, Kumar J. Clinical features and outcome of SARS-CoV-2 infection in children: A systematic review and meta-analysis. Indian Pediatr. 2020;57:820-6.
94. Ma X, Liu S, Chen L, Zhuang L, Zhang J, Xin Y. The clinical characteristics of pediatric inpatients with SARS-CoV-2 infection: A meta-analysis and systematic review. J Med Virol. 2021;93:234-0.
95. Sharathkumar AA, Faustino EVS, Takemoto CM. How we approach thrombosis risk in children with COVID-19 infection and MIS-C. Pediatr Blood Cancer. 2021;68(7):e29049.
96. Hoogenboom WS, Alamuri TT, McMahon DM, Balanchivadze N, Dabak V, Mitchell WB, et al. Clinical outcomes of COVID-19 in patients with sickle cell disease and sickle cell trait: A critical appraisal of the literature. Blood Rev 2022;53:100911.
97. Severance TS, Rahim MQ, French J 2nd, Baker RM, Shriner A, Khaitan A, et al. COVID-19 and hereditary spherocytosis: A recipe for hemolysis. Pediatr Blood Cancer. 2021;68:e28548.
98. Huang C, Wang Y, Li X, Ren L, Zhao J, Hu Y, et al. Clinical features of patients infected with 2019 novel coronavirus in Wuhan, China. Lancet. 2020;395:497-506.
99. Chen H, Guo J, Wang C, Luo F, Yu X, Zhang W, et al. Clinical characteristics and intrauterine vertical transmission potential of COVID-19 infection in nine pregnant women: A retrospective review of medical records. Lancet. 2020;395:809-15.
100. Schoenmakers S, Snijder P, Verdijk RM, Kuiken T, Kamphuis SSM, Koopman LP, et al. Severe acute respiratory syndrome coronavirus 2 placental infection and inflammation leading to fetal distress and neonatal multi-organ failure in an asymptomatic woman. J Pediatric Infect Dis Soc. 2021;10(5):556-61.
101. Chi J, Gong W, Gao Q. Clinical characteristics and outcomes of pregnant women with COVID-19 and the risk of vertical transmission: A systematic review. Arch Gynecol Obstet. 2020;303(2):337-45.
102. Li L, Zhou Q, Xu J. Changes of laboratory cardiac markers and mechanisms of cardiac injury in coronavirus disease 2019. Biomed Res Int. 2020;2020:7413673.
103. He W, Chen L, Chen L, Yuan G, Fang Y, Chen W, et al. COVID-19 in persons with haematological cancers. Leukemia. 2020;34:1637-45.
104. Dai M, Liu D, Liu M, Zhou F, Li G, Chen Z, et al. Patients with cancer appear more vulnerable to SARS-CoV-2: A multicenter study during the COVID-19 outbreak. Cancer Discov. 2020;10:783-91.

105. Piñana JL, Martino R, Garcia-Garcia I, Parody R, Morales MD, Benzo G, et al. Risk factors and outcome of COVID-19 in patients with hematological malignancies. Exp Hematol Oncol. 2020;9:21.
106. Debliquis A, Harzallah I, Mootien JY, Poidevin A, Labro G, Mejri A, et al. Haemophagocytosis in bone marrow aspirates in patients with COVID-19. Br J Haematol. 2020;190:e70-3.
107. Rapkiewicz AV, Mai X, Carsons SE, Pittaluga S, Kleiner DE, Berger JS, et al. Megakarocytes and platelet-fibrin thrombi characterize multi-organ thrombosis at autopsy in COVID-19; A case series. Eclinical Med. 2020;24:100434.
108. Khan AM, Ajmal Z, Raval M, Tobin E. Concurrent Diagnosis of acute myeloid leukemia and COVID-19: A management challenge. Cureus. 2020;12:e9629.
109. Brissot, E, Labopin M, Baron F, Bazarbachi A, Bug G, Ciceri F, et al. Management of patients with acute leukemia during the COVID-19 outbreak: Practical guidelines from the acute leukemia working party of the European Society for Blood and Marrow Transplantation. Bone Marrow Transplant. 2020;56:532-5.
110. Ljungman P, Mikulska M, De La Camara R, Basak GW, Chabannon C, Corbacioglu S, et al. The challenge of COVID-19 and hematopoietic cell transplantation; EBMT recommendations for management of hematopoietic cell transplant recipients, their donors, and patients undergoing CAR T-cell therapy. Bone Marrow Transplant. 2020;55:2071-6.
111. Kanellopoulos A, Ahmed MZ, Kishore B, Lovell R, Horgan C, Paneesha S, et al. COVID-19 in bone marrow transplant recipients: Reflecting on a single centre experience. Br J Haematol. 2020;190:e67-70.
112. Alfishawy M, Elbendary A, Mohamed M, Nassar M. COVID-19 mortality in transplant recipients. Int J Organ Transplant Med. 2020;11:145-62.

CHAPTER 6

Mature T- and NK-cell Neoplasms: Updates on Molecular Genetic Features

Sudha Sharma

■ INTRODUCTION

Mature T- and NK-cell neoplasms (MTNKNs) comprise 10–15% of all non-Hodgkin lymphomas (NHLs). These are derived from NK cells or mature, post-thymic T-cells. Both T- and NK-cells develop from a common lymphoid progenitor, depending upon the type of transcription factors expressed. NK cell lineage is developed if transcription factors ID2 and E4BP4 are expressed, while expression of transcription factors of NOTCH and RUNX members results in the development of T-cell lineage.[1] From the last many years, significant work is being done for understanding the biology of MTNKNs, which has a role in their diagnosis and prognosis, with a possible therapeutic potential in future. In the light of these findings, the 2017 WHO Classification was introduced, which was the revised 4th edition of 2008 classification of hematolymphoid tumors (WHOHAEM4).[2] The diagnosis was primarily based on clinical and immunohistologic characteristics. Recent genomic studies have improved understanding regarding the pathology of these neoplasms and have paved the way for providing better therapies.

The 5th edition of WHO Classification of hematolymphoid tumors (WHOHAEM5), 2022, has introduced a new terminology "T-cell and NK-cell lymphoid proliferations and lymphomas" **(Table 1)**, which include a class of tumor-like lesions with T-cell predominance and precursor T-lymphoblastic neoplasms.

Based on the disease localization, cell of origin, clinical features, and cytology MTNKNs have been divided into nine families.[3] The MTNKNs have been categorized together as some of these may be difficult to differentiate and present as hybrid or indeterminate phenotype.

TABLE 1: Mature T- and NK-cell neoplasms. Comparison between the revised World Health Organization (WHO) Classification, 2017, and WHO Classification 2022.[2,3]

WHO revised 4th edition 2017	WHO 5th edition 2022
Mature T- and NK-cell leukemias	
T-cell prolymphocytic leukemia	T-prolymphocytic leukemia
T-cell large granular lymphocytic leukemia	T-large granular lymphocytic leukemia
Chronic lymphoproliferative disorder of NK cells	NK-large granular lymphocytic leukemia
Adult T-cell leukemia/lymphoma	Adult T-cell leukemia/lymphoma
Sezary syndrome	Sezary syndrome
Aggressive NK-cell leukemia	Aggressive NK-cell leukemia
Primary cutaneous T-cell lymphoid proliferations and lymphomas	
Primary cutaneous CD4+ small/medium T-cell lymphoproliferative disorder	Primary cutaneous CD4+ small/medium T-cell lymphoproliferative disorder
Primary cutaneous acral CD8+ T-cell lymphoma	Primary cutaneous acral CD8+ lymphoproliferative disorder
Mycosis fungoides	Mycosis fungoides
Primary cutaneous CD30+ T-cell lymphoproliferative disorder: Lymphomatoid papulosis	Primary cutaneous CD30+ T-cell lymphoproliferative disorder: Lymphomatoid papulosis
Primary cutaneous CD30+ T-cell lymphoproliferative disorder: Primary cutaneous anaplastic large cell lymphoma	Primary cutaneous CD30+ T-cell lymphoproliferative disorder: Primary cutaneous anaplastic large cell lymphoma
Subcutaneous panniculitis-like T-cell lymphoma	Subcutaneous panniculitis-like T-cell lymphoma
Primary cutaneous gamma/delta T-cell lymphoma	Primary cutaneous gamma/delta T-cell lymphoma
Primary cutaneous CD8+ aggressive epidermotropic cytotoxic T-cell lymphoma	Primary cutaneous CD8+ aggressive epidermotropic cytotoxic T-cell lymphoma
Not included	Primary cutaneous peripheral T-cell lymphoma, NOS
Intestinal T- and NK-cell lymphoid proliferations and lymphomas	
Indolent T-cell lymphoproliferative disorder of the gastrointestinal tract	Indolent T-cell lymphoma of the gastrointestinal tract
Not included	Indolent NK-cell lymphoproliferative disorder of the gastrointestinal tract

Continued

Continued

WHO revised 4th edition 2017	WHO 5th edition 2022
Enteropathy-associated T-cell lymphoma	Enteropathy-associated T-cell lymphoma
Monomorphic epitheliotropic intestinal T-cell lymphoma	Monomorphic epitheliotropic intestinal T-cell lymphoma
Intestinal T-cell lymphoma, NOS	Intestinal T-cell lymphoma, NOS
Anaplastic large cell lymphoma	
Anaplastic large cell lymphoma, ALK+	ALK+ anaplastic large cell lymphoma
Anaplastic large cell lymphoma, ALK−	ALK− anaplastic large cell lymphoma
Breast implant-associated anaplastic large cell lymphoma	Breast implant-associated anaplastic large cell lymphoma
Nodal T-follicular helper (TFH) cell lymphomas	
Angioimmunoblastic T-cell lymphoma	Nodal TFH cell lymphoma, angioimmunoblastic-type
Follicular T-cell lymphoma	Nodal TFH cell lymphoma, follicular-type
Nodal peripheral T-cell lymphoma with TFH phenotype	Nodal TFH cell lymphoma, NOS
Other peripheral T-cell lymphomas	
Hepatosplenic T-cell lymphoma	Hepatosplenic T-cell lymphoma
Peripheral T-cell lymphoma, NOS	Peripheral T-cell lymphoma, NOS
EBV+ NK/T-cell lymphomas	
Not included (covered under peripheral T-cell lymphoma, NOS)	EBV+ nodal T- and NK-cell lymphoma
Extranodal NK/T-cell lymphoma, nasal type	Extranodal NK/T-cell lymphoma
EBV+ T- and NK-cell lymphoid proliferations and lymphomas of childhood	
Severe mosquito bite allergy	Severe mosquito bite allergy
Hydroa vacciniforme-like lymphoproliferative disorder	Hydroa vacciniforme lymphoproliferative disorder
Chronic active EBV infection of T- and NK-cell type, systemic form	Systemic chronic active EBV disease
Systemic EBV+ T-cell lymphoma of childhood	Systemic EBV+ T-cell lymphoma of childhood

SUBCLASSIFICATION OF MATURE T- AND NK-CELL NEOPLASMS

Mature T- and NK-cell Leukemias

These include proliferation of T- and NK-cells presenting as leukemic disease. This family includes:

T-prolymphocytic Leukemia

T-prolymphocytic leukemia (T-PLL) is suspected when there are >5 × 10^9/L lymphocytes with appropriate phenotype. These cells are monoclonal and show post-thymic mature T-cell immunophenotype. They are positive for CD4, CD2, CD5, and CD7 and negative for CD8, TdT, CD1a, CD16, and CD56. Structural variants with breakpoint in MTCP1 or TCL1A locus can be seen.[4]

T-large Granular Lymphocytic Leukemia

Peripheral blood showing large granular lymphocytes with moderate-to-abundant cytoplasm and azurophilic granules >2 × 10^9/L, should lead to suspicion of T-large granular lymphocytic leukemia (T-LGLL). These cells should be clonal. Polymerase chain reaction (PCR) should be performed using T-cell receptor (TCR)-γ probe.

T-large granular lymphocytic leukemia cells have a mature post-thymic phenotype and are positive for CD3, TCRαβ, CD8, CD16, CD45RA, and CD57 and are negative for CD4, $CD5^{dim}$, CD27, CD28, and CD45RO. Expression of CD57 and CD16 can be seen in >80% of T-LGLL:[5]

- $CD8^+$ T-LGLL associated with STAT3 mutation
- $CD4^+$ T-LGLL associated with STAT5B mutation
- Gamma/delta T-LGLL has poor prognosis and neutropenia[6]

NK-large Granular Lymphocytic Leukemia

These were called "chronic lymphoproliferative disorder (LPD) of NK cells" in WHOHAEM4. However, in WHOHAEM5, they have been renamed as NK-large granular lymphocytic leukemia (NK-LGLL). Most of the cases show a cytotoxic $CD16^{high}$ $CD56^{low}$ $CD57^{+/-}$ profile and are $CD5^{dim}$/$CD7^{dim}$, whereas normal NK cells show a heterogeneous CD16 expression and are $CD2^+$/$CD5^-$/$CD7^+$. KIR phenotyping is an important advancement in the diagnosis of NK-LGLL. A restricted activated KIR expression is seen in NK-LGLL cells. Mutational screening is more accurate, most common being *STAT3* function and *TET2* mutation.[7]

Adult T-cell Leukemia/Lymphoma

Adult T-cell leukemia/lymphoma (ATLL) is a rare T-cell lymphoproliferative neoplasm of mature $CD4^+$ $CD25^+$ T cells caused by human T-lymphotrophic virus 1 (HTLV-1). There are four main types: acute, lymphomatous, chronic, and smoldering forms. The characteristic cell type seen in peripheral blood smear is the "flower cell" or "cloverleaf," which shows condensed chromatin and convoluted nucleus. HTLV-1 infection can be confirmed by enzyme-linked immunosorbent assay (ELISA) or western blot, ELISA being more sensitive. No specific chromosomal abnormalities have been associated. Novel events have been identified stressing the importance of immune evasion like recurrent alterations in HLA-A and HLA-B, structural variations disrupting the 3′-untranslated region of CD274 (PD-L1), CTLA4::CD28, and ICOS::CD28 fusions. Indolent forms are associated with STAT3 mutations.[8-10]

Sezary Syndrome

Genomic signature analysis demonstrate the role of UV exposure and cellular aging in sezary syndrome (SS). Peripheral smear shows sezary cells that are large lymphocytes with cerebriform nucleus. Diagnosis can be confirmed by immunophenotyping. *TCR* gene rearrangement by PCR, Southern blot, or NGS can detect monoclonality. The International Society for Cutaneous Lymphomas has given the criteria for diagnosis of SS. Either >1,000 sezary cells/μL or a monoclonal population with CD4/CD8 ≥10% and/or CD4$^+$ CD7 ≥40%, and CD4$^+$ CD26 ≥30% are required for the diagnosis. The malignant cells are CD4$^+$ T cells with a memory phenotype (CD3$^+$ CD4$^+$ CD45RO$^+$ CD8$^-$) and CD7$^-$ in most cases. Rarely CD3$^+$ CD4$^-$ CD8$^+$ phenotype can be seen. Cases where CD30 positivity is seen in at least 10% of the neoplastic cells have shown response to drug brentuximab vedotin (linked to anti-CD30 monoclonal antibody).[11,12]

Aggressive NK-cell Leukemia

Aggressive NK-cell leukemia (ANKL) shows abnormal NK-cell proliferation and is associated with Epstein–Barr virus (EBV). They are more common in males. Genome-wide sequencing studies have found new mutations in *JAK/STAT* and *RAS/MAPK* pathway genes, immune checkpoint molecules PD-L1/PD-L2, and epigenetic modifiers (TET2, CREBBP, KMT2D) involved in the disease pathogenesis.[13]

Primary Cutaneous T-cell Lymphoid Proliferations and Lymphomas

These are cutaneous lymphomas and LPDs and include nine entities. No extracutaneous disease is seen at the time of diagnosis. The most common among these is mycosis fungoides (MF; 50%) followed by primary cutaneous CD30-positive T-cell LPD (25–30%).

Primary Cutaneous CD4$^+$ Small/Medium T-cell Lymphoproliferative Disorder

Clinical presentation is that of a plaque or tumor on face, upper trunk, or neck. CD4$^+$ small/medium-sized pleomorphic T cells are seen which express follicular helper T-cell markers PD-1, BCL6, and CXCL13. Admixed B cells, small reactive CD8$^+$ T cells, histiocytes, and giant cells can also be seen. Prognosis is excellent.[14]

Primary Cutaneous Acral CD8$^+$ Lymphoproliferative Disorder

This was previously classified as lymphoma. However, WHOHAEM5 has renamed it as LPD, because of its low proliferation rate, indolent behavior and excellent prognosis. The classical presentation is that of a slow growing, solitary papule on the ear. It can also present in acral sites like foot and nose. Histologically, immature cells can be seen separated from epidermis by a grenz zone. These cells are CD3$^+$, CD8$^+$ and CD4$^-$, CD30$^-$. Loss of pan-T-cell antigens (CD2, CD5, CD7) can be seen. They are positive for TIA-1, but negative for other cytotoxic proteins like perforin and granzyme B. CD68 can show Golgi zone dot-like staining.[14]

Mycosis Fungoides

Mycosis fungoides is the cutaneous counterpart of SS and constitutes 50% of all primary cutaneous lymphomas. The patients present at 55–60 years of age with skin lesions resembling "cigarette paper" appearance, due to epidermotropic lymphoid cells. In later stages, the lesions become shiny and form plaques, as the infiltrates extend into the dermis. The patients can also present with erythema, itching, and lymphadenopathy. Diagnosis is confirmed by demonstration of monoclonal skin-homing memory T cells. New biomarkers like KIRDL2 (CD158k) and PD-1 (CD279) have been discovered for detection of MF. Gene expression analysis shows overexpression of TWIST1, EPH4, NKp46, DNM3, PLS3, and CD158k/KIRDL2, and reduction of STAT4 expression.[14,15]

Primary Cutaneous CD30+ T-cell Lymphoproliferative Disorder: Lymphomatoid Papulosis

Primary cutaneous CD30+ LPD constitute 25% of cutaneous T cell lymphomas (CTCLs), and include lymphomatoid papulosis (LyP) and cutaneous anaplastic large cell lymphoma (ALCL). LyP shows recurrent papules and macules with superficial ulceration, which regress with time, without treatment. Five subtypes have been described (types A–E). A new subtype has been described with chromosomal rearrangements involving *DUSP-IRF4* locus on 6p25.3. Recognition of subtypes is important to prevent misdiagnosis as other aggressive lymphomas.[14,15]

Primary Cutaneous CD30+ T-cell Lymphoproliferative Disorder: Primary Cutaneous Anaplastic Large Cell lymphoma

Cutaneous anaplastic large cell lymphoma (cALCL) is usually seen in extremities and presents as nodule, plaque or tumor, with ulceration. Regional lymph nodes may be involved. Extracutaneous dissemination occurs in 10–15% patients. They do not resolve on their own. Unlike systemic ALCL, c-ALCL does not show *ALK* gene translocation. So ALK positivity suggests cutaneous involvement of a systemic ALK+ ALCL. Rearrangements of *DUSP22-IRF4* locus are seen in 25% of c-ALCL but do not have prognostic significance. *TP63* gene rearrangements are rarely found in c-ALCL. A novel recurrent *NPM1-TYK2* gene fusion resulting in constitutive STAT signaling has been described in both C-ALCL and LyP.[14,15]

Subcutaneous Panniculitis-like T-cell Lymphoma

This is a rare CTCL, presenting at a younger age of 35 years and has an indolent course. Tumor cells are limited to subcutaneous fat. It is characterized by CD8+ cytotoxic T cells expressing αβ TCRs and CD4−, CD8+, and CD56⁻ phenotypes. Approximately 20% cases can be complicated by hemophagocytic syndrome.[16]

Primary Cutaneous Gamma/Delta T-cell Lymphoma
This is a rare but aggressive malignancy, usually affecting the extremities of adults. Clonal proliferation of activated mature gamma-delta T cells is seen with a cytotoxic phenotype.[17]

Primary Cutaneous CD8⁺ Aggressive Epidermotropic Cytotoxic T-cell Lymphoma
This is a characterized by rapidly forming annular plaques with ulceration and have a poor prognosis. Initially, this entity was named as pagetoid reticulosis. On histopathology, medium sized, monomorphous atypical lymphocytes are seen infiltrating the epidermis in a pagetoid pattern.[18]

Primary Cutaneous Peripheral T-cell Lymphoma, NOS: New Entity
This is a rare form of CTCL and is a diagnosis of exclusion. It is characterized by solitary red-violaceous tumor-like nodule. Five-year survival is <20% due to rapid spread and systemic involvement. Diagnosis may be difficult due to varying immunophenotype. Most common immunophenotype is CD4⁺ with loss of T-cell antigens. There is absence of CD30. CD56 may rarely be positive.[19]

Intestinal T- and NK-cell Lymphoid Proliferations and Lymphomas
Indolent NK-cell LPD of the gastrointestinal tract (GIT) has been added as a new entity in WHOHAEM5, and indolent T-cell LPD of the GIT is now called "indolent T-cell lymphoma of the GIT."

Indolent T-cell Lymphoma of the Gastrointestinal Tract
Previously called "indolent T-cell LPD of the GIT," this neoplasm has been renamed as lymphoma because of its association with disseminated disease and morbidity.[20,21] However, because of their long course they are termed "indolent". Newer genetic correlation has been found between T-cell subsets. The CD4⁺, CD4⁺/CD8⁺, and CD4⁻/CD8⁻ subsets have been associated with mutations in epigenetic modifier genes (e.g., *TET2*, *KMT2D*) and alterations in *JAK-STAT* pathway genes. Some CD4⁺ cases can show STAT3::JAK2 fusions. In contrast, some CD8⁺ cases have been shown to harbor structural alterations involving the *IL2* gene.[22,23]

Indolent NK-cell Lymphoproliferative Disorder of the Gastrointestinal Tract
It was initially thought of as a reactive process and was called NK-cell enteropathy or lymphomatoid gastropathy, but recent findings prove its neoplastic nature. However, lesions usually regress spontaneously and do not

progress, hence the name "lymphoproliferative disorder". Differentiation from extranodal NK/T-cell lymphoma (ENKTL) can be done by EBV association, superficial and small lesions and expansile growth. Presence of bright eosinophilic granules in the paranuclear region can provide morphologic clue to diagnosis.

JAK3-STAT5 pathway activation has a role in pathogenesis. Recurrent JAK3 mutations (K563_C565del; NP_000206) have been found in these cases.[24,25] Recently, rare cases of tumor involving the vagina, gallbladder, and surrounding lymph nodes have been reported.[26,27]

Enteropathy-associated T-cell Lymphomas

Enteropathy-associated T-cell lymphoma (EATL) is the most common type of intestinal T-cell lymphoma occurring in North European regions. It has an aggressive course and is linked to celiac disease (CD). Risk factors include elderly age group, males, and homozygosity for HLA-DQ2. Small intestine is the most common site involved (>90% cases occur in ileum and jejunum).

Histopathology is the gold standard for diagnosis, with pleomorphic cells having propensity of intraepithelial spread. The adjacent intestinal mucosa shows features of CD. The neoplastic lymphocytes are positive for CD3, CD7, CD103 and negative for CD5, CD4, CD8. Expression of cytotoxic granule-associated proteins (perforin, TIA1, granzyme B) is seen. CD30 positivity has been seen in EATLs with large cell morphology. All cases show *TCR*-β or *TCR*-γ gene rearrangement.[28]

Monomorphic Epitheliotropic Intestinal T-cell Lymphoma

Type II EATL is now known as monomorphic epitheliotropic intestinal T-cell lymphoma (MEITL). It is more common in Asians and Hispanics and no association with CD is noted. Patients present with abdominal pain and intestinal perforation. In contrast to EATL, MEITL is composed of medium-sized, monomorphic cells with round nuclei and pale cytoplasm, infiltrating the intestinal epithelium. No necrosis or inflammation is seen.

Monomorphic epitheliotropic intestinal T-cell lymphoma is usually CD3$^+$, CD8$^+$, and CD56$^+$, but CD5$^-$, CD30$^-$, and CD103$^-$. Both EATL and MEITL have an activated cytotoxic T-cell immunophenotype. Activating mutations of JAK/STAT signaling pathway and activating hotspot mutations in *GNAI2* gene have been seen.[29]

Intestinal T-cell Lymphoma, NOS

It is a T-cell lymphoma of the intestines that does not show morphologic and immunophenotypic features of classic EATL or MEITL, hence a diagnosis of exclusion.

Anaplastic Large Cell Lymphoma

Anaplastic large cell lymphomas are mature T-cell lymphomas composed of pleomorphic cells including the "hallmark cells." They are strongly positive

for CD30 and frequently show defective T-lineage marker expression. WHOHAEM5 has categorized them into three entities[3]:
1. ALK-positive ALCL (ALK+ ALCL)
2. ALK-negative ALCL (ALK- ALCL)
3. Breast implant-associated ALCL (BIA-ALCL)

The pathogenesis of primary cutaneous ALCL is different from systemic ALCL and has a favorable outcome. Hence, it has been classified under primary cutaneous T-cell lymphoid proliferations and lymphomas.

ALK-positive Anaplastic Large Cell Lymphoma

ALK+ ALCLs are seen in young age and have better outcome than ALK- ALCL with a 5-year survival of 70–85%. They are characterized by rearrangement of *ALK* gene on chromosome 2p23, with *NMP1* on chromosome 5q35.1 being the most common partner gene. Rearrangement of ALK leads to *ALK* gene fusion and protein production, causing aberrant ALK expression, which can be detected by immunohistochemistry (IHC).[30] The ALK fusion proteins have constitutive tyrosine kinase activity that leads to cell proliferation by activating signaling pathways like JAK/STAT, PI3K/AKT, Ras/ERK, etc.[31] Secondary chromosomal imbalances like loss of 4q, 11q, 6q, 13q, and 17p and gain of 1q, 8q, 7p, and 17 can be seen.[32]

In addition to ALK and CD30 positivity, they can express transcripts related to JAK/STAT pathway activation, cytotoxic molecules, T-helper 17 cell-associated molecules, *HIF1-α* target genes, *IL-10*-induced genes, and *H-ras/K-ras*-induced genes.[33] Differential miRNA expression has been described among ALK+ and ALK- ALCL. miR-101 and miR-17-92 cluster, have been suggested to be a therapeutic target in ALK+ ALCL.[34] Activation of notch pathway is more common in ALK+ ALCL, and may act as a therapeutic target.[35]

ALK-negative Anaplastic Large Cell Lymphoma

ALK- ALCLs have a worse 5-year survival of 50%. However, recent studies show that it a heterogeneous disease.[36] Morphologically it is similar to ALK+ ALCL, except that ALK is negative on IHC. It occurs more commonly in elderly age group and involves the lymph nodes. ALK- ALCL has been associated with mainly two recurrent gene rearrangements detected by fluorescence in situ hybridization (FISH). When there is no rearrangement, it is called "triple negative ALCL."

DUSP22 on chromosome 6p25.3: This rearrangement is seen in 18–30% of systemic ALK- ALCL and have not been seen in ALK+ ALCL.[37] These lymphomas show sheets of monotonous, medium-sized cells with nuclear pseudoinclusions ("doughnut" cells).[38] On IHC, there is absence of phosphorylated STAT3 (pSTAT3), cytotoxic markers and PD-L1 expression.[36] A recent study has shown a unique profile of *DUSP22*-R ALK- ALCL with downregulation of *JAK/STAT* pathway genes, global DNA hypomethylation, overexpression of cancer testis antigen genes, and preservation of immunogenic mechanisms.[39] *DUSP22* rearranged ALCLs have a much better outcome, similar to that of ALK⁺ ALCL, hence aggressive treatment is not required in these cases.[36] All cases of ALK⁻ ALCLs should be subjected to FISH for *DUSP22* rearrangement.

TP63 on chromosome 3q28: These are seen in 2–8% of ALK⁻ ALCLs. The presence of *TP63* rearrangements in ALK⁻ ALCL imparts a very poor prognosis, worse than triple negative cases. The clinical significance of co-occurring *DUSP22* and *TP63* rearrangements, present rarely, is not known.[36]

ALK⁻ ALCL requires JAK/STAT pathway activation; however, they show *STAT3* and *JAK1* mutations as opposed to oncogenic fusions of tyrosine kinases seen in ALK⁺ ALCL.[40] Presence of oncogenic truncated *ERBB4* transcripts, impart a Hodgkin lymphoma-like morphology.[41] *PRDM1* inactivation, loss of 17p, *STAT3*, and *TP53* mutations are associated with a worse survival.[42] High IL-2Rα levels indicate poorer outcome but have also been suggested to be a novel therapeutic target.[43]

Breast Implant-associated Anaplastic Large Cell Lymphoma

This is a rare subtype, which arises in association with breast implants as a result of chronic antigenic stimulation, and has a very good prognosis. It is seen in superficial capsule or peri-implant seroma fluid. Morphologically and phenotypically, it is similar to ALK⁻ ALCL. Adverse prognostic factors include mass formation, extra-capsular extension, or lymph node involvement.[44]

Partial chromosome 20q loss has been shown to be characteristic for BIA-ALCL.[45] Copy number alterations (CNAs) of regions containing JAK/STAT pathway and epigenetic regulator genes can be seen.[46] BIA-ALCL has not been associated with ALK, DUSP22, or TP63 rearrangements; however, one case has shown *STAT3–JAK2* fusion.[47] More than 50% cases show PD-L1 expression.[48]

Nodal T-follicular Helper Cell Lymphomas

- Nodal T-follicular helper (TFH) cell lymphoma, angioimmunoblastic-type
- Nodal TFH cell lymphoma, follicular-type
- Nodal TFH cell lymphoma, NOS

All these three entities are CD4⁺ T-cell lymphomas with TFH cell origin as proved by the presence of common clinical, immunophenotypic, and genomic features. TFH cell origin is confirmed when at least two TFH markers are positive, most common being CD10, PD-1, BCL6, ICOS, and CXCL13.

Nodal T-follicular Helper Cell Lymphoma, Angioimmunoblastic-type

These arise in elderly age group and are associated with poor prognosis. Patients can present with skin rash and immune dysregulation. Histopathology shows small-to-intermediate cells with clear cytoplasm. Background shows polymorphous inflammatory cells with expansion of follicular dendritic cell (FDC) meshwork. EBV+ B cells can be seen.[49] Gain of chromosomes 5 and 21 and mutation of epigenetic modifiers like *TET2*, *DNMT3A*, and *IDH2* are present commonly. *TET2* mutations can be seen in 70–80% cases.[50] *RHOA* mutations (p.G17V point mutation) are present in 50–70% cases and are associated with stronger expression of TFH marker, higher vessel density, and proliferation of FDC meshwork.[51] *IDH2* mutations at R172 position are seen in 20–30% cases, and can act as a therapeutic target. These cases have medium-to-large clear tumor cells with strong CD10 and CXCL13 expression.[52] Additional clonal hematopoietic neoplasms like MDS, AML, and B-cell lymphoproliferative disease can also be seen.[53]

Nodal T-follicular Helper Cell Lymphoma, Follicular-type

This is a rare neoplasm with follicular arrangement and composed of neoplastic T cells with TFH phenotype. Extrafollicular FDC meshworks or any significant vascular proliferation are not seen. t(5;9) (q33;q22) *ITK-SYK* fusion is specific and is seen in 20–40% cases.[54] *TET2*, *DNMT3A*, and *RHOA* G17V mutations are seen similar to nodal TFH cell lymphoma, angioimmunoblastic-type.[55] Rarely *IDH2* R172 mutations have also been seen.[56]

RHOA G17V and *IDH2* mutations have been associated with TFH lymphomas. Presence of these mutations indicates the diagnosis of TFH lymphoma in the presence of appropriate clinical and immunohistochemical features. It also has therapeutic relevance because TFH lymphomas are sensitive to epigenetic modifier therapy like histone deacetylase (HDAC) inhibitors and hypomethylating agents.[57]

Nodal T-follicular Helper Cell Lymphoma, NOS

These patients present with disseminated disease and autoimmune phenomena. Morphologically, there are sheets of neoplastic T cells with TFH phenotype. Background shows no significant vascular proliferation, inflammation, or FDC meshwork expansion.

There is similarity in genomic complexity, gene expression profiling (GEP), and mutations among NOS category and angioimmunoblastic-type. Mutations in *DNMT3A*, *TET2*, *RHOA* G17V, and T cell receptor (TCR) signaling genes can be seen in both.[55]

Other Peripheral T-cell Lymphomas

Hepatosplenic T-cell Lymphoma

Hepatosplenic T-cell lymphoma (HSTCL) arises from lymphocytes expressing γ/δ TCR and are derived from double-negative (CD4⁻/CD8⁻) thymic precursors. Histopathology shows small-to-medium-sized mature T cells infiltrating liver and splenic sinusoids. Erythrophagocytosis can be seen. On IHC, double negative T cells are seen (CD4⁻, CD8⁻). Occasionally, CD8 may be expressed. Surface CD2, CD3, and CD7 are positive while CD1a, CD5, Cd10, and TdT are negative. Majority of the cases express the γδ TCR and CD56. Isochromosome 7q [i(7q)] and trisomy 8 are commonly present. Frequent epigenetic alterations seen are mutations in *SETD2, INO80, TET3,* and *SMARCA2*.[58]

Peripheral T-cell Lymphoma, NOS
Peripheral T-cell lymphoma (PTCL) is a diagnosis of exclusion, affects adults and has an aggressive course. Two biological variants of PTCL-NOS have been described based on the transcriptional program of T-helper-1 and T-helper-2 cells: PTCL-GATA3 and PTCL-TBX21. The molecular genetic profile of PTCLGATA3 is uniform, whereas PTCL-TBX21 is heterogeneous.[59]

Epstein–Barr Virus-positive NK/T-cell Lymphomas

Nodal T- and NK-cell Lymphoma
Previously it was described as a subtype of PTCL NOS; however, now it is a distinct entity. It occurs commonly in East Asians. Patients have lymph node enlargement and have a poor prognosis. Extranodal involvement may or may not be present. There is morphological resemblance to diffuse large B-cell lymphoma. EBV is positive and it shows a cytotoxic T-cell phenotype. *TET2* is the most commonly mutated gene.[60]

Extranodal NK/T-cell Lymphoma
WHOHAEM5 has dropped the term "nasal-type" from its name. Outcome has improved markedly with use of l-asparaginase-based chemotherapy alongwith radiotherapy. As immune evasion is an important pathway for survival of ENKTL, immune checkpoint inhibitor therapy can be used in relapse or refractory disease.[61]

Epstein–Barr Virus-positive T- and NK-cell Lymphoid Proliferations and Lymphomas of Childhood
These are rare disorders mainly occurring in native Americans and Asians; however, rarely they can occur in adults. They vary from indolent forms like severe mosquito bite allergy (SMBA) and hydroa vacciniforme lymphoproliferative disorder (HVLPD), to systemic disease with fever, lymphadenopathy, hepatosplenomegaly with or without cutaneous features like systemic chronic active EBV disease (CAEBVD) and systemic EBV-positive T-cell lymphoma of childhood.[62]

■ CONCLUSION

Mature T- and NK-cell leukemias (MTNKLs) are rare and aggressive group of neoplasms. Application of genomic techniques has further clarified regarding their pathobiology, based on which the classification has been modified, prognostication improved and new therapies are being developed. However, due to poor outcome of patients with MTNKL, more research is needed to better treat this aggressive disease.

REFERENCES

1. Sun JC, Lanier LL. NK cell development, homeostasis and function: parallels with CD8+ T cells. Nat Rev Immunol. 2011;11(10):645-57.
2. Swerdlow SH, Campo E, Harris NL, Jaffe ES, Pileri SA, Stein H, et al. WHO Classification of Tumours of Haematopoietic and Lymphoid Tissues, revised 4th edition. Lyon, France: IARC Press; 2017.
3. Alaggio R, Amador C, Anagnostopoulos I. The 5th edition of the World Health Organization classification of haematolymphoid tumours: Lymphoid neoplasms. Leukemia. 2022;36(7):1720-48.
4. Staber PB, Herling M, Bellido M, Jacobsen ED, Davids MS, Kadia TM, et al. Consensus criteria for diagnosis, staging, and treatment response assessment of T-cell prolymphocytic leukemia. Blood. 2019;134:1132-43.
5. Park SH, Lee YJ, Kim Y, Hyun-Ki Kim, Lim JH, Jo JC. T-large granular lymphocytic leukemia. Blood Res. 2023;58(Suppl 1):S52-7.
6. Barilà G, Teramo A, Calabretto G, Vicenzetto C, Gasparini VR, Pavan L, et al. Stat3 mutations impact on overall survival in large granular lymphocyte leukemia: A single-center experience of 205 patients. Leukemia. 2020;34:1116-24.
7. Drillet G, Pastoret C, Moignet A, Lamy T, Marchand T. Toward a better classification system for NK-LGL disorders. Front Oncol. 2022;12:821382.
8. Kataoka K, Nagata Y, Kitanaka A, Shiraishi Y, Shimamura T, Yasunaga JI, et al. Integrated molecular analysis of adult T cell leukemia/lymphoma. Nat Genet. 2015;47:1304-15.
9. Kogure Y, Kameda T, Koya J, Yoshimitsu M, Nosaka K, Yasunaga JI, et al. Wholegenome landscape of adult T-cell leukemia/lymphoma. Blood. 2022;139:967-82.
10. Kataoka K, Shiraishi Y, Takeda Y, Sakata S, Matsumoto M, Nagano S, et al. Aberrant PD-L1 expression through 3'-UTR disruption in multiple cancers. Nature. 2016;534:402-6.
11. Jones CL, Degasperi A, Grandi V, Amarante TD, Genomics England Research Consortium; Mitchell TJ, et al. Spectrum of mutational signatures in T-cell lymphoma reveals a key role for UV radiation in cutaneous T-cell lymphoma. Sci Rep. 2021;11:3962.
12. Miyashiro D, Sanches JA. Mycosis fungoides and Sézary syndrome: clinical presentation, diagnosis, staging, and therapeutic management. Front Oncol. 2023;13:1141108.
13. El Hussein S, Patel KP, Fang H, Thakral B, Loghavi S, Kanagal-Shamanna R, et al. Genomic and immunophenotypic landscape of aggressive NK-cell leukemia. Am J Surg Pathol. 2020;44:1235-43.
14. Willemze R, Cerroni L, Kempf W, Berti E, Facchetti F, Swerdlow SH. The 2018 update of the WHO-EORTC classification for primary cutaneous lymphomas. Blood. 2019;133(16):1703-14.
15. Pulitzer M. Cutaneous T-cell lymphoma. Clin Lab Med. 2017;37(3):527-46.
16. Lin EC, Liao JB, Fang YH, Hong CH. The pathophysiology and current treatments for the subcutaneous panniculitis-like T cell lymphoma: An updated review. Asia-Pac J Clin Oncol. 2023;19:27-34.
17. Violetti SA, Maronese CA, Venegoni L, Merlo V, Berti E. Primary cutaneous gamma-delta T cell lymphomas: A case series and overview of the literature. Dermatopathology (Basel). 2021;8(4):515-24.
18. Guitart J, Martinez-Escala ME, Subtil A, Duvic M, Pulitzer MP, Olsen EA, et al. Primary cutaneous aggressive epidermotropic cytotoxic T-cell lymphomas: Reappraisal of a provisional entity in the 2016 WHO classification of cutaneous lymphomas. Mod Pathol. 2017;30(5):761-72.
19. Aderhold K, Carpenter L, Brown K, Donato A. Primary cutaneous peripheral T-cell lymphoma not otherwise specified: A rapidly progressive variant of cutaneous T-cell lymphoma. Case Rep Oncol Med. 2015;2015:429068.

20. Margolskee E, Jobanputra V, Lewis SK Alobeid B, Green PHR, Bhagat G. Indolent small intestinal CD4+ T-cell lymphoma is a distinct entity with unique biologic and clinical features. PLoS One. 2013;8:e68343.
21. Perry AM, Warnke RA, Hu Q, Gaulard P, Copie-Bergman C, Alkan S, et al. Indolent T-cell lymphoproliferative disease of the gastrointestinal tract. Blood. 2013;122:3599-606.
22. Sharma A, Oishi N, Boddicker RL, Hu G, Benson HK, Ketterling RP, et al. Recurrent STAT3-JAK2 fusions in indolent T-cell lymphoproliferative disorder of the gastrointestinal tract. Blood. 2018;131:2262-6.
23. Soderquist CR, Patel N, Murty VV, Betman S, Aggarwal N, Young KH, et al. Genetic and phenotypic characterization of indolent T-cell lymphoproliferative disorders of the gastrointestinal tract. Haematologica. 2020;105:1895-906.
24. Xiao W, Gupta GK, Yao J, Jang YJ, Xi L, Baik J, et al. Recurrent somatic JAK3 mutations in NK-cell enteropathy. Blood. 2019;134:986-91.
25. Mansoor A, Pittaluga S, Beck PL, Wilson WH, Ferry JA, Jaffe ES. NK-cell enteropathy: A benign NK-cell lymphoproliferative disease mimicking intestinal lymphoma: Clinicopathologic features and follow-up in a unique case series. Blood. 2011; 117:1447-52.
26. Krishnan R, Ring K, Williams E, Portell C, Jaffe ES, Gru AA. An enteropathy-like indolent NK-cell proliferation presenting in the female genital tract. Am J Surg Pathol. 2020;44:561-5.
27. Dargent JL, Tinton N, Trimech M, de Leval L. Lymph node involvement by enteropathy-like indolent NK-cell proliferation. Virchows Arch. 2021;478:1197-202.
28. Somali ZA, Hamadani M, Dabaja MK, Sureda A, Fakih RE, Aljurf M. Enteropathy-associated T cell lymphoma. Curr Hematol Malignancy Rep 2021;16:140-7.
29. Veloza L, Cavalieri D, Missiaglia E, Ledoux-Pilon A, Bisig B, Pereira B, et al. Monomorphic epitheliotropic intestinal T-cell lymphoma comprises morphologic and genomic heterogeneity impacting outcome. Haematologica. 2023;108(1):181-95.
30. Morris SW, Kirstein MN, Valentine MB, Dittmer KG, Shapiro DN, Saltman DL, et al. Fusion of a kinase gene, ALK, to a nucleolar protein gene, NPM, in non-Hodgkin's lymphoma. Science. 1994;263(5151):1281-4.
31. Bai RY, Ouyang T, Miething C, Morris SW, Peschel C, Duyster J. Nucleophosmin-anaplastic lymphoma kinase associated with anaplastic large-cell lymphoma activates the phosphatidylinositol 3-kinase/Akt antiapoptotic signaling pathway. Blood. 2000;96(13):4319-27.
32. Zettl A, Rudiger T, Konrad MA, Chott A, Simonitsch-Klupp I, Sonnen R, et al. Genomic profiling of peripheral T-cell lymphoma, unspecified, and anaplastic large T-cell lymphoma delineates novel recurrent chromosomal alterations. Am J Pathol. 2004;164(5):1837-48.
33. Piva R, Agnelli L, Pellegrino E, Todoerti K, Grosso V, Tamagno I, et al. Gene expression profiling uncovers molecular classifiers for the recognition of anaplastic large-cell lymphoma within peripheral T-cell neoplasms. J Clin Oncol. 2010;28(9):1583-90.
34. Merkel O, Hamacher F, Laimer D, Sifft E, Trajanoski Z, Scheideler M, et al. Identification of differential and functionally active miRNAs in both anaplastic lymphoma kinase (ALK)+ and ALK- anaplastic large-cell lymphoma. Proc Natl Acad Sci USA. 2010;107(37): 16228-33.
35. Larose H, Prokoph N, Matthews JD, Schlederer M, Högler S, Alsulami AF, et al. Whole exome sequencing reveals NOTCH1 mutations in anaplastic large cell lymphoma and points to Notch both as a key pathway and a potential therapeutic target. Haematologica. 2021;106(6):1693-704.
36. Parrilla Castellar ER, Jaffe ES, Said JW, Swerdlow SH, Ketterling RP, Knudson RA, et al. ALK-negative anaplastic large cell lymphoma is a genetically heterogeneous disease with widely disparate clinical outcomes. Blood. 2014;124(9):1473-80.

37. Pedersen MB, Hamilton-Dutoit SJ, Bendix K, Ketterling RP, Bedroske PP, Luoma IM, et al. DUSP22 and TP63 rearrangements predict outcome of ALK-negative anaplastic large cell lymphoma: a Danish cohort study. Blood. 2017;130(4):554-7.
38. King RL, Dao LN, McPhail ED, Jaffe ES, Said J, Swerdlow SH, et al. Morphologic Features of ALK-negative Anaplastic Large Cell Lymphomas With DUSP22 Rearrangements. Am J Surg Pathol. 2016;40(1):36-43.
39. Luchtel RA, Dasari S, Oishi N, Pedersen MB, Hu G, Rech KL, et al. Molecular profiling reveals immunogenic cues in anaplastic large cell lymphomas with DUSP22 rearrangements. Blood. 2018;132(13):1386-98.
40. Crescenzo R, Abate F, Lasorsa E, Tabbo F, Gaudiano M, Chiesa N, et al. Convergent mutations and kinase fusions lead to oncogenic STAT3 activation in anaplastic large cell lymphoma. Cancer cell. 2015;27(4):516-32.
41. Scarfo I, Pellegrino E, Mereu E, Kwee I, Agnelli L, Bergaggio E, et al. Identification of a new subclass of ALK-negative ALCL expressing aberrant levels of ERBB4 transcripts. Blood. 2016;127(2):221-32.
42. Boi M, Rinaldi A, Kwee I, Bonetti P, Todaro M, Tabbò F, et al. PRDM1/BLIMP1 is commonly inactivated in anaplastic large T-cell lymphoma. Blood. 2013;122(15):2683-93.
43. Liang HC, Costanza M, Prutsch N, Zimmerman MW, Gurnhofer E, Montes-Mojarro IA, et al. Super-enhancerbased identification of a BATF3/IL-2R-module reveals vulnerabilities in anaplastic large cell lymphoma. Nat Commun. 2021;12(1):5577.
44. Ferrufino-Schmidt MC, Medeiros LJ, Liu H, Clemens MW, Hunt KK, Laurent C, et al. Clinicopathologic features and prognostic impact of lymph node involvement in patients with breast implant-associated anaplastic large cell lymphoma. Am J Surg Pathol. 2018;42(3):293-305.
45. Los-de Vries GT, de Boer M, van Dijk E, Stathi P, Hijmering NJ, Roemer MGM, et al. Chromosome 20 loss is characteristic of breast implant-associated anaplastic large cell lymphoma. Blood. 2020;136(25):2927-32.
46. Laurent C, Nicolae A, Laurent C, Bras FL, Haioun C, Fataccioli V, et al. Gene alterations in epigenetic modifiers and JAK-STAT signaling are frequent in breast implant-associated ALCL. Blood. 2020;135(5):360-70.
47. Quesada AE, Zhang Y, Ptashkin R, Ho C, Horwitz S, Benayed R, et al. Next generation sequencing of breast implant-associated anaplastic large cell lymphomas reveals a novel STAT3-JAK2 fusion among other activating genetic alterations within the JAK-STAT pathway. Breast J. 2021;27(4):314-21.
48. Tabanelli V, Corsini C, Fiori S, Agostinelli C, Calleri A, Orecchioni S, et al. Recurrent PDL1 expression and PDL1 (CD274) copy number alterations in breast implant-associated anaplastic large cell lymphomas. Hum Pathol. 2019;90:60-9.
49. de Leval L, Parrens M, Le Bras F, Jais JP, Fataccioli V, Martin A, et al. Angioimmunoblastic T-cell lymphoma is the most common T-cell lymphoma in two distinct French information data sets. Haematologica. 2015;100(9):e361-4.
50. Odejide O, Weigert O, Lane AA, Toscano D, Lunning MA, Kopp N, et al. A targeted mutational landscape of angioimmunoblastic T-cell lymphoma. Blood. 2014;123(9):1293-6.
51. Nagao R, Kikuti YY, Carreras J, Kikuchi T, Miyaoka M, Matsushita H, et al. Clinicopathologic analysis of angioimmunoblastic T-cell Lymphoma with or without RHOA G17V mutation using formalin-fixed paraffin-embedded sections. Am J Surg Pathol. 2016;40(8):1041-50.
52. Wang C, McKeithan TW, Gong Q, Zhang W, Bouska A, Rosenwald A, et al. IDH2R172 mutations define a unique subgroup of patients with angioimmunoblastic T-cell lymphoma. Blood. 2015;126(15):1741-52.

53. Lewis NE, Petrova-Drus K, Huet S, Epstein-Peterson ZD, Gao Q, Sigler AE, et al. Clonal hematopoiesis in angioimmunoblastic T-cell lymphoma with divergent evolution to myeloid neoplasms. Blood Adv. 2020;4(10):2261-71.
54. Streubel B, Vinatzer U, Willheim M, Chott A. Novel t(5;9)(q33;q22) fuses ITK to SYK in unspecified peripheral T-cell lymphoma. Leukemia. 2006;20(2):313-8.
55. Dobay MP, Lemonnier F, Missiaglia E, Bastard C, Vallois D, Jais JP, et al. Integrative clinicopathological and molecular analyses of angioimmunoblastic T-cell lymphoma and other nodal lymphomas of follicular helper T-cell origin. Haematologica. 2017;102(4):e148-51.
56. Debackere K, van der Krogt JA, Tousseyn T, Ferreiro JAF, Roosbroeck KV, Marcelis L, et al. FER and FES tyrosine kinase fusions in follicular T-cell lymphoma. Blood. 2020;135(8):584-8.
57. Ghione P, Faruque P, Mehta-Shah N, Seshan V, Ozkaya N, Bhaskar S, et al. T follicular helper phenotype predicts response to histone deacetylase inhibitors in relapsed/refractory peripheral T-cell lymphoma. Blood Adv. 2020;4(19):4640-7.
58. Pro B, Allen P, Behdad A. Hepatosplenic T-cell lymphoma: A rare but challenging entity. Blood. 2020;136(18):2018-26.
59. Iqbal J, Wright G, Wang C, Rosenwald A, Gascoyne RD, Weisenburger DD, et al. Gene expression signatures delineate biological and prognostic subgroups in peripheral T-cell lymphoma. Blood. 2014;123:2915-23.
60. Wai CMM, Chen S, Phyu T, Fan S, Leong SM, Zheng W, et al. Immune pathway upregulation and lower genomic instability distinguish EBV-positive nodal T/NK cell lymphoma from ENKTL and PTCL-NOS. Haematologica. 2022;107(8):1864-79.
61. Tse E, Au-Yeung R, Kwong YL. Recent advances in the diagnosis and treatment of natural killer/T-cell lymphomas. Expert Rev Hematol. 2019;12:927-35.
62. Hong M, Ko YH, Yoo KH, Koo HH, Kim SJ, Kim WS, et al. EBV-Positive T/NK-cell lymphoproliferative disease of childhood. Korean J Pathol. 2013;47:137-47.

CHAPTER 7

Pediatric Leukemias: Recent Updates

Sumayya Shah, Afshan Atta

INTRODUCTION

There have been numerous changes made to the classification of hematological cancers which have been collated in the latest 5th edition of the World Health Organization (WHO) Classification of Hematolymphoid Tumors. While a detailed discussion of all the updates would not be possible here, we will limit ourselves to those relevant to leukemias which affect the pediatric age group, that is, from birth to 17 years.

ACUTE LYMPHOBLASTIC LEUKEMIA

Pediatric acute lymphoblastic leukemia (ALL) is the success story of oncology and with innovations in diagnosis and therapeutic armamentarium, outlook is getting further refined and better with emphasis to minimize and mitigate the undesired long-term sequelae.

The last decade has witnessed great advances in our understanding of the genetic and biological basis of childhood ALL, the development of experimental models to probe mechanisms and evaluate new therapies, and the development of more efficacious treatment stratification. Genomic analysis has revolutionized our understanding of the molecular taxonomy of ALL, and these advances have led the push to implement genome and transcriptome characterization in the clinical management of ALL to facilitate more accurate risk stratification, and in some cases, targeted therapy.

Heritable Susceptibility to Acute Lymphoblastic Leukemia

Various studies denote that there is a genetic predisposition (Knudson hypothesis) to ALL, at least in a subgroup of cases. This evidence includes the presence of:
- Rare constitutional syndromes with greater risk for ALL such as Down syndrome (B-cell ALL) and ataxia-telangiectasia (T-cell ALL).

- Familial cancer syndromes such as Li-Fraumeni syndrome.[1]
- Non-coding DNA polymorphisms that subtly influence the risk of ALL. Genome-wide association studies (GWAS) have identified at least 13 loci associated with ALL.[2-4]
- Genes harboring germline nonsilent variants presume to contribute toward the risk of sporadic ALL.

Prenatal Origin of Leukemia

Several lines of investigation indicate that a subset of childhood leukemia cases arise before birth. Chromosomal translocations, particularly *ETV6-RUNX1* may be detected at birth in blood spots and cord blood, years before the clinical onset of leukemia providing support for a multistep process of leukemogenesis. This is supported by genomic analysis of monozygotic, monochorionic twins concordant for leukemia showing genetic identity of initiating lesions and discordance for secondary genetic alterations indicating intertwin intrauterine transmission of leukemia. Evidence for in utero origin is strongest for *KMT2A*-rearranged and *ETV6-RUNX1* ALL.[5-7]

Genetics of B-cell Acute Lymphoblastic Leukemia

The most common form of ALL, B-cell ALL, comprises greater than 20 subtypes of variable prevalence according to age that are associated with distinct gene expression profiles and are driven by three main types of initiating genetic alteration:
1. Chromosomal aneuploidy
2. Rearrangements that deregulate oncogenes or encode chimeric transcription factors[8-10]
3. Point mutation

High hyperdiploidy (>50 chromosomes) is present in up to 30% childhood ALL and is associated with mutations in the RAS-pathway and has favorable outcome.[11] Low hypodiploidy (31–39 chromosomes) is present in approximately 1% of childhood ALL but in >10% of adult ALL. It is characterized by the deletion of *IKZF2* and by near-universal *TP53* which are inherited in approximately half the cases.[12,13] Near haploidy (24–30 chromosomes) is present in approximately 2% of pediatric ALL and is associated with RAS mutation (NF1) and deletion of *IKZF3*.[14] Both low hypodiploid and near-haploid ALL are associated with unfavorable outcomes. ALL with intra chromosomal amplification of chromosome 21 *(iAMP21)* is most common in older children and is associated with poor prognosis. t(12;21) (p13;q22) encoding *ETV 6-RUNX1* is the most common translocation in children and is associated with favorable prognosis.[15-17] Philadelphia chromosome formation due to t(9;22) (q34;q11.2) translocation encodes *BCR-ABL1* and is associated with unfavorable outcome, despite the fact that the prognosis has now been improved with help of combined chemotherapy and tyrosine kinase inhibition **(Table 1)**.

TABLE 1: Genetic alterations, clinical features, age distribution, and genetic-based therapy among pediatric B- and T-acute lymphoblastic leukemia.

Category	Age	Description	Potential therapeutic implications
B-cell precursor acute lymphoblastic leukemia (ALL)			
Hyperdiploidy with more than 50 chromosomes	Children >> adults	Excellent prognosis; mutations in RAS signaling pathway and histone modifiers	Reduction of intensity
Near-haploid	Children-adults	24–31 chromosomes; poor prognosis; RAS-activating mutations; inactivation of *IKZF3*	BCL2 inhibitors
Low hypodiploid	Children < adults	32–39 chromosomes; poor prognosis; TP53 mutations (somatic and germline)	BCL2 inhibitors
iAMP21	Older children	Complex alterations of chromosome 21; requires high-risk therapy for good outcomes	Intensification of therapy
t(12;21) (p13;q22) encoding *ETV6-RUNX1*	Children >> adults	Excellent prognosis; cryptic rearrangement that is detectable by FISH	Reduction of intensity
ETV6-RUNX1–like	Children > adults	Absence of *ETV6-RUNX1* fusion; mutations in both *ETV6* and *IKZF1*	Reduction of intensity
t(1;19)(q23;p13) encoding *TCF3-PBX1*	Children-adults	Increased incidence in African Americans; favorable prognosis	
t(9;22)(q34;q11.2) encoding BCR-ABL1	Children << adults	Historically poor prognosis, improved with tyrosine kinase inhibitors; common deletions of *IKZF1*	ABL1 inhibitors, FAK inhibitors, rexinoids, BCL2 inhibitors
Ph-like	Children < adults	Kinase-activating lesions; poor outcome; potentially amenable to kinase inhibition	ABL1 inhibitors, JAK inhibitors, PI3K inhibitors, BCL2 inhibitors
CRLF2 rearranged (*IGH-CRLF2*; *P2RY8-CRLF2*)	Children < adults	Common in Down syndrome and Ph-like ALL; associated with *IKZF1* deletion and *JAK1/2* mutation	JAK inhibitors, BCL2 inhibitors
KMT2A (MLL) rearranged	Infants >> children-adults	Common in infant ALL; dismal prognosis; few co-operating mutations, commonly in RAS signaling pathway	DOT1L inhibitors, menin inhibitors, proteasome inhibitors, HDAC inhibitors, BCL2 inhibitors

Continued

Continued

Category	Age	Description	Potential therapeutic implications
DUX4 rearranged and *ERG* deregulated	Children-adults	Distinct gene expression profile; most have focal ERG deletions and favorable outcome despite *IKZF1* alterations	Reduction of intensity
MEF2D rearranged	Children-adults	Distinct gene expression profile; potential sensitivity to HDAC inhibition	HDAC inhibitors
ZNF384 rearranged	Children	Pro-B-ALL phenotype; expression of myeloid markers; *FLT3* increased expression	FLT3 inhibitors
PAX5alt	Children > adults	PAX5 fusions, mutation, or amplifications; prognosis intermediate	
PAX5 P80R	Children < adults	Frequent signaling pathway alterations	Kinase inhibitors
IKZF1 N159Y	Children-adults	Rare; unknown prognosis	FAK inhibitors, rexinoids
NUTM1 rearranged	Children	Exclusively in children; rare; prognosis excellent	HDAC inhibitors, bromodomain inhibitors
t(17;19)(q22;p13) encoding TCF3-HLF	Children-adults	Rare; dismal prognosis	BCL2 inhibitors
Rearranged *BCL2/MYC*	Children << adults	Poor prognosis	
T-lineage acute lymphoblastic leukemia			
TAL1 deregulation	Children-adults	Enrichment of mutation in PI3K signaling pathway	PI3K inhibitors, nelarabine, BCL2 inhibitors nelarabine, BCL2 inhibitors
TLX3 deregulation	Children-adults	Poor prognosis; frequent co-operating mutation in ubiquitination and ribosomal genes	
HOXA deregulation	Children-adults	Frequent mutations in JAK-STAT pathway, *KMT2A* rearrangements	JAK inhibitors, nelarabine, BCL2 inhibitors
TLX1 deregulation	Children-adults	Favorable prognosis	Nelarabine, BCL2 inhibitors
LMO2/LYL1 deregulation	Children-adults	Poor prognosis; enriched for ETP-ALL, frequent co-operating mutation in JAK-/STAT	JAK inhibitors, nelarabine, BCL2 inhibitors

Continued

Continued

Category	Age	Description	Potential therapeutic implications
NKX2-1 deregulation	Children-adults	Frequent co-operating mutation in ribosomal genes	Nelarabine, BCL2 inhibitors
NUP214-ABL1 with 9q34 amplification	Children-adults	Neutral prognosis, in contrast to kinase-driven B-ALL; potentially amenable to tyrosine kinase inhibition	ABL1 inhibitors, nelarabine, BCL2 inhibitors
Early T-cell precursor ALL	Children-adults	Poor prognosis; genetically heterogeneous with mutations in hematopoietic regulators, cytokine and RAS signaling, and epigenetic modifiers	JAK inhibitors, BCL2 inhibitors

(FISH: fluorescence in situ hybridization; ALL: acute lymphoblastic leukemia; HDAC: histone deacetylase)
Source: Inaba H, Mullighan CG. Pediatric acute lymphoblastic leukemia. Haematologica 2020; 105(11):2524-39.

Kinase-driven Subtypes

Of therapeutic relevance are the two-kinase-driven subtypes; Philadelphia chromosome-positive and Philadelphia chromosome like ALL. Their frequency increases with age and they account for 25% and 20% respectively of adult ALL.[18]

Genetic Basis of T-cell Acute Lymphoblastic Leukemia

Childhood T-cell ALL is characterized by recurrent alterations in 10 pathways, but in most cases, three pathways are abnormally regulated.
1. Expression of transcription factors of T-cell lineage.
2. Signaling of NOTCH/MYC.
3. Cell cycle control.[19-21]

■ MIXED-PHENOTYPE ACUTE LEUKEMIA

It is uncommon, representing only 2–5% of pediatric leukemias. Mixed-phenotype acute leukemia (MPAL) is defined as acute leukemia expressing a combination of antigens not restricted to a single lineage with the following categories; B/myeloid NOS and T/myeloid NOS in addition to two genetic subgroups of MPAL; that with t(9;22) (q34.1;q11.2), *BCR–ABL 1* and that with t(v;11q23.3), *KMT2A* rearranged. Genetic characterization of pediatric MPAL revealed that rearrangement of ZNF 384 is common in B/myeloid MPAL and biallelic WT1 alterations are common in T/myeloid MPAL. Such genetic alterations are consistent with the results of a retrospective multinational study showing that ALL type therapy is more effective than acute myeloid leukemia (AML) or combined type treatment in patients with MPAL.

Risk Assignment for Treatment (Table 2)
Adverse Prognostic Factors
- Age (infant or ≥ 10 years)
- WBC count (≥50 × 10^5/L)
- Involvement of the CNS
- T-cell immunophenotype
- Race (Black or Hispanic)
- Male sex

TABLE 2: Risk factors in pediatric acute lymphoblastic leukemia.		
Factor	**Better**	**Worse**
Patient and clinical characteristics		
Age at diagnosis	1 to <10 years	<1 year or ≥10 years
Sex	Female	Male
Race	Caucasian Asian	African American, Hispanic
Down syndrome	No	Yes
WBC counts at diagnosis	<50 × 10^9/L	≥50 × 10^9/L
CNS involvement at diagnosis	CNS 1	CNS 2 and CNS 3, traumatic tap with blasts
Testicular involvement	No	Yes
Immunophenotype	B-ALL	T-ALL
Cytogenetic and genetics		
	High hyperdiploidy (51–65 chromosomes)	Hypodiploidy (<44 chromosomes)
	ETV6-RUNX1: t(12;21)(p13.2;q22.1)	*KMT2A* rearrangement: t(v;11q23.3)
	NUMT1 rearrangement	*BCR-ABL1*: t(9;22)(q34.1;q11.2) (Ph+)
		BCR-ABL1-like (Ph-like)
		TCF3-HLF: t(17;19)(q22;p13)
		MEF2D rearrangement
		Intrachromosomal amplification of chromosome 21 (iAMP21)
		BCL2 or *MYC* rearrangements
Minimal residual disease		
	Negative	Positive
	Continuously decreasing and becoming negative	Increasing and/or persistently positive while monitored

(WBC: white blood cell; CNS: central nervous system; ALL: acute lymphoblastic leukemia; Ph: philadelphia chromosome)

Source: Inaba H, Mullighan CG. Pediatric acute lymphoblastic leukemia. Haematologica 2020; 105(11):2524-39.

Better Prognosis Factors
- Hyperdiploidy (>50 chromosomes)
- *ETV6-RUNX1*
- Low WBC counts

Worst Prognostic Factors
- Hypodiploidy (< 44 chromosomes)
- Ph-positive or Ph-like ALL/*KMT2A/MEF2D or BCL2/MYC* rearrangements

Treatment

In the last decade, molecularly targeted agents and immunotherapy have emerged as novel therapeutic strategies. Immunotherapy can be provided as antibody-based therapy, e.g., blinatumomab or inotuzumab ozogamicin or T-cell-based therapy, i.e., chimeric antigen receptor T (CAR-T) cells that have enhanced the response rate and the results in patients with relapsed/refractory B-ALL. Antibodies and CAR-T cells against T-ALL are also under investigation **(Fig. 1)**.

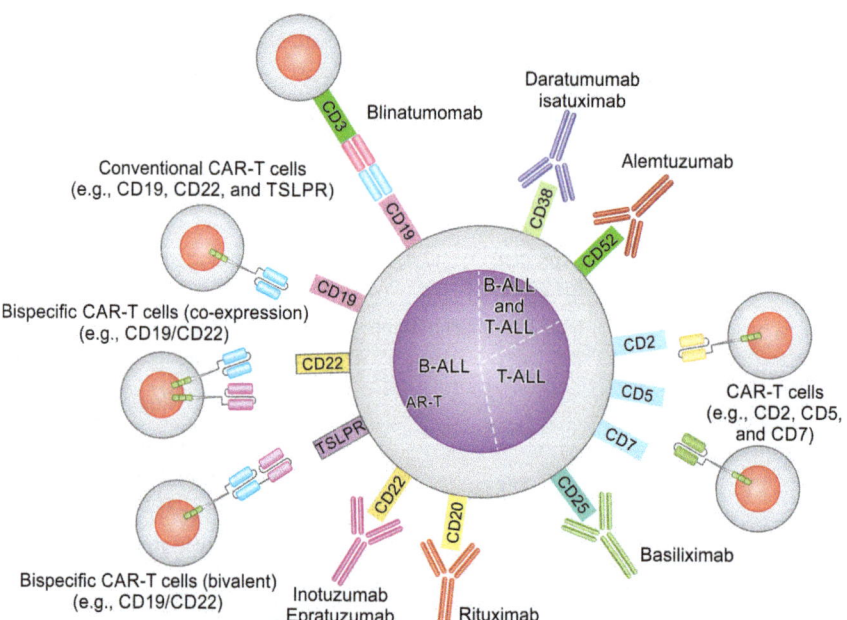

FIG. 1: Immunotherapy in acute lymphoblastic leukemia.
(CAR-T cells: chimeric antigen receptor T cells; ALL: acute lymphoblastic leukemia; TSLPR: thymic stromal lymphopoietin receptor.
Source: Inaba H, Mullighan CG. Pediatric acute lymphoblastic leukemia. Haematologica 2020;105(11): 2524-39.

ACUTE MYELOID LEUKEMIA

The risk of developing AML in most cases is biological rather than environmental with the only established pediatric AML cause being in utero exposure to ionizing radiation.[22-24] Other exposures for example, maternal chemical exposure and parental age have only limited evidence supporting their association with AML.[25] Down syndrome is the most common genetic risk factor followed by diseases associated with DNA repair deficiencies, such as Fanconi anemia and ataxia telangiectasia. The AML to ALL ratio is 1:4 except in neonatal period.

Biology of Pediatric Acute Myeloid Leukemia

The latest WHO classification allows for a much finer differentiation, with more accurate prognostic correlations. The major categories are AML with defining genetic abnormalities and AML, defined by differentiation **(Box 1)**.

BOX 1 | Acute myeloid leukemia.

Acute myeloid leukemia with defining genetic abnormalities
- Acute promyelocytic leukemia with *PML::RARA* fusion
- Acute myeloid leukemia with *RUNX1::RUNX1T1* fusion
- Acute myeloid leukemia with *CBFB::MYH11* fusion
- Acute myeloid leukemia with *DEK::NUP214* fusion
- Acute myeloid leukemia with *RBM15::MRTFA* fusion
- Acute myeloid leukemia with *BCR::ABL1* fusion
- Acute myeloid leukemia with *KMT2A* rearrangement
- Acute myeloid leukemia with *MECOM* rearrangement
- Acute myeloid leukemia with *NUP98* rearrangement
- Acute myeloid leukemia with *NPM1* mutation
- Acute myeloid leukemia with *CEBPA* mutation
- Acute myeloid leukemia, myelodysplasia-related
- Acute myeloid leukemia with other defined genetic alterations

Acute myeloid leukemia, defined by differentiation
- Acute myeloid leukemia with minimal differentiation
- Acute myeloid leukemia without maturation
- Acute myeloid leukemia with maturation
- Acute basophilic leukemia
- Acute myelomonocytic leukemia
- Acute monocytic leukemia
- Acute erythroid leukemia
- Acute megakaryoblastic leukemia

Source: Khoury JD, Solary E, Abla O, Akkari Y, Alaggio R, Apperley JF, et al. The 5th edition of the World Health Organization Classification of Haematolymphoid Tumours: Myeloid and Histiocytic/Dendritic Neoplasms. Leukemia. 2022;36:1703-19.

Transient Abnormal Myelopoiesis

It is seen in neonatal period, more commonly in cases of Down syndrome. About 10% of children with Down syndrome develop transient abnormal myelopoiesis (TAM).[26-28] Majority remit by 3 months. Dysplastic features are common. Mutations in *GATA-1* gene is incriminated.

Core-binding Factor Leukemia

Two common cytogenetic abnormalities make up the largest group of core-binding factor (CBF) leukemias; t(8;21) (q22;q22) and inv(16) (p13.1q 22) representing approximately 15% and 6% of pediatric AML cases, respectively.

Acute Promyelocytic Leukemia with PML::RARA Fusion Gene

Almost every case (95%) of acute promyelocytic leukemia (APL) has a characteristic t(15;17) (q22;q21) translocation which results in the fusion of promyelocytic leukemia (PML) (role in transcriptional regulation and tumor suppression) and *RARA* genes (role in differentiation process). When these two genes fuse, the resultant protein prevents both physiological functions and conversely the fusion protein binds to DNA and acts in a dominant negative fashion to repress gene expression as well as nuclear body formation. Though APL is considered to be universally fatal, this unique biology allows the use of targeted therapies that makes APL have a more favorable prognosis.

Therapy-related Myeloid Neoplasms

It is less common in children as by the time therapy-related myeloid neoplasms (t-AML) develops, the patient has reached adulthood. Though t-AML is not defined by any specific set of genetic abnormalities, there are trends that are arising. The use of certain chemotherapy drugs, especially anthracyclines and etoposide are highly correlated with the development of t-AML with chromosomal abnormalities involving 11q23.

Acute Myeloid Leukemia with CEPBA Mutation

The CCAAT enhancer-binding protein family (C/EBP) is made up of several related transcription factors, the α isoform of which is commonly mutated in pediatric AML.

Treatment and Prognostic Considerations for Pediatric AML

When treating AML, there are many factors that need to be considered:
- Urgency
- Efficacy

Though advances have been made in the treatment of pediatric AML, the most effective therapies are profoundly toxic even when administered properly. Therefore, it is imperative that measures be taken to maximize efficacy and minimize toxicity.

Favorable Prognostic Indicators

Core binding factor AML represents one of the largest AML subgroups associated with favorable prognosis. Similarly, APL with the standard cytogenetics is also associated with good outcome.

Adverse Prognostic Indicators

Certain translocations including t(10;11) (p12;q23), t(6;9) (p23;q34), inv(3) (q21126.2) are poor prognostic markers. t-AML is always considered to have adverse prognosis.

MYELOPROLIFERATIVE NEOPLASMS

These include all the diseases mentioned in previous editions with the addition of juvenile myelomonocytic leukemia (JMML) **(Box 2)**. They have a chronic phase (CP) which transforms into an accelerated phase (AP) and then a blast phase (BP) with acquisition of more and more cytogenetic and/or molecular mutations.

Chronic Myeloid Leukemia

This is the most common of the myeloproliferative neoplasms (MPNs), the hallmark of which is the *BCR::ABL1* fusion gene resulting from t(9;22) (q34;q11). Majority of the cases present in CP which then progresses to BP, with or without passing through AP. With the advent of tyrosine kinase inhibitors (TKIs) and disease monitoring, longer progression-free intervals have become the norm with an overall 10-year survival rate of 80–90%. With resistance due to *ABL1* kinase mutations and/or additional cytogenetic mutations and development of BP recognized as important disease characteristics,[29,30] AP has become superfluous and has been removed in this classification with more stress placed on high-risk features associated with CP progression and TKI resistance. BP criteria include (1) ≥20% myeloblasts in peripheral blood or bone marrow; or (2) extramedullary proliferation of blasts; or (3) increased lymphoblasts in peripheral blood or bone marrow.

BOX 2 | **Myeloproliferative neoplasms.**

- Chronic myeloid leukemia
- Polycythemia vera
- Primary myelofibrosis
- Essential thrombocythemia
- Chronic neutrophilic leukemia
- Chronic eosinophilic leukemia
- Juvenile myelomonocytic leukemia
- Myeloproliferative neoplasm, not otherwise specified

Source: Khoury JD, Solary E, Abla O, Akkari Y, Alaggio R, Apperley JF, et al. The 5th edition of the World Health Organization Classification of Haematolymphoid Tumours: Myeloid and Histiocytic/Dendritic Neoplasms. Leukemia. 2022;36:1703-19.

The exact cutoff percentage of lymphoblasts and significance of increased lymphoblasts is not yet known.

BCR::ABL1-negative Myeloproliferative Neoplasms

There have been some small changes in the diagnostic criteria of polycythemia vera (PV), primary myelofibrosis (PMF) and essential thrombocythemia (ET).

Measurement of increased red cell mass using ^{51}Cr-labeled red cells has been omitted as a diagnostic criterion since this test is rarely done in routine practice. Increased hemoglobin/hematocrit with panmyelosis and pleomorphic mature megakaryocytes in the marrow along with *JAK2 V617F* or *JAK2 exon 12* mutations are still major diagnostic criteria. The criteria for diagnosing ET, PMF, and chronic neutrophilic leukemia (CNL) remain the same.

Major changes have been made in the diagnosis of chronic eosinophilic leukemia (CEL): (1) persistent hypereosinophilia for 4 weeks instead of 6 months. (2) Both clonality and atypical bone marrow morphology (e.g., erythroid or megakaryocytic dysplasia) required. (3) Increased blasts as a substitute for clonality have been abolished. These updates further clarify the difference between CEL and conditions such as idiopathic hypereosinophilic syndrome and hypereosinophilia of unknown significance.[31] With refinement of diagnostic criteria and greater understanding of CEL in relation to other diseases with eosinophilia, the adjunct "not otherwise specified" has been eliminated.

Myeloproliferative neoplasm, not otherwise specified (MPN-NOS) is used for cases with morphological, laboratory, and molecular features of MPN which do not fit into a particular subtype or fit into more than one subtype.

Juvenile Myelomonocytic Leukemia

Juvenile myelomonocytic leukemia has now been classified as a myeloproliferative neoplasm of childhood with some revisions to its diagnostic criteria which include (1) *KMT2A* rearrangements excluded, (2) monosomy 7 removed as a cytogenetic criterion, and (3) greater weightage given to diagnostic molecular tests especially those that indicate RAS-pathway activation. Risk stratification and therapeutic approach depend on the genetics of each case with those showing germline CBL mutations occasionally undergoing spontaneous remission while those having somatic mutations involving *PTPN11* and germline pathogenic variants involving neurofibromatosis type 1 behaving aggressively. The classification of JMML as an MPN signifies the lack of true dysplasia in this condition.

■ MYELODYSPLASTIC NEOPLASMS

Myelodysplastic syndromes have been renamed as myelodysplastic neoplasms, although still abbreviated as MDS, emphasizing their malignant disposition, and bringing them in line with MPN. They are now divided into those having defining genetic abnormalities and those that are morphologically defined **(Table 3)**. This rearrangement bases risk stratification on schemes like the Revised International Prognostic Scoring System for MDS (IPSS-R) by focusing on genetic basis of disease.[32] Also, clearer terms are used to better differentiate MDS with low blasts (MDS-LB) and MDS with increased blasts (MDS-IB) with the maintenance of previous cutoff values.

TABLE 3: Classification and defining features of myelodysplastic neoplasms (MDS).			
	Blasts	**Cytogenetics**	**Mutations**
MDS with defining genetic abnormalities			
MDS with low blasts and isolated 5q deletion (MDS-5q)	<2% PB and <5% BM	5q deletion alone, or with 1 other abnormality other than monosomy 7 or 7q deletion	
MDS with low blasts and SF3B1 mutation[a] (MDS-SF3B1)		Absence of 5q deletion, monosomy 7, or complex karyotype	SF3B1
MDS with biallelic TP53 inactivation (MDS-biTP53)	<20% PB and BM	Usually complex	Two or more TP53 mutations, or 1 mutation with evidence of TP53 copy number loss or cnLOH
MDS, morphologically defined			
MDS with low blasts (MDS-LB)	<2% PB and <5% BM		
MDS, hypoplastic[b] (MDS-h)			
MDS with increased blasts (MDS-IB)			
MDS-IB1	2–4% PB or 5–9% BM		
MDS-IB2	5–19% PB or 10–19% BM or Auer rods		
MDS with fibrosis (MDS-f)	2–19% PB; 5–19% BM		

[a]Detection of ≥15% ring sideroblasts may substitute for SF3B1 mutation. Acceptable related terminology: MDS with low blasts and ring sideroblasts.
[b]By definition, ≤25% bone marrow cellularity, age adjusted.
(PB: peripheral blood; BM: bone marrow; cnLOH: copy neutral loss of heterozygosity)
Source: Khoury JD, Solary E, Abla O, Akkari Y, Alaggio R, Apperley JF, et al. The 5th edition of the World Health Organization Classification of Haematolymphoid Tumours: Myeloid and Histiocytic/Dendritic Neoplasms. Leukemia 2022;36:1703-19.

Myelodysplastic Syndrome with Defining Genetic Abnormalities

This comprises MDS with low blasts and isolated 5q deletion (MDS-5q), MDS with low blasts and *SF3B1* mutation (MDS-SF3B1), and MDS with biallelic *TP53* inactivation (MDS-biTP53).

MDS-5q diagnostic criteria remain the same. An additional *SF3B1* or *TP53* mutation (not multi-hit) does not alter a diagnosis of MDS-5q, although their presence is considered to change the behavior and/or prognosis of disease.

MDS-SF3B1 is now considered a separate entity which includes nearly all cases of MDS with ≥5% ring sideroblasts.[33] For cases with wild-type SF3B1 and ≥15% ring sideroblasts, the term MDS with low blasts and ring sideroblasts can still be used, allowing uncommon MDS cases with driver mutations in other *RNA* splicing genes to be covered as well.

Myelodysplastic Syndrome, Morphologically Defined

Hypoplastic MDS (MDS-h) has now been identified as a distinct disease subtype in the latest WHO classification. It involves a T-cell-mediated immune attack on hematopoietic stem cells with oligoclonal proliferation of CD8+ cytotoxic T-cells producing TNF-α and/or IFN-γ. There are many similarities seen among MDS-h, paroxysmal nocturnal hemoglobinuria (PNH) and aplastic anemia (AA), including an association with clonal hematopoiesis (CH).[34-36] MDS-h also needs to be differentiated from patients having germline pathogenic mutations in *GATA2*, *DDX41*, Fanconi anemia (FA) or telomerase complex genes as these also have hypoplastic marrows and progress to MDS and/or AML but do not respond to immunosuppressive agents unlike MDS-h which shows a good response to anti-thymocyte globulin (ATG), a drug typically used in AA.

Specifying single lineage or multiple lineage dysplasia has become redundant as the number of cell lines involved keeps changing and reflects clonal evolution rather than different MDS subtypes. The category of MDS, unclassifiable has also been eliminated due to upgradation of the MDS classification scheme and inclusion of clonal cytopenia of undetermined significance (CCUS).

Myelodysplastic Syndrome and Acute Myeloid Leukemia

There have been several calls to redefine the blast percentage in bone marrow which differentiates MDS-IB2 from AML for various reasons and due to new therapies that are effective in patients currently diagnosed as MDS or AML with 10–30% blasts.[37-39] Some of the practical problems justifying this review include (1) myeloid neoplasms exist on a biological spectrum, making any blast cutoff discretionary; (2) blast counts differ due to sampling variations/error and subjective assessments; and (3) there is no gold standard for blast enumeration and orthogonal tests often give mismatched results. Combining MDS-IB2 and AML and lowering the blast percentage to 10% (forming a new

TABLE 4: Childhood myelodysplastic neoplasms (MDS).	
	Blasts
Childhood MDS with low blasts	<2% PB; <5% BM
Hypocellular	
Not otherwise specified	
Childhood MDS with increased blasts	2–19% PB; 5–19% BM

(PB: peripheral blood; BM: bone marrow)
Source: Khoury JD, Solary E, Abla O, Akkari Y, Alaggio R, Apperley JF, et al. The 5th edition of the World Health Organization Classification of Haematolymphoid Tumours: Myeloid and Histiocytic/Dendritic Neoplasms. Leukemia 2022;36:1703-19.

group of MDS/AML) had the same objections as above as well as danger of overtreatment. Therefore, a 20% blast cutoff was maintained to distinguish MDS from AML except for cases of AML with defining genetic mutations, which can have any blast percentage. However, from a treatment and clinical trial design viewpoint, MDS-IB2 is considered equivalent to AML.

Childhood Myelodysplastic Neoplasms

These are clonal hematopoietic stem cell cancers found in children and adolescents resulting in ineffective hematopoiesis, cytopenia(s) and risk of evolution into AML. This group does not include JMML, myeloid proliferations of Down syndrome and post-cytotoxic therapy MDS. The qualifier, childhood, signifies that this type of MDS is biologically separate from adult MDS,[40,41] the exact pathogenesis still incompletely understood.

"Refractory cytopenia of childhood (RCC)" is now known as childhood MDS with low blasts (cMDS-LB) and has two subtypes: childhood MDS with low blasts, hypocellular; and childhood MDS with low blasts, not otherwise specified (NOS) **(Table 4)**. Cases need to be carefully assessed for dysplasia in hematopoietic cell lines as majority (80%) show bone marrow hypocellularity and features resembling severe AA and other bone marrow failure syndromes (BMFS).[42] Patients with monosomy 7, 7q deletion or complex karyotype are treated with hematopoietic stem cell transplant due to high risk of evolution to AML while patients with normal karyotype or trisomy 8 have an indolent course.

Childhood MDS with increased blasts (cMDS-IB) shows ≥5% blasts in bone marrow or ≥2% blasts in peripheral blood. Acquired cytogenetic aberrations andthway mutations are more common in it compared with cMDS-LB.[43,44]

MYELODYSPLASTIC/MYELOPROLIFERATIVE NEOPLASMS

The latest edition of the WHO classification has significant modifications in the chronic myelomonocytic leukemia (CMML) diagnostic criteria as well as terminology changes for other MDS/MPN types **(Box 3)**.

> **BOX 3 Myelodysplastic/myeloproliferative neoplasms.**
>
> - Chronic myelomonocytic leukemia
> - Myelodysplastic/myeloproliferative neoplasm with neutrophilia
> - Myelodysplastic/myeloproliferative neoplasm with SF3B1 mutation and thrombocytosis
> - Myelodysplastic/myeloproliferative neoplasm, not otherwise specified
>
> *Source*: Khoury JD, Solary E, Abla O, Akkari Y, Alaggio R, Apperley JF, et al. The 5th edition of the World Health Organization Classification of Haematolymphoid Tumours: Myeloid and Histiocytic/Dendritic Neoplasms. Leukemia 2022;36:1703-19.

Chronic Myelomonocytic Leukemia

The absolute monocyte count for sustained peripheral blood monocytosis is reduced from $1.0 \times 10^9/L$ to $0.5 \times 10^9/L$, helping encompass cases previously named as oligomonocytic CMML.[45-47] Dysplasia in at least one lineage plus clonal cytogenetic or molecular abnormality is required for diagnosis when absolute monocyte count is between $0.5 \times 10^9/L - 1.0 \times 10^9/L$. Abnormal separation of peripheral blood monocyte subsets has been introduced as a new supporting criterion **(Box 4)**.[48,49] Further research is required to classify those with unexplained clonal monocytosis[50] who do not fulfil the new CMML diagnostic criteria.

Chronic myelomonocytic leukemia has two subtypes, divided based on white cell count: (1) myelodysplastic CMML (MD-CMML) with WBC count $<13 \times 10^9/L$; and (2) myeloproliferative CMML (MP-CMML) with WBC count $\geq 13 \times 10^9/L$. The latter usually shows activating RAS-pathway mutations and adverse prognosis.[51] The subgroup of CMML-0 has been removed due to no/limited prognostic significance.[52,53]

Terminology Updates

Diagnostic criteria of other MDS/MPNs remain mostly the same. Atypical chronic myeloid leukemia (CML) has been renamed as MDS/MPN with neutrophilia, thus emphasizing the MDS/MPN nature of the disease and avoiding confusion with CML. MDS/MPN with ring sideroblasts and thrombocytosis has been replaced by the term MDS/MPN with SF3B1 mutation and thrombocytosis but can still be used for cases with wild-type *SF3B1* mutation and ≥15% ring sideroblasts. MDS/MPN, unclassifiable is now known as MDS/MPN, not otherwise specified, being part of an attempt to omit the paradoxical qualifying term of "unclassifiable" from the whole classification.

■ MASTOCYTOSIS

It has three types: (1) systemic mastocytosis (SM), (2) cutaneous mastocytosis (CM), and (3) mast cell sarcoma (MCS) **(Box 5)**.[54]

> **BOX 4** **Diagnostic criteria of chronic myelomonocytic leukemia (CMML).**
>
> *Prerequisite criteria:*
> - Persistent absolute (≥0.5 × 10⁹/L) and relative (≥10%) peripheral blood monocytosis
> - Blasts constitute <20% of the cells in the peripheral blood and bone marrow[a]
> - Not meeting diagnostic criteria of chronic myeloid leukemia or other myeloproliferative neoplasms[b]
> - Not meeting diagnostic criteria of myeloid/lymphoid neoplasms with tyrosine kinase fusions[c]
>
> *Supporting criteria:*
> - Dysplasia involving ≥1 myeloid lineages[d]
> - Acquired clonal cytogenetic or molecular abnormality
> - Abnormal partitioning of peripheral blood monocyte subsets[e]
>
> *Requirements for diagnosis:*
> - Prerequisite criteria must be present in all cases
> - If monocytosis is ≥1 × 10⁹/L: One or more supporting criteria must be met
> - If monocytosis is ≥0.5 and <1 × 10⁹/L: Supporting criteria 1 and 2 must be met
>
> *Subtyping criteria:*
> - Myelodysplastic CMML (MD-CMML): WBC <13 × 10⁹/L
> - Myeloproliferative CMML (MP-CMML): WBC ≥13 × 10⁹/L
>
> *Subgrouping criteria (based on percentage of blasts and promonocytes):*
> - CMML-1: <5% in peripheral blood and <10% in bone marrow.
> - CMML-2: 5–19% in peripheral blood and 10–19% in bone marrow.
>
> [a]Blasts and blast equivalents include myeloblasts, monoblasts, and promonocytes.
> [b]Myeloproliferative neoplasms (MPN) can be associated with monocytosis at presentation or during the course of the disease; such cases can mimic CMML. In these instances, a documented history of MPN excludes CMML. The presence of MPN features in the bone marrow and/or high burden of MPN-associated mutations (JAK2, CALR or MPL) tends to support MPN with monocytosis rather than CMML.
> [c]Criteria for myeloid/lymphoid neoplasms with tyrosine kinase fusions should be specifically excluded in cases with eosinophilia.
> [d]Morphologic dysplasia should be present in ≥10% of cells of a hematopoietic lineage in the bone marrow.
> [e]Based on detection of increased classical monocytes (>94%) in the absence of known active autoimmune diseases and/or systemic inflammatory syndromes.
>
> *Source:* Khoury JD, Solary E, Abla O, Akkari Y, Alaggio R, Apperley JF, et al. The 5th edition of the World Health Organization Classification of Haematolymphoid Tumours: Myeloid and Histiocytic/Dendritic Neoplasms. Leukemia 2022;36:1703-19.

There have been some changes in SM diagnostic criteria. CD30 and any *KIT* mutation have been introduced as minor diagnostic criteria. Basal serum tryptase level >20 ng/mL is also a minor criterion.[55] This level is to be adjusted in patients of hereditary alpha-tryptasemia. Bone marrow mastocytosis is a new SM subtype marked by the absence of skin lesions and B-findings and a basal serum tryptase level <125 ng/mL. There have been some improvements in B (burden of disease) and C-findings (cytoreduction requiring), most important of which is that *KIT D816V* mutation with variant

> **BOX 5** **Mastocytosis types and subtypes.**
>
> *Cutaneous mastocytosis:*
> - Urticaria pigmentosa/maculopapular cutaneous mastocytosis
> - Monomorphic
> - Polymorphic
> - Diffuse cutaneous mastocytosis
> - Cutaneous mastocytoma
> - Isolated mastocytoma
> - Multilocalized mastocytoma
>
> *Systemic mastocytosis:*
> - Bone marrow mastocytosis
> - Indolent systemic mastocytosis
> - Smoldering systemic mastocytosis
> - Aggressive systemic mastocytosis
> - Systemic mastocytosis with an associated hematologic neoplasm
> - Mast cell leukemia
>
> *Mast cell sarcoma*
>
> *Note:* Well-differentiated systemic mastocytosis (WDSM) represents a morphologic variant that may occur in any SM type/subtype, including mast cell leukemia.
>
> *Source:* Khoury JD, Solary E, Abla O, Akkari Y, Alaggio R, Apperley JF, et al. The 5th edition of the World Health Organization Classification of Haematolymphoid Tumours: Myeloid and Histiocytic/Dendritic Neoplasms. Leukemia 2022;36:1703-19.

allele frequency (VAF) ≥10% in bone marrow or peripheral blood leukocytes is now considered a B-finding.

Well-differentiated systemic mastocytosis (WDSM) is acknowledged as a morphological pattern that can be seen in any SM subtype, showing round, well-granulated mast cells widely infiltrating the marrow. In many such patients, *KIT 816* mutation is not found and the abnormal mast cells are positive for CD30 and negative for CD25 and CD2.[56]

MYELOID/LYMPHOID NEOPLASMS WITH EOSINOPHILIA AND TYROSINE KINASE GENE FUSIONS

These cancers cover extensive histologic types ranging from MPN, MDS, MDS/MPN, AML, and MPAL as well as B- or T-lymphoblastic leukemia/lymphoma (ALL). Till now, they included fusions of genes, such as *PDGFRA*, *PDGFRB*, and *FGFR1* with various partners. Now, a new category of MLN-TK with JAK2 rearrangement, involving *JAK2* fusion with genes other than *PCM1*, has been identified.[57,58] Rare cases of *FLT3* rearrangement have been seen and included in this category as well as MLN-TK with ETV6::ABL1 fusion.[59]

MLN-TK with other defined tyrosine kinase fusions includes all remaining genetic abnormalities involving tyrosine kinase genes which are very rare and thus very little is known about them **(Box 6)**.[60,61]

> **BOX 6** **Genetic abnormalities defining myeloid/lymphoid neoplasms with eosinophilia and tyrosine kinase gene fusions.**
>
> - *PDGFRA* rearrangement
> - *PDGFRB* rearrangement
> - *FGFR1* rearrangement
> - *JAK2* rearrangement
> - *FLT3* rearrangement
> - *ETV6::ABL1* fusion
>
> Other defined tyrosine kinase fusions:
> - *ETV6::FGFR2; ETV6::LYN; ETV6::NTRK3; RANBP2::ALK; BCR::RET; FGFR1OP::RET*
>
> *Source*: Khoury JD, Solary E, Abla O, Akkari Y, Alaggio R, Apperley JF, et al. The 5th edition of the World Health Organization Classification of Haematolymphoid Tumours: Myeloid and Histiocytic/Dendritic Neoplasms. Leukemia 2022;36:1703-19.

GENETIC TUMOR SYNDROMES WITH PREDISPOSITION TO MYELOID NEOPLASIA

The new WHO classification recognizes five hematologic subtypes of FA based on blast percentage, *RAS*-pathway gene mutations and/or classic phenotype suggestive of a RASopathy.[62]

CONCLUSION

Understanding and unmasking biology and potential target sites is a process continuum. Focused efforts and innovative research is slowly but surely rewarding. We started in fifties with vincristine, methotrexate, 6-mercaptopurine with incorporation of radiotherapy and in 2023 we discuss where and how to incorporate biosimilars, CAR T cell, and other targeted therapies in pipeline. Focus of our discussion is now how to mitigate side effects and make these modalities patient friendly.

This chapter highlights and underscore recent advances in pediatric leukemia with a desired objective and goal to make it a confident success story with no neurocognitive sequelae.

REFERENCES

1. Holmfeldt L, Wei L, Diaz-Flores E, Walsh M, Zhang J, Ding L, et al. The genomic landscape of hypodiploid acute lymphoblastic leukemia. Nat Genet. 2013;45(3):242-52.
2. Gu Z, Churchman ML, Roberts KG, Moore I, Zhou X, Nakitandwe J, et al. PAX5-driven subtypes of B-progenitor acute lymphoblastic leukemia. Nat Genet. 2019;51(2):296-307.
3. Churchman ML, Qian M, Te Kronnie G, Zhang R, Yang W, Zhang H, et al. Germline genetic IKZF1 variation and predisposition to childhood acute lymphoblastic leukemia. Cancer Cell. 2018;33(5):937-48.
4. Kuehn HS, Boisson B, Cunningham-Rundles C, Reichenbach J, Stray-Pedersen A, Gelfand EW, et al. Loss of B cells in patients with heterozygous mutations in IKAROS. N Engl J Med. 2016;374(11):1032-43.

5. Zhang J, McCastlain K, Yoshihara H, Xu B, Chang Y, Churchman ML, et al. Deregulation of DUX4 and ERG in acute lymphoblastic leukemia. Nat Genet. 2016;48(12):1481-9.
6. Brown AL, Arts P, Carmichael CL, Babic M, Dobbins J, Chong CE, et al. RUNX1-mutated families show phenotype heterogeneity and a somatic mutation profile unique to germline predisposed AML. Blood Adv. 2020;4(6):1131-44.
7. Feurstein S, Godley LA. Germline ETV6 mutations and predisposition to hematological malignancies. Int J Hematol. 2017;106(2):189-95.
8. Gocho Y, Yang JJ. Genetic defects in hematopoietic transcription factors and predisposition to acute lymphoblastic leukemia. Blood. 2019;134(10):793-7.
9. Papaemmanuil E, Hosking FJ, Vijayakrishnan J, Price A, Olver B, Sheridan E, et al. Loci on 7p12.2, 10q21.2 and 14q11.2 are associated with risk of childhood acute lymphoblastic leukemia. Nat Genet. 2009;41(9):1006-10.
10. Trevino LR, Yang W, French D, Hunger SP, Carroll WL, Devidas M, et al. Germline genomic variants associated with childhood acute lymphoblastic leukemia. Nat Genet. 2009;41(9):1001-5.
11. Roberts KG, Mullighan CG. The biology of B-progenitor acute lymphoblastic leukemia. Cold Spring Harb Perspect Med. 2020;10(7):a034835.
12. Carroll AJ, Shago M, Mikhail FM, Raimondi S, Hirsch BA, Loh MI, et al. Masked hypodiploidy: hypodiploid acute lymphoblastic leukemia (ALL) mimicking hyperdiploid ALL in children: a report from the Children's Oncology Group. Cancer Genet. 2019;238:62-8.
13. Hunger SP, Galili N, Carroll AJ, Crist WM, Link MP, Cleary ML. The t(1;19)(q23;p13) results in consistent fusion of E2A and PBX1 coding sequences in acute lymphoblastic leukemias. Blood. 1991;77(4):687-93.
14. Crist WM, Carroll AJ, Shuster JJ, Behm FG, Whitehead M, Vietti TJ, et al. Poor prognosis of children with pre-B acute lymphoblastic leukemia is associated with the t(1;19)(q23;p13): a Pediatric Oncology Group study. Blood. 1990;76(1):117-22.
15. de Smith AJ, Lavoie G, Walsh KM. Predisposing germline mutations in high hyperdiploid acute lymphoblastic leukemia in children. Genes Chromosomes Cancer. 2019;58(10):723-30.
16. Hochhaus A, Larson RA, Guilhot F, Radich JP, Branford S, Hughes TP, et al. Long-term outcomes of imatinib treatment for chronic myeloid leukemia. N Engl J Med. 2017;376(10):917-27.
17. Kalmanti L, Saussele S, Lauseker M, Müller MC, Dietz CT, Heinrich L, et al. Safety and efficacy of imatinib in CML over a period of 10 years: data from the randomized CML-study IV. Leukemia. 2015;29(5):1123-32.
18. Paulsson K, Lilljebjorn H, Biloglav A, Olsson L, Rissler M, Castor A, et al. The genomic landscape of high hyperdiploid childhood acute lymphoblastic leukemia. Nat Genet. 2015;47(6):672-6.
19. Perez-Andreu V, Roberts KG, Harvey RC, Yang W, Cheng C, Pei D, et al. Inherited GATA3 variants are associated with Ph-like childhood acute lymphoblastic leukemia and risk of relapse. Nat Genet. 2013;45(12):1494-98.
20. Qian M, Xu H, Perez-Andreu V, Roberts KG, Zhang H, Yang W, et al. Novel susceptibility variants at the ERG locus for childhood acute lymphoblastic leukemia in Hispanics. Blood. 2019;133(7):724-9.
21. Qian M, Zhao X, Devidas M, Yang W, Gocho Y, Smith C, et al. Genomewide association study of susceptibility loci for T-cell acute lymphoblastic leukemia in children. J Natl Cancer Inst. 2019;111(12):1350-7.
22. Greaves M. Pre-natal origins of childhood leukemia. Rev Clin Exp Hematol. 2003;7(3):233-45.

23. Greaves MF, Maia AT, Wiemels JL, Ford AM. Leukemia in twins: lessons in natural history. Blood. 2003;102(7):2321-33.
24. Ma Y, Dobbins SE, Sherborne AL, Chubb D, Galbiati M, Cazzaniga G, et al. Developmental timing of mutations revealed by whole-genome sequencing of twins with acute lymphoblastic leukemia. Proc Natl Acad Sci USA. 2013;110(18):7429-33.
25. Bueno C, Tejedor JR, Bashford-Rogers R, González-Silva L, Valdés-Mas R, Agraz-Doblás A, et al. Natural history and cell of origin of TC F3-ZN F384 and PTPN11 mutations in monozygotic twins with concordant BCPALL. Blood. 2019;134(11):900-5.
26. de Smith AJ, Lavoie G, Walsh KM, Aujla S, Evans E, Hansen HM, et al. Predisposing germline mutations in high hyperdiploid acute lymphoblastic leukemia in children. Genes Chromosomes Cancer. 2019;58(10):723-30.
27. Pouliot GP, Degar J, Hinze L, Kochupurakkal B, Vo CD, Burns MA, et al. Fanconi- BRCA pathway mutations in childhood T cell acute lymphoblastic leukemia. PLoS One. 2019;14(11):e0221288.
28. Winer P, Muskens IS, Walsh KM, Vora A, Moorman AV, Wiemels JL, et al. Germline variants in predisposition genes in children with Down syndrome and acute lymphoblastic leukemia. Blood Adv. 2020;4(4):672-5.
29. Wang W, Cortes JE, Tang G, Khoury JD, Wang S, Bueso-Ramos CE, et al. Risk stratification of chromosomal abnormalities in chronic myelogenous leukemia in the era of tyrosine kinase inhibitor therapy. Blood. 2016;127(22):2742-50.
30. Soverini S, Bavaro L, De Benedittis C, Martelli M, Iurlo A, Orofino N, et al. Prospective assessment of NGS-detectable mutations in CML patients with non-optimal response: the NEXT-in-CML study. Blood. 2020;135(8):534-41. Erratum in Blood. 2022;139(10):1601.
31. Fang H, Ketterling RP, Hanson CA, Pardanani A, Kurtin PJ, Chen D, et al. A test utilization approach to the diagnostic workup of isolated eosinophilia in otherwise morphologically unremarkable bone marrow: a single institutional experience. Am J Clin Pathol. 2018;150(5):421-31.
32. Greenberg PL, Tuechler H, Schanz J, Sanz G, Garcia-Manero G, Solé F, et al. Revised international prognostic scoring system for myelodysplastic syndromes. Blood. 2012;120(12):2454-65.
33. Malcovati L, Stevenson K, Papaemmanuil E, Neuberg D, Bejar R, Boultwood J, et al. SF3B1-mutant MDS as a distinct disease subtype: a proposal from the International Working Group for the Prognosis of MDS. Blood. 2020;136(2):157-70.
34. Yoshizato T, Dumitriu B, Hosokawa K, Makishima H, Yoshida K, Townsley D, et al. Somatic mutations and clonal hematopoiesis in aplastic anemia. N Engl J Med. 2015;373(1):35-47.
35. Nazha A, Seastone D, Radivoyevitch T, Przychodzen B, Carraway HE, Patel BJ, et al. Genomic patterns associated with hypoplastic compared to hyperplastic myelodysplastic syndromes. Haematologica. 2015;100(11):e434-7.
36. Fattizzo B, Ireland R, Dunlop A, Yallop D, Kassam S, Large J, et al. Clinical and prognostic significance of small paroxysmal nocturnal hemoglobinuria clones in myelodysplastic syndrome and aplastic anemia. Leukemia. 2021;35(11):3223-31.
37. Estey E, Hasserjian RP, Döhner H. Distinguishing AML from MDS: a fixed blast percentage may no longer be optimal. Blood. 2022;139(3):323-32.
38. DiNardo CD, Garcia-Manero G, Kantarjian HM. Time to blur the blast boundaries. Cancer. 2022;128(8):1568-70.
39. Chen X, Fromm JR, Naresh KN. "Blasts" in myeloid neoplasms – how do we define blasts and how do we incorporate them into diagnostic schema moving forward? Leukemia. 2022;36(2):327-32.

40. Pastor V, Hirabayashi S, Karow A, Wehrle J, Kozyra EJ, Nienhold R, et al. Mutational landscape in children with myelodysplastic syndromes is distinct from adults: specific somatic drivers and novel germline variants. Leukemia. 2017;31(3):759-62.
41. Schwartz JR, Ma J, Lamprecht T, Walsh M, Wang S, Bryant V, et al. The genomic landscape of pediatric myelodysplastic syndromes. Nat Commun. 2017;8(1):1557.
42. Baumann I, Führer M, Behrendt S, Campr V, Csomor J, Furlan I, et al. Morphological differentiation of severe aplastic anaemia from hypocellular refractory cytopenia of childhood: reproducibility of histopathological diagnostic criteria. Histopathology. 2012;61(1):10-7.
43. Sahoo SS, Pastor VB, Goodings C, Voss RK, Kozyra EJ, Szvetnik A, et al. Clinical evolution, genetic landscape and trajectories of clonal hematopoiesis in SAMD9/SAMD9L syndromes. Nat Med. 2021;27(10):1806-17.
44. Sahoo SS, Kozyra EJ, Wlodarski MW. Germline predisposition in myeloid neoplasms: Unique genetic and clinical features of GATA2 deficiency and SAMD9/SAMD9L syndromes. Best Pract Res Clin Haematol. 2020;33(3):101197.
45. Montalban-Bravo G, Kanagal-Shamanna R, Guerra V, Ramos-Perez J, Hammond D, Shilpa P, et al. Clinical outcomes and influence of mutation clonal dominance in oligomonocytic and classical chronic myelomonocytic leukemia. Am J Hematol. 2021;96:E50-E53.
46. Calvo X, Garcia-Gisbert N, Parraga I, Gibert J, Florensa L, Andrade-Campos M, et al. Oligomonocytic and overt chronic myelomonocytic leukemia show similar clinical, genomic, and immunophenotypic features. Blood Adv. 2020;4(20):5285-96.
47. Geyer JT, Tam W, Liu YC, Chen Z, Wang SA, Bueso-Ramos C, et al. Oligomonocytic chronic myelomonocytic leukemia (chronic myelomonocytic leukemia without absolute monocytosis) displays a similar clinicopathologic and mutational profile to classical chronic myelomonocytic leukemia. Mod Pathol. 2017;30(9):1213-22.
48. Patnaik MM, Timm MM, Vallapureddy R, Lasho TL, Ketterling RP, Gangat N, et al. Flow cytometry based monocyte subset analysis accurately distinguishes chronic myelomonocytic leukemia from myeloproliferative neoplasms with associated monocytosis. Blood Cancer J. 2017;7(7):e584.
49. Selimoglu-Buet D, Wagner-Ballon O, Saada V, Bardet V, Itzykson R, Bencheikh L, et al. Characteristic repartition of monocyte subsets as a diagnostic signature of chronic myelomonocytic leukemia. Blood. 2015;125(23):3618-26.
50. Cargo C, Cullen M, Taylor J, Short M, Glover P, Van Hoppe S, et al. The use of targeted sequencing and flow cytometry to identify patients with a clinically significant monocytosis. Blood. 2019;133(12):1325-34.
51. Carr RM, Vorobyev D, Lasho T, Marks DL, Tolosa EJ, Vedder A, et al. RAS mutations drive proliferative chronic myelomonocytic leukemia via a KMT2APLK1 axis. Nat Commun. 2021;12(1):2901.
52. Xicoy B, Triguero A, Such E, García O, Jiménez MJ, Arnán M, et al. The division of myelomonocytic leukemia (CMML)-1 into CMML-0 and CMML-1 according to 2016 World Health Organization (WHO) classification has no impact in outcome in a large series of patients from the Spanish group of MDS. Leuk Res. 2018;70:34-6.
53. Loghavi S, Sui D, Wei P, Garcia-Manero G, Pierce S, Routbort MJ, et al. Validation of the 2017 revision of the WHO chronic myelomonocytic leukemia categories. Blood Adv. 2018;2(15):1807-16.
54. Valent P, Akin C, Gleixner KV, Sperr WR, Reiter A, Arock M, et al. Multidisciplinary challenges in mastocytosis and how to address with personalized medicine approaches. Int J Mol Sci. 2019;20(12):2976.
55. Valent P, Akin C, Hartmann K, Alvarez-Twose I, Brockow K, Hermine O, et al. Updated diagnostic criteria and classification of mast cell disorders: a consensus proposal. Hemasphere. 2021;5(11):e646.

56. Alvarez-Twose I, Jara-Acevedo M, Morgado JM, García-Montero A, Sánchez-Muñoz L, Teodósio C, et al. Clinical, immunophenotypic, and molecular characteristics of well-differentiated systemic mastocytosis. J Allergy Clin Immunol. 2016;137(1):168-78.
57. Schwaab J, Naumann N, Luebke J, Jawhar M, Somervaille TCP, Williams MS, et al. Response to tyrosine kinase inhibitors in myeloid neoplasms associated with PCM1-JAK2, BCR-JAK2 and ETV6-ABL1 fusion genes. Am J Hematol. 2020;95(7):824-33.
58. Tang G, Sydney Sir Philip JK, Weinberg O, Tam W, Sadigh S, Lake JI, et al. Hematopoietic neoplasms with 9p24/JAK2 rearrangement: a multicenter study. Mod Pathol. 2019;32(4):490-8.
59. Yao J, Xu L, Aypar U, Meyerson HJ, Londono D, Gao Q, et al. Myeloid/lymphoid neoplasms with eosinophilia/basophilia and ETV6-ABL1 fusion: cell-of-origin and response to tyrosine kinase inhibition. Haematologica. 2021;106(2):614-8.
60. Carll T, Patel A, Derman B, Hyjek E, Lager A, Wanjari P, et al. Diagnosis and treatment of mixed phenotype (T-myeloid/lymphoid) acute leukemia with novel ETV6-FGFR2 rearrangement. Blood Adv. 2020;4(19):4924-8.
61. Telford N, Alexander S, McGinn OJ, Williams M, Wood KM, Bloor A, et al. Myeloproliferative neoplasm with eosinophilia and T-lymphoblastic lymphoma with ETV6-LYN gene fusion. Blood Cancer J. 2016;6(4):e412.
62. Bhoj EJ, Yu Z, Guan Q, Ahrens-Nicklas R, Cao K, Luo M, et al. Phenotypic predictors and final diagnoses in patients referred for RASopathy testing by targeted next-generation sequencing. Genet Med. 2017;19(6):715-8.

CHAPTER 8

CAR-T Cell in the Treatment of Hematological Malignancies

Karthik Rengaraj, Uday Prakash Kulkarni, Aby Abraham

■ INTRODUCTION

The B and T lymphocytes, parts of the adaptive immune system, recognize foreign antigens through various mechanisms. B-cell receptors are antibodies on the surface of cells that recognize antigens. B cells secrete antibodies and do not interact with the immunologic target directly, unlike T-cell receptors (TCRs), which recognize only specific peptides processed and presented by antigen-presenting cells and bound to the major histocompatibility complex. Chimeric antigen receptor T cells are a manufactured combination of the antigen specificity of antibody-mediated immunity with the lethal cytotoxicity of the effector T cells.

■ ORIGIN OF CAR-T CELL THERAPY

For many years, oncologists have harnessed the body's immune system in the fight against cancer. Allogenic hematopoietic stem cell transplant (HSCT) is considered the earliest form of immunotherapy,[1] along with donor lymphocyte infusions and its potential to induce lasting remission, which has always been the solution for cure.[2] Bispecific T-cell-recruiting antibodies (BiTEs) augment the interaction between the tumor cell and immune effector cells, such as with CD19 and CD3 antibody.[3] These BiTEs have two antibody receptors directed against a tumor antigen and a T-cell-activating receptor leading to a T-cell-mediated kill.

The early CAR construct, called T-body,[4] exchanged the variable regions of the TCR with the antibody **(Fig. 1)** and was developed by Zelig Eshhar and Gideon Gross in 1989–1993 in Israel. However, they were only experimental and not effective.[4] Dr Carl June, David Porter, and Stephan Grupp developed the first clinically effective CAR-T cells[5] initially against chronic lymphocytic leukemia (CLL) in the year 2011[6] and later acute lymphoblastic leukemia (ALL) in 2012.[7]

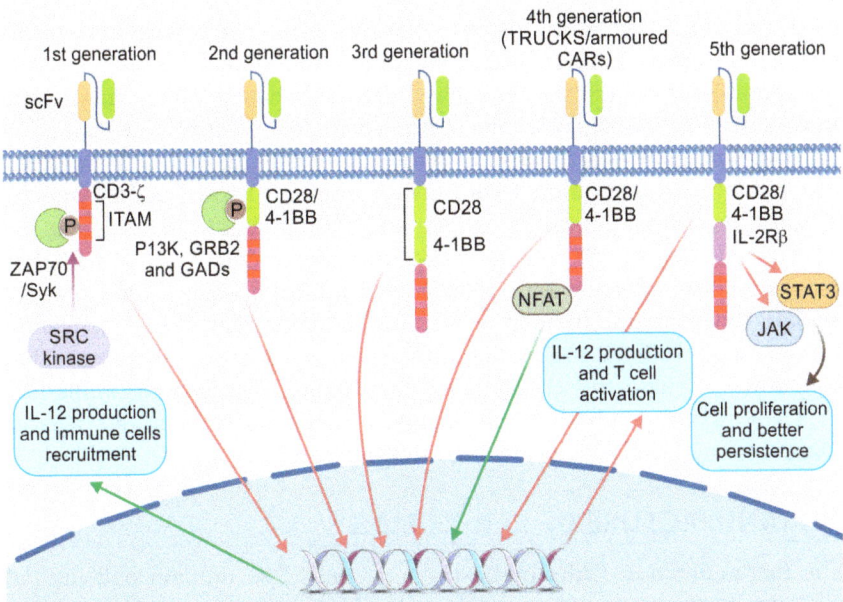

FIG. 1: Cartoon artwork depiction of CAR-T construct.
Source: Reproduced from Lu J, Jiang G. The journey of CAR-T therapy in haematological malignancies. Mol Cancer. 2022;21:194.

■ BIOLOGY OF IMMUNE RECEPTORS AND CARS

Antibodies are 10–15 nm proteins made of two heavy and light chains, represented genetically on different chromosomes. Each antibody has a region that recognizes the antigen with a variable light chain and a variable heavy chain. The three-dimensional structure formed by combining these two domains includes a complementary binding region to the antigen called the fragment variable (Fv) region. The remaining antibody, consisting of one heavy chain and one light chain, makes up the constant region, which, together with the Fv region, forms the fragment antigen binding (Fab) region. The heavy chain domains are linked beyond the hinge region called the fragment crystallizable (Fc) region. When an antigen is bound to the Fv region of the antibody, the Fc region serves as the beacon to recruit innate immune cells and eliminate the antigen. Though antigen recognition is precise and involves direct interactions, antibodies rely on other immune effector cells to elicit an immune response.

T-cell receptors are structurally like antibodies externally but differ intracellularly. The alpha-beta ($\alpha\beta$) T cell, the most crucial T-cell subset, also contains two alpha and beta chains, like heavy and light chains of B-cell receptors, which are similar in size and together form an antigen-binding site except that TCR is bound by a transmembrane region which anchors it to the cell.

Six proteins at the base of a TCR collectively called the CD3 complex—CD3delta (δ), CD3gamma (γ), two CD3epsilon (ε), and two CD3zeta (ζ) chains, comprise the internal machinery of a TCR. Antigen binding to a TCR phosphorylates the tyrosine in each of the CD3 chains. CD3ζ contains the maximum tyrosine kinases; hence, it plays a significant role in mediating downstream pathways leading to activation of the T cell, cell-mediated cytotoxicity, and replication. CD8 T cells, commonly known as the cytotoxic T cells, identify the presented antigen and kill the target cells, whereas the CD4 T cells help the B cells to make antibodies. Along with TCRs, other costimulatory molecules help identify and bind the antigen and transmit signals downstream, thereby preventing inappropriate T-cell activation but making it difficult to identify immune antigens, especially tumors that can down-regulate the costimulatory molecules. Without costimulation, TCR stimulation leads to T-cell anergy, a mechanism to protect against inappropriate T-cell activity and autoimmunity.

■ MANUFACTURE OF CAR-T CELLS

The first-generation CARs harboring only the CD3ζ domain had limited signaling capacity and did not produce durable T-cell responses or sustained cytokine release. Adding costimulatory signaling domains (e.g., CD28 or 4-1BB) led to increased activation, better survival, and successful expansion of the modified T cells.[8] These second-generation constructs as "living drugs" form the basis of the currently approved CAR-T cell therapy.[1] Third-generation CAR-T cells have the added benefit of two costimulatory signals, which are expressed on the modified cells (e.g., CD28 and 4-1BB). The mechanism of fourth-generation CARs, also called TRUCKs (T-cell redirected for universal cytokine-mediated killing), to increase the duration of the activation signal is by additional genes which can secrete specific cytokines (e.g., IL-12). Fifth-generation CARs harbor IL-2 receptors that stimulate downstream signaling via the JAK-/STAT pathway to maintain T-cell persistence **(Fig. 2)**.

The manufacture of CAR-T cells is a multifaceted and meticulous procedure that begins with the apheresis of white blood cells from the patient **(Table 1)**. Density gradients and magnetic separation methods can achieve the isolation of T cells to remove red blood cells and platelets. Closed systems using different mechanisms enable further separation into different T-cell subsets. CAR-T cells are subsequently activated using anti-CD3 antibodies, artificial antigen-presenting cells, or by passing through readily available nano matrix conjugated with CD3/CD28 agonists (TransActä, from Miltenyi Biotec) to ensure in vitro proliferation.

The activated T-cell-enriched product is then transducted with viral vectors carrying the required genes. Lentiviral vectors have a relatively safer genomic integration profile than gamma-retroviral vectors and are hence preferred in CAR T-cell trials.[9] The transposon system is a novel plasmid-based integration system (called sleeping beauty transposon system) that inserts

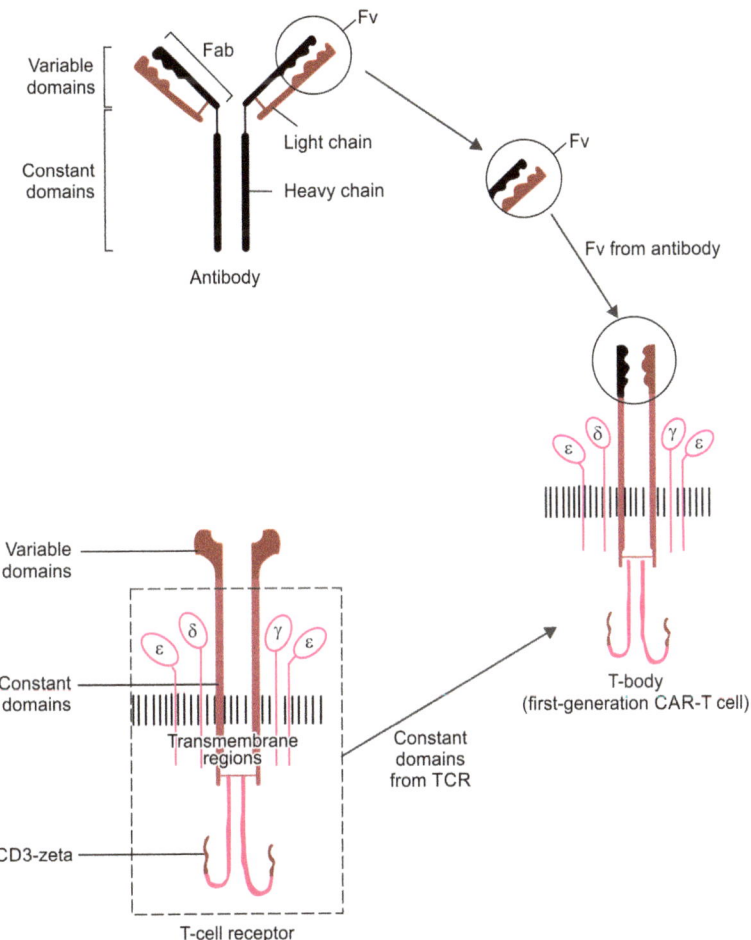

FIG. 2: Cartoon depiction of CAR-T construct.
Source: With permission from http://creativecommons.org/licenses/by/4.0/

anti-CD19 CARs into T cells through electroporation.[10] However, newer gene-transfer methods require caution as previous CAR-T cell lymphomas have been reported using a transposon system for gene transfer.[11]

The T cells are then cultured to produce therapeutic doses of CAR-T cells, which can be either freshly collected (in case of in-house manufacture) or as cryopreserved cells in case of decentralized manufacture of CAR-T cells and are delivered to the treatment center to be thawed and infused to the patient. The final step is the infusion of the CAR-T cells into the patient who has been treated with lymphodepleting chemotherapy (most commonly fludarabine-cyclophosphamide) to promote proliferative advantage to the CAR-modified T cells. Predominant costs of CAR-T cell manufacturing depend on

TABLE 1: CAR-T cell production process.		
Steps	CAR-T cell production	Process
1	Patient leukapheresis	WBC harvested from the donor by apheresis
2	T-cell selection	T cells are selected by magnetic immunobeads
3	T-cell activation	Cytokine cocktail including IL-2, IL-7, and IL-13
4	Transduction of gene	Using lentiviral or nonviral vectors
5	CAR-T expansion	CAR-T cells expansion ex vivo by cell culture to final dose
6	Lymphodepleting chemotherapy	Fludarabine-cytarabine conditioning to reduce T regulatory cells and prevent rejection
7	CAR-T cell infusion	After premedication with antihistaminic, antipyretics
8	Post CAR-T cell	• Watchful for CRS/ICANS • Acyclovir prophylaxis from day +1 till 1 year. Mould prophylaxis with fluconazole in low risk and posaconazole in high risk* from day +1 till unsupported ANC >0.5 for 3 days. Septran prophylaxis after count recovery till 1 year

*High risk of mould prophylaxis-leukemia, post HSCT, neutropenia >14 days, Grade 3/4 CRS/ICANS, HLH/MAS and >3 days of corticosteroids.

(CRS: cytokine release syndrome; HLH: hemophagocytic lymphohistiocytosis; HSCT: hematopoietic stem cell transplant; ICANS: immune effector cell-associated neurotoxicity syndrome; MAS: macrophage activation syndrome; WBC: white blood cell)

transporting the apheresis product for processing and vector transduction in centralized laboratories and exporting the clinical grade CAR-T product back for infusion to the patient. Decentralized production of CAR-T cells using closed systems (like CliniMACS Prodigy) can reduce production costs and improve access to CAR-T cell therapy in developing nations.[12] VELCART, a product of the decentralized manufacture of CAR-T cells at the Christian Medical College, Vellore, has been shown as an example **(Fig. 3)**.

■ DISEASE-SPECIFIC CAR-T THERAPIES (TABLE 2)

Acute Lymphoblastic Leukemia

The initial CAR-T cell product approved by the United States Food and Drug Administration (FDA) was Tisagenlecleucel (Kymriah, Novartis) for relapsed B-cell ALL in August 2017 based on the ELIANA trial.[13] CD19 is the most frequently targeted antigen because of its universal expression in B-cell leukemia and lymphomas. It is highly expressed compared with other potential targets like CD20 or CD22. It is restricted to only the B-cell lineage among normal cells, which may lead to B-cell aplasia as a side effect but can be alleviated by monthly immunoglobulin infusions.[14] The second product that received approval was brexucabtagene autoleucel based on ZUMA-3[15] in adults and ZUMA-4[16] in the pediatric population.

CHAPTER 8: CAR-T Cell in the Treatment of Hematological Malignancies

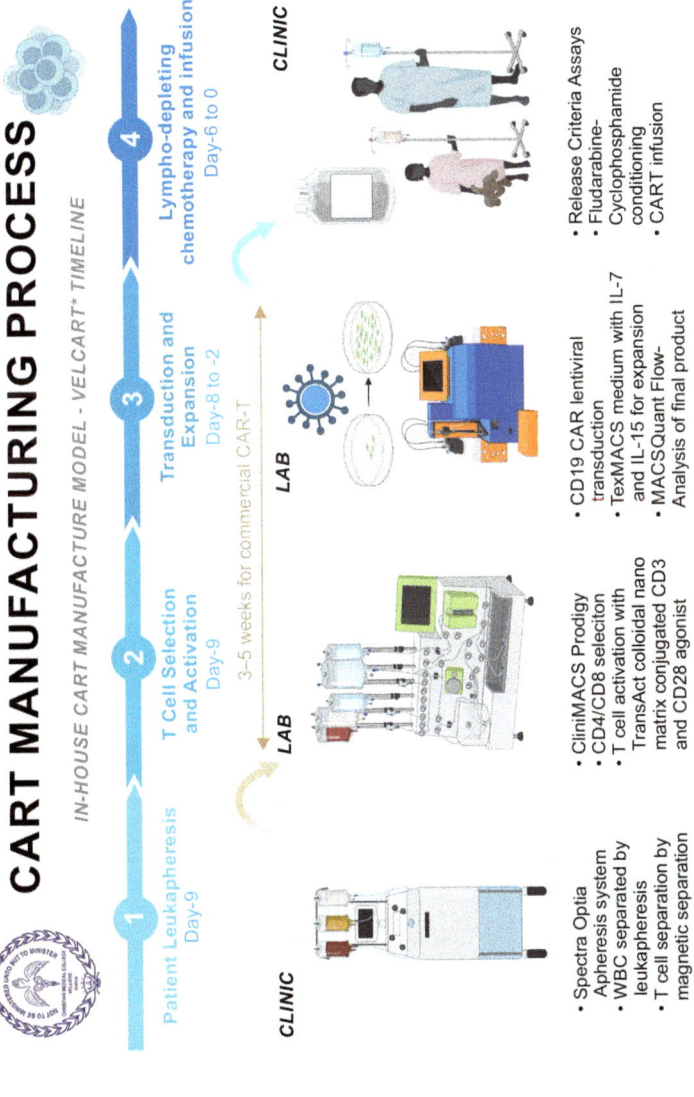

*CAR-T product of Christian Medical College, Vellore, Tamil Nadu, India.
FIG. 3: CAR-T manufacturing process. In-house manufacturing model of VELCART.
Source: Created with BioRender.

TABLE 2: Approved CAR-T cell products and indications.

CAR-T product	Target antigen	Construct	TRIAL approved	Target population	CRS and ICANS rate*	ORR and OS-12m
Tisagenlecleucel (KYMRIAH, Novartis)	CD19	FMC63 Costimulation: 4-1BB Vector: Lentivirus	ELIANA[13]	Children ≤25 years, refractory B-ALL or at second-relapse	CRS 77%, ICANS 40%	ORR at 3m-81%, EFS 50%, OS 76%
			JULIET[19]	Adults with R/R DLBCL as third line therapy	CRS 22%, ICANS 12%	ORR at 12m-52%, RFS at 12m-65%
Axicabtagene ciloleucel (YESCARTA, Gilead-Kite)	CD19	FMC63 Costimulation: CD28 Vector: Retrovirus	ZUMA-1[17]	Adults with R/R DLBCL, PMBCL, or TFL as third-line therapy	CRS 13%, ICANS 28%	ORR 82%, OS at 18m-52%
			ZUMA-7[18]	Adults R/R DLBCL as second line therapy	CRS 6%, ICANS 21%	ORR 83%, OS at 2 years—61%
Lisocabtagene maraleucel (Lisocel, Bristol-Myers Squibb/Celgene Company) (BREYANZI)	CD19	FMC63 Costimulation: 4-1BB/CD zeta Vector: Lentivirus	TRANSCEND NHL 001 trial[22]	Adults with R/R DLBCL as third-line therapy	CRS 1%, ICANS 4%	CR rate—74%, OS at 18m 73%
Brexucabtagene autoleucel (TECARTUS)	CD19	FMC63 Costimulation: CD28/CD3zeta Vector: Lentivirus	ZUMA-2 trial[21]	>18 years relapsed/refractory MCL after five previous therapies; including BTK inhibitor therapy	CRS 15%, ICANS 31%	ORR 85%, 12m PFS 61%, 12m OS 83%
			ZUMA-3[15] and ZUMA-4[16]	ALL in children and adults	CRS 24%, ICANS 25%	CR at 16.4m 71%

Continued

Continued

CART product	Target antigen	Construct	TRIAL approved	Target population	CRS and ICANS rate*	ORR and OS-12m
Idecabtagene Vicleucel (ABECMA)	BCMA	BCMA scFv Co-stimulation: 4-1BB/CD3 zeta Vector: Lentivirus	KarMMa [24]	>18 years, at least 3 previous regimens including IMiDs, a proteasome inhibitor, and an anti-CD38 antibody; or had PD, within 60 days of the last dose	CRS 84%, [5% (grade >3)] ICANS 18%, [3% (grade >3)]	At 13.3m ORR 73%, Median PFS 8.8m
Ciltacabtagene autoleucel (CARVYKTI)	BCMA	BCMA scFv Costimulation: 4-1BB/CD3 zeta Vector: Lentivirus	CARTITUDE [49]	>18 years, at least 3 previous regimens including IMiDs, a proteasome inhibitor, and an anti-CD38 antibody; or had PD, within 12 months of the last dose	CRS 95%, [4% (grade >3)] ICANS 21%, [9% (grade >3)]	ORR 97%, 12m PFS 77%, 12m OS 89%

*CRS grading variable among different trials.

[ALL: acute lymphoblastic leukemia; BTK: bruton tyrosine kinase; DLBCL: diffuse large B-cell lymphoma; IMiDs: immunomodulatory drugs; MCL: mantle cell lymphoma; PMBCL: primary mediastinal B-cell Lymphoma; R/R: relapsed and refractory; scFv: single chain fragment variable (V_H+V_L); TFL: transformed follicular lymphoma]

Non-Hodgkin's Lymphoma

Axicabtagene ciloleucel [Yescarta, Kite (Gilead)], though the second CAR-T-cell product approved, was the first to be approved for patients with diffuse large B-cell lymphoma (DLBCL) in October 2017 for use in relapsed/refractory DLBCL which is refractory to more than two lines of therapy or relapses within 12 months based on ZUMA-1[17] and later approved for second-line based on ZUMA-7 trial.[18] Tisagenlecleucel was approved for use based on the JULIET trial[19] in patients with relapsed and refractory DLBCL who were >18 years of age and refractory to two lines of therapy with rituximab and anthracycline. Phase I trials in India have cost-effectively shown similar efficacy with feasibility in LMIC countries like India.[12,20] Brexucabtagene autoleucel received approval in July 2020 based on the results of the Phase II open-label single-arm multicenter ZUMA-2 trial for the treatment of mantle cell lymphoma which had relapsed or is refractory to five lines of therapy, including a BTKi.[21] Lisocabtagene maraleucel is approved for relapsed refractory B-cell lymphomas as the third-line based on the TRANSFORM trial.[22]

Chronic Lymphocytic Leukemia

Despite CAR-T cells showing efficacy in CLL, there are currently no FDA-approved indications for use in CLL. The efficiency of CAR-T cells in CLL is less compared with the dramatic effects in other B-cell malignancies, probably due to T-cell dysfunction in CLL patients with incomplete immune synapse formation with antigen-presenting.[23] Lenalidomide, an immunomodulatory drug that improves immune synapse formation, is being explored as a potential CAR-T cell adjunct.

Multiple Myeloma

Studies have shown encouraging results for CAR-T cells targeting B-cell maturation antigen (BCMA) in multiple myeloma. Two agents approved for this purpose are idecabtagene vicleucel (ide-cel) based on the KarMMa trial[24] and ciltacabtagene autoleucel (cilta-cel) based on the CARTITUDE trial.[25] Anti-BCMA CAR-T cell therapies did not show a plateau in the survival curve, with most patients experiencing a relapse.[26] Individuals who experience a relapse following BCMA-directed therapies have few treatment alternatives. Newer targets such as G protein-coupled receptor, class C, group 5, member D (GPRC5D)[27] or FCRL5 (fragment crystallizable receptor-like protein 5) are emerging as potential targets in BCMA refractory cases.

Solid Malignancies

Though under development, CAR-T cell therapy for solid malignancies poses various challenges, including translocating to the disease sites, which requires migrating through the endothelium and tissue stroma before infiltrating into tumors. Solid tumors have a more heterogeneous antigen expression, which hinders T-cell homing. CAR-T cells must survive a harsh tumor microenvironment (TME) characterized by hypoxia, oxidative stress, nutrient-deprived state, and acidic pH. The cancer cells express many immunosuppressive cytokines and inhibitory molecules. These molecules coordinate with inhibitory receptors on T cells, attracting regulatory T cells and creating an immune-tolerant environment.[28] Various techniques are being studied to address these challenges with the aim of developing potent CAR-T cells.

CAR-T CELL TOXICITY

CAR-T cell therapy is associated with a different constellation of toxicities compared to conventional chemotherapy and HSCT, which requires early recognition and expertise in management **(Table 3)**. Some grade of toxicity is experienced by over 90% of patients and should be taken into account with factors related to the patient, disease, and CAR-T construct.

Cytokine Release Syndrome

Cytokine release syndrome (CRS) is the most common complication after CAR-T cell therapy. The incidence of CRS in patients treated with tisagenlecleucel is 77% for ALL[13] and 57% for non-Hodgkin's lymphoma (NHL).[19] The incidence of CRS in patients with NHL treated with axicabtagene ciloleucel is 93%.[17] However, CRS grading varies between trials, and the number of patients with more than grade 3 CRS remains less.

Pathophysiology

The mechanism of CRS is caused by the interaction between CAR-T cells and their target. This leads to the activation and expansion of CAR-T cells, as well as the lysis of both normal and tumor cells.[29] When released, cytokines such as IFN-γ and TNF-α activate monocytes and macrophages. The activation of macrophages leads to higher levels of proinflammatory cytokines (including IL-6, IL-1, and IL-10) and other mediators, such as inducible nitric oxide

TABLE 3: CAR-T cell toxicities.	
Early toxicities (0–90 days)	**Late toxicities (>90 days)**
Cytokine release syndrome	Autoimmune disorders
Neurotoxicity (CRES and ICANS)	Graft-versus-host disease
Tumor lysis syndrome	Hypogammaglobulinemia
Cytopenia	Second malignancies
Infections	
(CRES: CAR-T-cell related encephalopathy syndrome; ICANS: immune effector cell-associated neurotoxicity syndrome)	

synthase (iNOS). This results in endothelial activation, recruitment of myeloid cells, and ultimately worsens CRS.[30]

Clinical Presentation

Cytokine release syndrome may occur within 3 weeks after infusion of CAR-T cells. The median onset time is 2 days, with a range of 1–12 days for axicabtagene ciloleucel[17] and 3 days for tisagenlecleucel in ALL patients and up to 9 days in NHL patients.[13,19] Clinical presentations of CRS vary from subtle prodromal syndrome to severe acute respiratory distress syndrome (ARDS) or refractory shock. Fever >38°C is the first and most common sign of CRS. It is possible to experience gastrointestinal symptoms like nausea, diarrhea, and vomiting. Severe CRS can be signaled by mild hypoxia or hypotension, leading to hemodynamic instability and organ dysfunction later. ASTCT CRS grading is the most used and is based on the more severe event of hypoxia or hypotension, which cannot be attributed to any other cause.[31] Fever may not be taken into account for grading once the patient has received treatment with steroids or anticytokine therapy, such as tocilizumab, and grading is predominantly based on hypoxia or hypotension.[31]

Cytokine Release Syndrome Management (Fig. 4)

Patients with early CRS should be closely monitored for signs of infection, and treated symptomatically with antipyretics and empirical antibiotics, especially in neutropenic patients following lymphodepleting chemotherapy.[32]

Tocilizumab, an IL-6 receptor antagonist, is approved for severe CRS, but indications vary by product. It is generally indicated for CRS grade >2. Patients <30 kg are treated with a dose of 12 mg/kg,[33] and those ≥30 kg with 8 mg/kg.[34] In case of no clinical improvement, tocilizumab can be repeated up to 4 times with a minimum interval of 8 hours between doses. In case of no response within 12–24 hours after starting tocilizumab or if CRS worsens, corticosteroids are given and gradually reduced over 3 days.[14] Siltuximab (Janssen) has not been tested as a first-line therapy for CRS. Nevertheless, its capability to bind to soluble IL-6 has been explored in refractory cases. In cases where both tocilizumab and corticosteroids are ineffective, consider alternative treatments such as etanercept (anti-TNFα) or anakinra (IL-1R inhibitor). However, these cases have high mortality rates.

CAR-T Cell-associated Neurotoxicity

The frequency of central nervous system (CNS) toxicity varies greatly, ranging from 0 to 87%. It is more frequently observed in immature B-cell diseases. In 90% of the patients, CNS toxicity occurs concomitantly or after the resolution of CRS, but the remaining 10% of CNS toxicity can arise without any evidence of CRS.

CHAPTER 8: CAR-T Cell in the Treatment of Hematological Malignancies

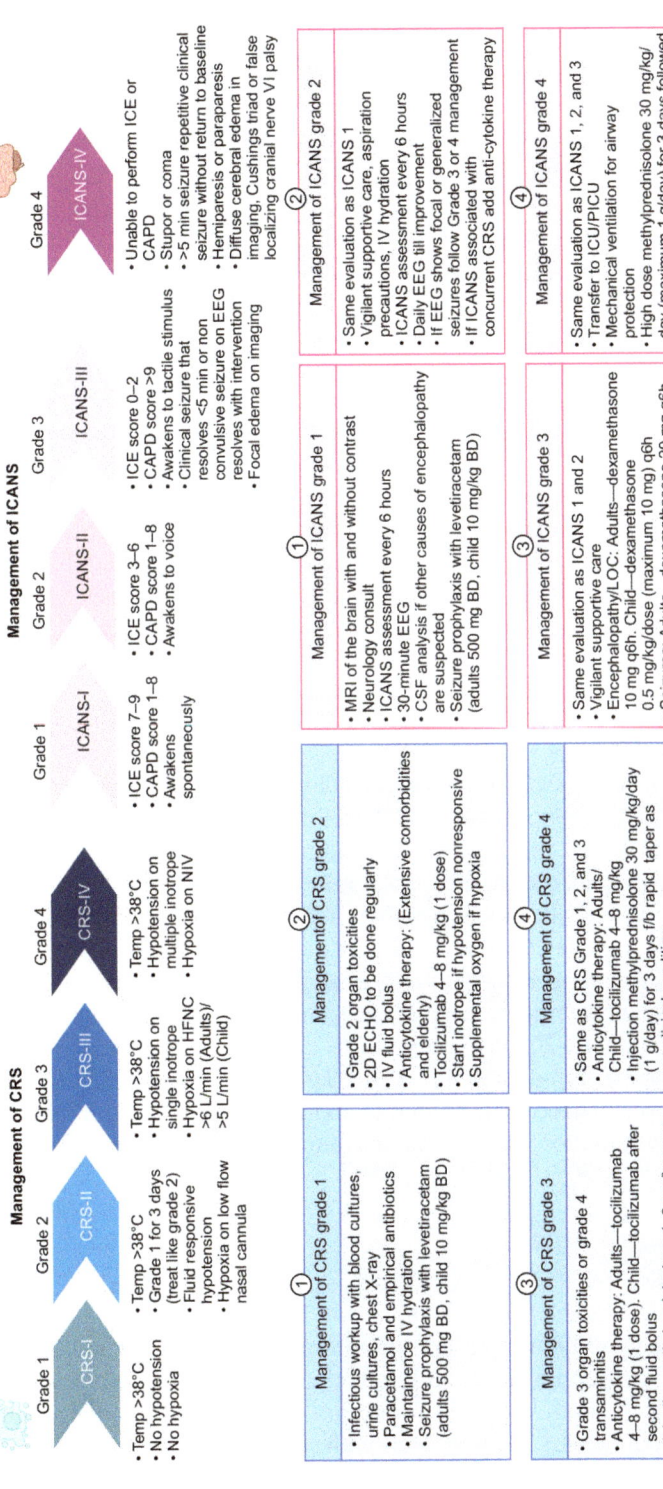

FIG. 4: Management of CRS and ICANS (pocket-card).

(CRS: cytokine release syndrome; ICANS: immune effector cell-associated neurotoxicity syndrome)

Source: Created with BioRender.

Pathophysiology

Initially, it was believed that the neurotoxicity was caused by the CAR-T cell itself. However, current research suggests that the root cause is the malfunctioning of the blood–brain barrier (BBB). The BBB comprises capillary endothelial cells, extracellular matrix (basal lamina), pericytes, microglia, and astrocytes. The dysfunction of the BBB function is linked to TNF-α, IL-6, and IL-1. The balance between ANG1 and ANG2, as well as neurotoxic substances like glutamate and quinolinic acid, which are elevated in severe forms of CAR-T cell neurotoxicity, also contribute to the impairment of the BBB function.

Clinical Presentation

Immune effector cell-associated neurotoxicity syndrome (ICANS) can cause symptoms such as lethargy, cognitive problems, agitation, tremors, aphasia, delirium, encephalopathy, seizures, and cerebral edema seen on radiological examinations.[14] The most commonly used grading system for ICANS is the ASTCT consensus, which takes into account various factors. For adults, the immune effector cell-associated encephalopathy (ICE) score is used, while for children under 12, the Cornell assessment of pediatric delirium (CAPD) score is used. The ICE score can assess the orientation to time, person, and place, simple mathematics, and the ability to name everyday objects.

ICANS Management

Immune effector cell-associated neurotoxicity syndrome grades 1 and 2 are managed with supportive care, baseline evaluation of metabolic parameters, and brain imaging with computed tomography/magnetic resonance imaging and electroencephalogram to look for any subclinical seizure activity. Levetiracetam is usually used as seizure prophylaxis in patients with any grade of CRS/ICANS. Tocilizumab usually does not traverse the BBB; hence, it is used only with concomitant CRS. High-dose steroids are the predominant treatment for grade 3 or more toxicity and are treated with dexamethasone, 10–20 mg every 6 hours, and grade 4 ICANS is treated with high-dose methylprednisolone, 30 mg/kg/day to a maximum of 1 g daily.[14] These patients need to be shifted to an intensive care unit for airway protection with intubation and ventilation and intensive management of seizure activity.

Tumor Lysis Syndrome

Tumor lysis syndrome (TLS) after CAR-T cell therapy is relatively less common, even in patients with high tumor burden and approximately <10%,[35] unlike chemotherapy or immunotherapy. Prophylactic measures for TLS include intravenous fluids and oral allopurinol or febuxostat before lymphodepleting chemotherapy. It is important to monitor and manage the signs and symptoms of TLS in accordance with standard guidelines.

Cytopenia and Infections

Cytopenia of grade ≥3 was the most common adverse effect after axicabtagene ciloleucel[17] and tisagenlecleucel[13,19] and can persist for several weeks following the CAR-T cell infusion. The cause of cytopenia is often multifactorial, involving the conditioning regimen, cytokines released during CRS, macrophage activation syndrome, and prior exposure to multiple chemotherapy treatments. Although neutropenia is common, myeloid growth factors like granulocyte macrophage colony-stimulating factor (GM-CSF) are not advised due to their link with severe neurotoxicity and ICANS development, as shown in Phase II studies.[36] Severe thrombocytopenia is also expected and was observed in 38% of patients treated in the ZUMA-1 trial and 11%[17] in the JULIET trial.[19] The reason for the differences is likely due to the higher dose of cyclophosphamide used in the ZUMA-1 trial. In the ELIANA trial, 41% of patients still had thrombocytopenia by day 28, which was not resolved.[13] It is unsafe to use thrombopoietin agonists due to cytokine toxicity concerns, and they are managed predominantly with transfusion support according to current transfusion guidelines.

Anti-CD19 CAR-T cells also target healthy B cells due to their on-target off-tumor effects. This may not require immediate treatment, but if B-cell aplasia persists or in the setting of life-threatening or recurrent infections, children are given regular immunoglobulin replacement. However, CD19 is absent in mature B cells (plasma cells), and adults who have already encountered many infections, as in developing nations, may retain immunoprotecting antibodies. As CRS and infections are very close differentials, all patients with CRS are treated with empirical antibiotics. According to published literature, around 25% of patients who underwent CD19-targeted CAR-T cell therapy developed an infection within 4 weeks of receiving the infusion. The first infection typically occurred within a median of 6 days from the CAR-T cell infusion.[32]

■ LIMITATIONS AND STRATEGIES

Antigen Escape

CAR-T cell products that target only one antigen may initially be effective, but over time the antigen may be lost, leading to decreased efficacy. This is known as antigen escape.[37] Around 30–70% of patients who experienced disease relapse after treatment showed reduced CD19 expression, while patients treated with BCMA-targeted CAR-T cells also exhibited downregulation or loss of BCMA expression. Potential strategies to overcome this phenomenon of antigen escape is to target multiple antigens with dual CAR constructs or tandem CARs, which is a single CAR construct that has two single chain fragment variables (scFvs) to simultaneously target various target antigens on the tumor.[38,39] Preliminary results using dual-targeted CAR-T cells (CD19/CD22 or CD19/BCMA) have shown promising results.[39,40]

On Target Off-tumor Effects

Antigen selection plays a significant role in CAR design for therapeutic efficacy and limiting "on-target off-tumor" toxicity. A potential strategy to overcome the on-target off-tumor toxicities is to target tumor-restricted post-translational modifications such as truncated "O" glycans in solid tumors. Utilization of direct delivery routes such as local administration is also being explored to eliminate the need to traffic to disease sites. Techniques to improve CAR-T cell trafficking involve stimulating chemokine receptors on the cells with tumor-derived chemokines, for example, integrin $\alpha v\beta 6$-CAR-T cells modified to express CXCR1 or CXCR2 have enhanced trafficking and significantly improved antitumor efficacy.[41]

Immunosuppressive Microenvironment

Poor T-cell expansion and short-term persistence are significant reasons for the lack of or attenuated response. It has been hypothesized that the development of T-cell exhaustion is triggered by coinhibitory pathways. It has been suggested that combining CAR-T cell therapy with checkpoint blockade could be the next step in overcoming immune escape mechanisms in tumors. A combination of PD-1 blockade and CD19 CAR-T cell therapy in heavily pretreated B-ALL resulted in improved persistence of CAR-T cells in a single-center study with potential for possible improvement in current outcomes.[42]

Possible strategies to reduce toxicity from CAR-T include:
- Targeting the higher antigen density on tumor cells by reducing the affinity of the antigen-binding domain results in high activation levels near the tumor and sparing of normal tissue with low antigen levels.
- CAR-T cell cytokine secretion can be modified by adjusting hinge and transmembrane regions of construct. Lower cytokine release and decreased CAR-T cell proliferation were observed with CD19-CAR, which had modified CD8-α hinge and transmembrane sequences.[43]
- Reduction of immunogenicity of the CAR-T construct by using human or humanized antibody fragments instead of murine-derived CARs may be beneficial.[44]
- Preclinical studies show reduced neurotoxicity and CRS rates with increased CAR-T cell activity with inhibition of GM-CSF receptor by lenzilumab[36] or by GM-CSF mutational inactivation.[45]
- Incorporating "off-switches" or suicide genes, which facilitate the selective kill of the engineered cells with the onset of severe toxicity by administering the "antidote". For example, CAR designs that express full-length CD20 or similar receptors facilitate the depletion of CAR-T cells by treatment with anti-CD20 agents like rituximab.[46] Still, as reversal may take longer due to slow kill, faster reversal agents were necessary. More closed switches with inducible CAS9[47] and protease-based small molecule-assisted shutoff CARs (SMASh-CARs), also called switch-off CARS (SWIFF-CARs)[48] cause rapid kill of CAR-T cells within 30 minutes.

Still, the most significant limitation of suicide strategies is the abrupt loss of therapy and potential disease progression, hence reserved as a last resort.

CONCLUSION

With its exciting potential and improved efficacy, CAR-T cell therapy has become the most researched advancement in oncology. The possibility of utility in the relatively frail and unfit, which is usually the case in multiple relapsed and refractory patients after multiple lines of chemotherapy, makes it an attractive option for cure in patients who would otherwise be counseled for palliation is an essential advancement in science.

REFERENCES

1. Subklewe M, von Bergwelt-Baildon M, Humpe A. Chimeric antigen receptor T cells: A race to revolutionize cancer therapy. Transfus Med Hemother. 2019;46(1):15-24.
2. Kolb HJ. Donor leukocyte transfusions for treatment of leukemic relapse after bone marrow transplantation. EBMT Immunology and Chronic Leukemia Working Parties. Vox Sang. 1998;74(Suppl 2):321-9.
3. Riethmuller G. Symmetry breaking: Bispecific antibodies, the beginnings, and 50 years on. Cancer Immun. 2012;12:12.
4. Gross G, Waks T, Eshhar Z. Expression of immunoglobulin-T-cell receptor chimeric molecules as functional receptors with antibody-type specificity. Proc Natl Acad Sci U S A. 1989;86(24):10024-8.
5. Styczyński J. A brief history of CAR-T cells: From laboratory to the bedside. Acta Haematol Polonica. 2020;51:2-5.
6. Porter DL, Levine BL, Kalos M, Bagg A, June CH. Chimeric antigen receptor-modified T cells in chronic lymphoid leukemia. New Engl J Med. 2011;365(8):725-33.
7. Grupp SA, Kalos M, Barrett D, Aplenc R, Porter DL, Rheingold SR, et al. Chimeric antigen receptor-modified T cells for acute lymphoid leukemia. New Engl J Med. 2013;368(16):1509-18.
8. Krause A, Guo HF, Latouche JB, Tan C, Cheung NK, Sadelain M. Antigen-dependent CD28 signaling selectively enhances survival and proliferation in genetically modified activated human primary T lymphocytes. J Exp Med. 1998;188(4):619-26.
9. Vannucci L, Lai M, Chiuppesi F, Ceccherini-Nelli L, Pistello M. Viral vectors: A look back and ahead on gene transfer technology. New Microbiol. 2013;36(1):1-22.
10. Singh H, Huls H, Kebriaei P, Cooper LJ. A new approach to gene therapy using Sleeping Beauty to genetically modify clinical-grade T cells to target CD19. Immunol Rev. 2014;257(1):181-90.
11. Micklethwaite KP, Gowrishankar K, Gloss BS, Li Z, Street JA, Moezzi L, et al. Investigation of product-derived lymphoma following infusion of piggyBac-modified CD19 chimeric antigen receptor T cells. Blood. 2021;138(16):1391-405.
12. Palani HK, Arunachalam AK, Yasar M, Venkatraman A, Kulkarni U, Lionel SA, et al. Decentralized manufacturing of antiCD19 CAR-T cells using CliniMACS Prodigy(R): Real-world experience and cost analysis in India. Bone Marrow Transplant. 2023;58(2):160-7.
13. Maude SL, Laetsch TW, Buechner J, Rives S, Boyer M, Bittencourt H, et al. Tisagenlecleucel in children and young adults with B-cell lymphoblastic leukemia. New Engl J Med. 2018;378(5):439-48.
14. Neelapu SS. Managing the toxicities of CAR T-cell therapy. Hematol Oncol. 2019;37(S1):48-52.

15. Shah BD, Ghobadi A, Oluwole OO, Logan AC, Boissel N, Cassaday RD, et al. KTE-X19 for relapsed or refractory adult B-cell acute lymphoblastic leukaemia: Phase 2 results of the single-arm, open-label, multicentre ZUMA-3 study. Lancet (London, England). 2021;398(10299):491-502.
16. Wayne AS, Huynh V, Hijiya N, Rouce RH, Brown PA, Krueger J, et al. Three-year results from phase I of ZUMA-4: KTE-X19 in pediatric relapsed/refractory acute lymphoblastic leukemia. Haematologica. 2023;108(3):747-60.
17. Neelapu SS, Locke FL, Bartlett NL, Lekakis LJ, Miklos DB, Jacobson CA, et al. Axicabtagene ciloleucel CAR T-cell therapy in refractory large B-cell lymphoma. New Engl J Med. 2017;377(26):2531-44.
18. Locke FL, Miklos DB, Jacobson CA, Perales MA, Kersten MJ, Oluwole OO, et al. Axicabtagene ciloleucel as second-line therapy for large B-cell lymphoma. New Engl J Med. 2022;386(7):640-54.
19. Schuster SJ, Bishop MR, Tam CS, Waller EK, Borchmann P, McGuirk JP, et al. Tisagenlecleucel in adult relapsed or refractory diffuse large B-cell lymphoma. New Engl J Med. 2019;380(1):45-56.
20. Jain H, Karulkar A, Sharma N, Sengar M, Jaiswal A, Shah S, et al. Phase I trial of humanized CD19 CART-cell therapy developed in India: Safe, active and feasible for outpatient therapy. Blood. 2022;140(Supplement 1):10332-4.
21. Wang M, Munoz J, Goy A, Locke FL, Jacobson CA, Hill BT, et al. KTE-X19 CAR T-cell therapy in relapsed or refractory mantle-cell lymphoma. New Engl J Med. 2020;382(14):1331-42.
22. Abramson JS, Solomon SR, Arnason J, Johnston PB, Glass B, Bachanova V, et al. Lisocabtagene maraleucel as second-line therapy for large B-cell lymphoma: Primary analysis of the phase 3 TRANSFORM study. Blood. 2023;141(14):1675-84.
23. Todorovic Z, Todorovic D, Markovic V, Ladjevac N, Zdravkovic N, Djurdjevic P, et al. CAR T cell therapy for chronic lymphocytic leukemia: Successes and shortcomings. Curr Oncol. 2022;29(5):3647-57.
24. Munshi NC, Anderson LD, Jr., Shah N, Madduri D, Berdeja J, Lonial S, et al. Idecabtagene vicleucel in relapsed and refractory multiple myeloma. New Engl J Med. 2021;384(8):705-16.
25. Martin T, Usmani SZ, Berdeja JG, Agha M, Cohen AD, Hari P, et al. Ciltacabtagene autoleucel, an anti-B-cell maturation antigen chimeric antigen receptor T-cell therapy, for relapsed/refractory multiple myeloma: CARTITUDE-1 2-year follow-Up. J Clin Oncol. 2023;41(6):1265-74.
26. Mailankody S, Landgren O. T-cell engagers - Modern immune-based therapies for multiple myeloma. New Engl J Med. 2022;387(6):558-61.
27. Mailankody S, Devlin SM, Landa J, Nath K, Diamonte C, Carstens EJ, et al. GPRC5D-targeted CAR T cells for myeloma. New Engl J Med. 2022;387(13):1196-206.
28. Milone MC, Xu J, Chen SJ, Collins MA, Zhou J, Powell DJ, Jr., Melenhorst JJ. Engineering enhanced CAR T-cells for improved cancer therapy. Nat Cancer. 2021;2(8):780-93.
29. Yanez L, Sanchez-Escamilla M, Perales MA. CAR T cell toxicity: Current management and future directions. Hemasphere. 2019;3(2):e186.
30. Hay KA, Hanafi LA, Li D, Gust J, Liles WC, Wurfel MM, et al. Kinetics and biomarkers of severe cytokine release syndrome after CD19 chimeric antigen receptor-modified T-cell therapy. Blood. 2017;130(21):2295-306.
31. Lee DW, Santomasso BD, Locke FL, Ghobadi A, Turtle CJ, Brudno JN, et al. ASTCT consensus grading for cytokine release syndrome and neurologic toxicity associated with immune effector cells. Biol Blood Marrow Transplant. 2019;25(4):625-38.
32. Hill JA, Li D, Hay KA, Green ML, Cherian S, Chen X, et al. Infectious complications of CD19-targeted chimeric antigen receptor-modified T-cell immunotherapy. Blood. 2018;131(1):121-30.

33. Mahadeo KM, Khazal SJ, Abdel-Azim H, Fitzgerald JC, Taraseviciute A, Bollard CM, et al. Management guidelines for paediatric patients receiving chimeric antigen receptor T cell therapy. Nat Rev Clin Oncol. 2019;16(1):45-63.
34. ACTEMRA® (tocilizumab) prescribing information. FDA. 2017. [Online]. Available from: https://www.accessdata.fda.gov/drugsatfda_docs/label/2017/125276s114lbl.pdf
35. Howard SC, Trifilio S, Gregory TK, Baxter N, McBride A. Tumor lysis syndrome in the era of novel and targeted agents in patients with hematologic malignancies: A systematic review. Ann Hematol. 2016;95(4):563-73.
36. Sterner RM, Sakemura R, Cox MJ, Yang N, Khadka RH, Forsman CL, et al. GM-CSF inhibition reduces cytokine release syndrome and neuroinflammation but enhances CAR-T cell function in xenografts. Blood. 2019;133(7):697-709.
37. Majzner RG, Mackall CL. Tumor antigen escape from CAR T-cell therapy. Cancer Discov. 2018;8(10):1219-26.
38. Dai H, Wu Z, Jia H, Tong C, Guo Y, Ti D, et al. Bispecific CAR-T cells targeting both CD19 and CD22 for therapy of adults with relapsed or refractory B cell acute lymphoblastic leukemia. J Hematol Oncol. 2020;13(1):30.
39. Spiegel JY, Patel S, Muffly L, Hossain NM, Oak J, Baird JH, et al. CAR T cells with dual targeting of CD19 and CD22 in adult patients with recurrent or refractory B cell malignancies: A phase 1 trial. Nat Med. 2021;27(8):1419-31.
40. Zhang H, Gao L, Liu L, Wang J, Wang S, Gao L, et al. A Bcma and CD19 bispecific CAR-T for relapsed and refractory multiple myeloma. Blood. 2019;134(Supplement_1):3147.
41. Whilding LM, Halim L, Draper B, Parente-Pereira AC, Zabinski T, Davies DM, Maher J. CAR T-cells targeting the integrin alphavbeta6 and co-expressing the chemokine receptor CXCR2 demonstrate enhanced homing and efficacy against several solid malignancies. Cancers (Basel). 2019;11(5):674.
42. Li AM, Hucks GE, Dinofia AM, Seif AE, Teachey DT, Baniewicz D, et al. Checkpoint Inhibitors augment CD19-directed chimeric antigen receptor (CAR) T cell therapy in relapsed B-cell acute lymphoblastic leukemia. Blood. 2018;132(Supplement 1):556.
43. Ying Z, Huang XF, Xiang X, Liu Y, Kang X, Song Y, et al. A safe and potent anti-CD19 CAR T cell therapy. Nat Med. 2019;25(6):947-53.
44. Sommermeyer D, Hill T, Shamah SM, Salter AI, Chen Y, Mohler KM, Riddell SR. Fully human CD19-specific chimeric antigen receptors for T-cell therapy. Leukemia. 2017;31(10):2191-9.
45. Sterner RM, Cox MJ, Sakemura R, Kenderian SS. Using CRISPR/Cas9 to knock out GM-CSF in CAR-T cells. J Vis Exp. 2019(149).
46. Philip B, Kokalaki E, Mekkaoui L, Thomas S, Straathof K, Flutter B, et al. A highly compact epitope-based marker/suicide gene for easier and safer T-cell therapy. Blood. 2014;124(8):1277-87.
47. Di Stasi A, Tey SK, Dotti G, Fujita Y, Kennedy-Nasser A, Martinez C, et al. Inducible apoptosis as a safety switch for adoptive cell therapy. New Engl J Med. 2011;365(18):1673-83.
48. Juillerat A, Tkach D, Busser BW, Temburni S, Valton J, Duclert A, et al. Modulation of chimeric antigen receptor surface expression by a small molecule switch. BMC Biotechnol. 2019;19(1):44.
49. Berdeja JG, Madduri D, Usmani SZ, Jakubowiak A, Agha M, Cohen AD, et al. Ciltacabtagene autoleucel, a B-cell maturation antigen-directed chimeric antigen receptor T-cell therapy in patients with relapsed or refractory multiple myeloma (CARTITUDE-1): A phase 1b/2 open-label study. Lancet (London, England). 2021;398(10297):314-24.

CHAPTER 9

Role of MicroRNA in the Pathogenesis of Plasma Cell Dyscrasias

Manveen Kaur, Anshu Palta

■ INTRODUCTION

Plasma cell dyscrasias encompass a diverse range of disorders marked by the generation of a monoclonal "M" protein by clonal plasma cells, potentially accompanied by organ manifestations or occurring independently.[1] Multiple myeloma (MM) represents one extreme within the spectrum of plasma cell dyscrasias, emerging from the malignant conversion of clonal plasma cells postgerminal center (GC), and displaying clinical characteristics associated with dysfunction in end organs. As the second most prevalent hematological malignancy, it contributes to around 10% of all hematological malignancies.[2] The opposite end of the spectrum is marked by an asymptomatic clonal expansion of plasma cells, referred to as monoclonal gammopathy of undetermined significance (MGUS). While MGUS is recognized as a premalignant phase, it is detected in around 3% of the general population aged 50 years and above.[3,4]

Monoclonal gammopathy of undetermined significance (MGUS) has the potential to advance into MM or other conditions like Waldenström's macroglobulinemia, primary amyloid light chain (AL) amyloidosis, or a lymphoproliferative disorder.[5] The majority of MM cases originates from the MGUS stage, and the progression rate from MGUS to MM or related disorders is approximately 1% annually. An intermediary phase known as smoldering MM (SMM) exists between MM and MGUS, observed in a subset of MM patients and clinically discernible with greater efficiency than MGUS. Extramedullary multiple myeloma *(EMM)* generally represents a more aggressive tumor, occasionally linked with secondary or primary plasma cell leukemia (PCL). These conditions arise when malignant cells lose their reliance on the bone marrow (BM). PCL is identified by the presence of ≥5% circulating plasma cells in the peripheral blood.[6,7] More recently, a distinct entity termed monoclonal gammopathy of clinical significance has been delineated, marked by involvement of a single organ.[8]

Historically, MM was considered to be a disease of the elderly, but recent studies have shown a progressive decline in the age group of patients affected by MM. The clinical manifestations of MM are attributable to the disease-induced damage to end organs, presenting as hypercalcemia, renal dysfunction, anemia, and lytic bone lesions. Confirming the diagnosis of MM necessitates a BM examination. Despite notable progress in the clinical management of MM, leading to enhanced survival and improved quality of life for patients, the condition remains classified as incurable. Further understanding of the pathogenesis of MM holds the potential to unveil additional treatment avenues for this challenging malignancy.

■ DIAGNOSTIC CRITERIA FOR PLASMA CELL DYSCRASIAS

Plasma cell dyscrasias involve the abnormal proliferation of monoclonal plasma cells, accompanied by the production of monoclonal immunoglobulins (Igs) or Ig fragments. These serve as tumor markers, detectable in the serum, urine, or both. Diagnosing and categorizing plasma cell dyscrasias hinge on the convergence of clinical, biochemical, radiological, and BM evidence. The most recent WHO classification for hematolymphoid tumors has established precise criteria for diagnosing various plasma cell dyscrasias. In 2022, the International Consensus Classification of Mature Lymphoid Neoplasms introduced subtle alterations in terminology and refined diagnostic criteria **(Table 1)**.[9,10]

■ PATHOGENESIS OF PLASMA CELL DYSCRASIAS

Origin of Plasma Cell Dyscrasias

The cellular origin of plasma cell dyscrasias is the post-GC B cell. Pre-GC B cells have the capacity to generate short-lived plasma cells residing in lymphoid tissues. Conversely, long-lived plasma cells emerge in the BM from plasmablasts, characterized by acquired somatic hypermutation of the Ig heavy chains and IgH switch recombination.[11,12] The progression from asymptomatic stage of MGUS to SMM to finally symptomatic MM/PCL occurs through the acquisition of various cytogenetic abnormalities, which begins by antigenic stimulation of plasma cells. The immunophenotype of plasma cells in MGUS, SMM, and MM diverges from that of normal BM plasma cells in the expression of CD38, CD138, CD19, CD45, and CD56. Unlike normal BM plasma cells, which strongly express CD38, CD138, CD19, and CD45 while being CD56 negative, abnormal plasma cells in these conditions typically exhibit reduced or dim expression of CD19 and CD45. They retain strong expression of CD38 and CD138 and show a bright expression of CD56 **(Fig. 1)**.[13,14]

TABLE 1: Classification and diagnostic criteria of plasma cell dyscrasias.

Disorder	Diagnostic criteria
• Non-IgM monoclonal gammopathy of undetermined significance (MGUS) • IgM MGUS—plasma cell type	a. Serum non-IgM type monoclonal protein <3 g/dL (<30 g/L) b. Clonal bone marrow plasma cells <10% c. Absence of end-organ damage (CRAB) such as hypercalcemia, renal insufficiency, anemia, and bone lesions (a + b + c)
Light chain MGUS	a. Abnormal free light chain (FLC) ratio (<0.26 or >1.65) b. Increased level of the appropriate involved light chain (increased kappa FLC in patients with ratio >1.65 and increased lambda FLC in patients ratio <0.26) c. No immunoglobulin heavy chain expression on immunofixation d. Absence of end-organ damage that can be attributed to the plasma cell proliferative disorder e. Clonal bone marrow plasma cells <10% f. Urinary monoclonal protein <500 mg/24 h (a + b + c + d + e)

Plasma cell myeloma/ multiple myeloma	a. Clonal bone marrow plasma cells ≥10% OR biopsy-proven plasmacytoma (bony or extramedullary)
	b. Any one or more of the following myeloma defining events:
	  ○ Evidence of end-organ damage that can be attributed to the underlying plasma cell disorder, specifically:
	    – Hypercalcemia: Serum calcium >0.25 mmol/L (>1 mg/dL) higher than the upper limit of normal or >2.75 mmol/L (>11 mg/dL)
	    – Renal insufficiency: Creatinine clearance <40 mL/min or serum creatinine >177 µmol/L (>2 mg/dL)
	    – Anemia: Hemoglobin value of >2 g/dL below the lower limit of normal, or a hemoglobin value <10 g/dL
	    – Bone lesions: One or more osteolytic lesions on skeletal radiography, computed tomography (CT), or positron emission tomography computed tomography (PET-CT)
	  ○ Clonal bone marrow plasma cell percentage ≥60%
	  ○ Involved: Uninvolved serum FLC ratio ≥100 (involved free light chain level must be ≥100 mg/L)
	  ○ >1 focal lesions on magnetic resonance imaging (MRI) studies (at least 5 mm in size)
	
	(a+ any one or more of b features)

Continued

Continued

Disorder	Diagnostic criteria
Plasma cell leukemia	a. All criteria required for the diagnosis of multiple myeloma b. ≥5% plasma cells counted on differential leucocyte count on peripheral blood film (PBF) **a + b**
Solitary plasmacytoma (osseous or extraosseous)	a. Biopsy-proven solitary lesion of bone or soft tissue with evidence of clonal plasma cells b. Normal bone marrow with no evidence of clonal plasma cells or with minimal marrow involvement (<10% clonal plasma cells) c. Normal skeletal survey and MRI (or CT) of spine and pelvis (except for the primary solitary lesion) d. Absence of end-organ damage such as hypercalcemia, renal insufficiency, anemia, or bone lesions (CRAB) that can be attributed to a lympho-plasma cell proliferative disorder **a + b + c + d**
Plasma cell neoplasms associated with paraneoplastic syndrome	
POEMS syndrome	Polyneuropathy, organomegaly, endocrinopathy, monoclonalgammapathy, skin changes
TEMPI syndrome	Telangiectasia, elevated erythropoietin and erythrocytosis, monoclonal gammopathy, perinephric fluid collection, and intrapulmonary shunting
AESOP syndrome	Adenopathy and extensive skin patch overlying plasmacytoma

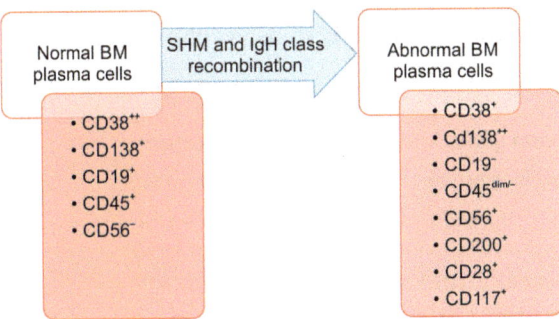

FIG. 1: Comparison of immunophenotype of PCs in plasma cell dyscrasias with normal BM PCs.
(BM: bone marrow; PC: plasma cell)

Cytogenetic Abnormalities in Plasma Cell Dyscrasias

Cytogenetic irregularities are prevalent in plasma cell dyscrasias, encompassing both numerical and structural anomalies such as deletions, translocations, trisomies, and complex chromosomal abnormalities. These abnormalities are detectable in approximately one-third of plasma cell dyscrasia cases through karyotyping and in over 90% of cases using fluorescence in situ hybridization (FISH). Cytogenetic analysis classifies plasma cell dyscrasias into two main groups: (i) the hyperdiploid group and (ii) the nonhyperdiploid group. Hyperdiploidy involves gains in three or more of the odd-numbered chromosomes 3, 5, 7, 9, 11, 15, 19, and 21. The most frequently observed chromosomal abnormalities entail translocations that affect the IgH locus on chromosome 14q32, with a majority of these translocations linked to a nonhyperdiploid status. Hyperdiploidy and IgH translocations are generally regarded as nearly mutually exclusive cytogenetic occurrences. IgH translocations become more prevalent, ranging from 55 to 70% of cases, as the disease progresses from MGUS to SMM to MM. Over 85% of PCL cases exhibit abnormalities in the *IgH* gene. IgL translocations are found in approximately 10% of MGUS/SMM tumors and 15-20% of MM cases. Translocations involving an IgK locus are rare, occurring in only 1-2% of MM. The common outcome of most IgH abnormalities is the overexpression of cyclin D, considered a pivotal event in the development of MGUS and MM.[15-19] Seven partner genes are important in IgH translocations in plasma cell dyscrasias as shown in **Box 1**.

Late/secondary events involved in progression of disease from MGUS to MM involve monosomy 13 or partial deletion of chromosome 13q14, rearrangements of *MYC* gene and activating mutations of *BRAF*, *KRAS*, and *NRAS* genes.[20] Mutations resulting in activation of the NFκB pathway and TP53 mutations, with or without del17p have also been implicated. Other late cytogenetic alterations include loss of chromosome 1p, gain of chromosome 1q, and secondary Ig translocations (**Fig. 2**).[7,20]

BOX 1 | **Partner genes involved in IgH translocations.**

- *CYCLIN D1* on chromosome 11q13 resulting in t(11;14)(q13;q32)
- *CYCLIN D2* on chromosome 12p13 resulting in t(12;14)(p13;q32)
- *CYCLIN D3* on chromosome 6p25 resulting in t(6;14)(p25;q32)
- *MAF* on chromosome 16q23; resulting in t(14;16)(q32;q23)
- *MAFB* on chromosome 20q11 resulting in t(14;20)(q32;q11)
- *MAFA* on chromosome 8q24 resulting in t(8;14)(q24;q32)
- *NSD2* or *MMSET* on chromosome 4p16 resulting in t(4;14) (p16;q32)

CHAPTER 9: Role of MicroRNA in the Pathogenesis of Plasma Cell Dyscrasias

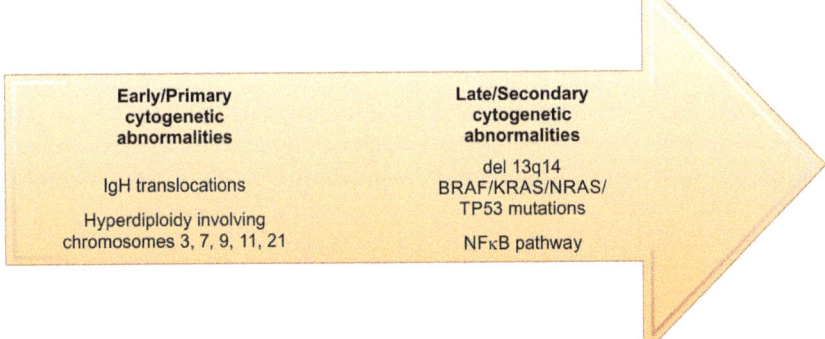

FIG. 2: Cytogenetic abnormalities in plasma cell dyscrasias.

What Drives the Proliferation of Plasma Cells in Bone Marrow?

The Role of Bone Marrow Microenvironment

Beyond the impact of cytogenetic abnormalities on the onset and advancement of plasma cell dyscrasias, the sustained proliferation of long-lived plasma cells, leading to the formation of MGUS and MM cells, is contingent on the BM microenvironment. The BM microenvironment comprises both cells and the extracellular matrix (ECM). Various components, such as BM stromal cells, fibroblasts, mesenchymal stem cells, osteoclasts, osteoblasts, vascular endothelial cells, and immune cells (including T-lymphocytes, dendritic cells, macrophages, and NK cells), actively facilitate the proliferation of plasma cells.[12,21] In addition, interactions between various adhesion molecules, cytokines, and their receptors are also involved in progression of the disease. Cytokines such as IL-6, CXCL12, IGF-1, vascular endothelial growth factor-A (VEGF-A), TNF-α, and TGF-β intervene the migration, proliferation, and survival of the PCs. Some of these act as antiapoptotic and chemotactic factors while others are involved in the proliferation of PCs via a positive feedback mechanism.[22]

The pathogenesis of MM and its associated clinical manifestations involve a delicate crosstalk between the clonal plasma cells and BM osteoclasts. While increased osteoclastic activity is associated with the development of osteopenia and lytic bone lesions in MM, MM cells are also known to promote the differentiation and activity of BM osteoclasts. Clonal PCs in the BM are also linked to an increase in the angiogenic factors such as VEGF, hepatocyte growth factor (HGF), and basic fibroblast growth factor (b-FGF). This increased angiogenesis is important for the progression of disease.[22,23]

■ EPIGENETIC ABNORMALITIES IN PLASMA CELL DYSCRASIAS

The progression of MM is attributed to a diverse set of secondary genetic abnormalities, yet none of these alterations singularly suffice to propel the disease forward. Recently, numerous epigenetic abnormalities have come to light in MM patients, potentially contributing to tumor heterogeneity. Consequently, these abnormalities may play a role not only in the onset of the disease but also in its progression and resistance to therapy.

Epigenetics can be defined as heritable changes in chromatin and DNA that alter genetic expression without any alteration of the DNA sequence.[24] Epigenetic abnormalities have been identified as primary event in pathogenesis of many cancers. Three main forms of epigenetic modifications include modifications of DNA (DNA methylation), modifications of DNA-binding proteins (histone modifications) and noncoding RNA [microRNA (miRNA)] expression.[15,24,25] Under typical conditions, epigenetic modifications, encompassing DNA methylation and post-translational histone modifications, are pivotal for maintaining proper chromatin structure and facilitating transcriptional regulation.

The most thoroughly investigated epigenetic mechanism is DNA methylation, which involves the addition of a methyl group at the 5' carbon of cytosine in DNA.[17-24] This modification primarily occurs at CpG islands and is facilitated by enzymes called DNA methyltransferases (DNMT). CpG islands are the sites at the 5' ends of DNA which are rich in cytosine–phosphate–guanine (CpG) dinucleotides. Around 60–80% of CpGs (out of a total of approximately 28 million CpGs) in the human genome undergo methylation. DNA methylation is accountable for functionally silencing genes by methylating cytosine residues situated in regulatory regions. In MM, abnormal DNA methylation manifests as genome-wide DNA hypomethylation and locus-specific hypermethylation, resulting in the diminished expression of tumor suppressor genes and certain tumor suppressor miRNAs.[26,27]

Histones are proteins crucial for packaging DNA into nucleosomes, forming chromatin, and further condensing into chromosomes. They play a pivotal role in gene expression regulation through their interaction with DNA, influenced by post-translational modifications on the N-terminal tails of histone proteins. These modifications encompass methylation, acetylation, phosphorylation, ubiquitination, sumoylation, and deamination. Anomalies in histone modification patterns are evident in various malignancies. In MM, a noteworthy and intriguing histone-modifying enzyme abnormality involves the upregulation of MMSET, leading to the epigenetic modification of certain miRNAs and consequent overexpression of the MYC proto-oncogene.[28,29]

■ MICRORNA IN HEALTH AND DISEASE

MicroRNAs constitute a category of small (19–25 nucleotides), noncoding RNAs that modulate mRNA expression by influencing transcription and translation.[26,28] Over 6,000 distinct miRNAs have been identified in humans, playing a crucial role in both normal physiology and the pathogenesis of various inflammatory conditions and malignancies.[24] Given that the number of protein-coding genes is nearly three times greater than the number of miRNAs, it is evident that each miRNA has the capacity to regulate the expression of multiple protein-coding genes.

The production of miRNA initiates with the transcription of the miRNA sequence by the RNA polymerase II enzyme, generating a precursor miRNA termed primary miRNA or pri-miRNA. These pri-miRNAs are then processed into smaller fragments called pre-miRNA and subsequently into mature single-stranded miRNA with the assistance of the enzyme Dicer. miRNAs combine with a multiprotein complex, forming the RNA-induced silencing complex (RISC). This complex leads to the post-transcriptional suppression of mRNA from protein-coding genes by binding to their 3'-untranslated region (UTR).[30,31]

The location of *miRNA* genes at the fragile sites of chromosomes makes them susceptible to a variety of genetic alterations such as deletions, amplifications, and translocations. Furthermore, disruptions in miRNA expression have been attributed to epigenetic modifications encompassing both DNA methylation and histone modifications. The initial indication of the involvement of miRNA in cancer pathogenesis was identified in chronic lymphocytic leukemia (CLL) by Calin et al. Their study demonstrated significantly reduced expression of two miRNAs, miR-15a and miR-16, in CLL.[32]

Many studies have documented role of miRNA in the initiation as well as progression and metastases of cancer. miRNAs can be classified as either tumor suppressive or oncogenic, depending on whether they target tumor suppressor genes or oncogenes. The latter, also known as oncomirs, are miRNAs that are amplified or overexpressed in cancers, while the tumor suppressor miRNAs are generally under expressed or downregulated.[15,33] Apart from their role in the pathogenesis, miRNAs have also been found to be helpful in the establishing the diagnosis and prognosis of certain malignancies. Their role as potential therapeutic targets, particularly in cancers refractory to the standard treatment, cannot be overemphasised. Moreover, identifying circulating miRNAs in the form of exosomes or extracellular vesicles may act as biomarkers for the early detection of cancer, potentially before it manifests clinically.[15,34]

■ ROLE OF MICRORNA IN PATHOGENESIS OF PLASMA CELL DYSCRASIAS

In the past two decades, there has been a growing recognition of the involvement of numerous miRNAs in the biology of plasma cell dyscrasias. The first ever evidence was provided by Masri and his colleagues in 2005, who demonstrated that the human myeloma cell lines and MM cells exhibited a miRNA profile distinct from that of the normal plasma cells.[35] In plasma cell dyscrasias, miRNAs may act both as tumor suppressor genes and as oncogenes. Monoclonal gammopathy of undetermined significance and MM plasma cells have also been shown to have differential miRNA expression, thus, pointing toward a role of miRNA in disease progression. The tumor-promoting effects of miRNAs are exerted by their role in modulation of BM microenvironment, proliferation of malignant clone, and angiogenesis.[26,36]

In the following discussion, we shall look at the differential miRNA expression profile of normal plasma cells versus abnormal plasma cells, and that of MGUS and MM. The upcoming section will concentrate on the potential mechanisms through which miRNAs experience dysregulation in plasma cell dyscrasias and the ways in which they contribute to the genesis of myeloma.

Pattern of MicroRNA Expression in Normal B-cell Maturation and Plasma Cells

The standard progression of B-cell maturation involves the transformation of naïve B cells into GC cells, which then mature into memory B cells and subsequently develop into antibody-producing mature plasma cells. Numerous miRNAs are theorized to play a role in the normal development of B cells. Different miRNAS may target transcription factors that control the B-cell maturation at various stages. miR-181a and b, miR-142, and miR-17~92 cluster play an essential role in the early B-cell development.[37-40] In their investigation into the expression of miRNAs in diffuse large B-cell lymphomas, Jima et al. illustrated that the small RNA transcriptome of the malignant B cells markedly differed from that of the normal B cells.[41] The miRNA expression could also identify the subgroups of DLBCL; activated B-cell (ABC) type versus germinal center (GCB) type similar to the gene expression profiling.

During the transition from GC cells to mature plasma cells, a differential expression of at least 33 different types of miRNAs has been found, most of which are overexpressed in GC cells and underexpressed in the plasma cells. Among these, notably significant ones comprise miR-9, miR-30b, and miR-30d, which diminish the expression of the Blimp1 protein by binding to the 3'-untranslated region of the *PRDM1* gene. The Blimp-1 protein is essential for the differentiation of plasma cells. Consequently, the downregulation of miR-9, miR-30b, and miR-30d facilitates the expression of Blimp-1, enabling the differentiation of mature B cells into plasma cells **(Fig. 3)**.[42,43]

MicroRNA Dysregulation in Plasma Cell Dyscrasias (MGUS and MM)

Numerous studies conducted in recent years underscore the significant role of miRNA, not only in the onset of plasma cell dyscrasias but also in the proliferation of malignant plasma cells. Consequently, miRNAs contribute to the progression of the disease from the asymptomatic MGUS stage to

CHAPTER 9: Role of MicroRNA in the Pathogenesis of Plasma Cell Dyscrasias

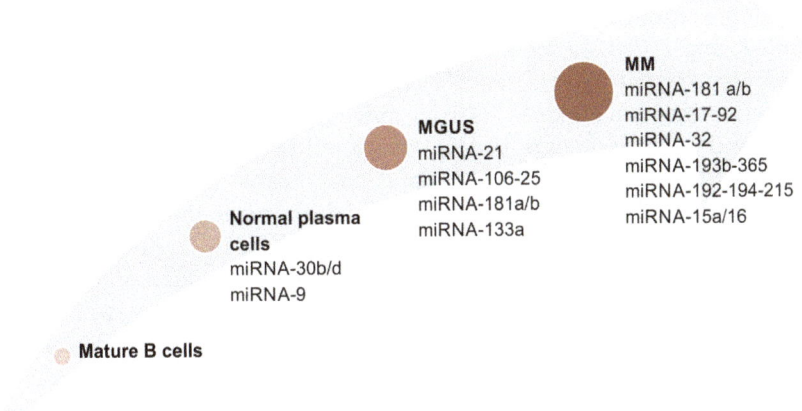

FIG. 3: Differential expression of miRNAs in normal plasma cells versus plasma cell dyscrasias. (MGUS: monoclonal gammopathy of undetermined significance; MM: multiple myeloma; miRNA: microRNA)

overt malignancy, such as MM. These miRNAs hold promise as potential diagnostic and prognostic markers. Specific miRNAs are associated with the development of drug resistance in MM. In the long run, many miRNAs could be utilized for targeted therapy in addressing this formidable hematological malignancy.[15,44,45]

Techniques like quantitative polymerase chain reaction (PCR), microarray, and next-generation sequencing have provided insights into the differential expression of miRNAs in MGUS and MM. Important examples of miRNAs that are overexpressed in MGUS include miR-21, miR-181 a/b, miR-106b-25, and miR-133a. In addition to these, miR-32 and miR-17-92 have been found to be upregulated both in MGUS and MM.[37,46] Pichiorri et al. demonstrated a signature of the upregulated miRNAs in MM consisting of miR-32, miR-21, miR-17~92, miR—106~25 and miR-181a/b.[47]

miR-21 causes sustained growth of the abnormal plasma cells, independent of IL-6. miR-21 and miR-106~25 clusters target *PTEN*, *BIM*, and *p21* tumor suppressor genes. miR-17~92 cluster is associated with the Myc proto-oncogene and is prominently expressed specifically in MM. This MM-specific miRNA is implicated in the upregulation of the *Myc* gene as MM progresses. Numerous studies have demonstrated that miR-17~92 also fosters the survival of malignant plasma cells by inhibiting the proapoptotic gene *BIM*.[48-50] miR-221 and miR-222 act as tumor promoters by inhibiting the expression of tumor suppressor gene, PTEN and proapoptotic gene, *PUMA*.[51,52] Elevated expression of these miRNAs is observed in MM but not in MGUS, and this upregulation has been linked to drug resistance in MM.

The heightened expression of miR-92 is implicated in the advancement of MM by activating the proto-oncogene c-jun.[53]

Some miRNAs such as miR-15 and 16, miR-328, miR-125b, miR-133a, miR-1, and miR-124a are down regulated in MGUS and MM as compared with the normal plasma cells.[54-56] Epigenetic modification in the form of hypermethylation of miR-34a/b/c, miR-124-1, miR-194-2, miR-192, miR-203, and miR-154 occurs in MM. These miRNAs are normally implicated in negative regulation of the genes responsible for cell survival and proliferation. Thus, methylation results in down regulation of these miRNAs in MM, ultimately leading to progression of disease by conferring a survival advantage to the malignant plasma cells. Hypermethylation of miR-34a/b/c interferes with the tumor suppressive function of *p53* gene. An additional miRNA that experiences decreased expression in MM is miR-29b, and its downregulation is linked to the proliferation of malignant cells and disrupted osteoclast function in the BM. The miR-29 family typically exerts a tumor-inhibitory effect by regulating cell proliferation, differentiation, and apoptosis through the PI3/AKT-3 pathway.[15,27,57-59]

Mechanisms of MicroRNA Dysregulation in Plasma Cell Dyscrasias

As previously explained, cytogenetic changes, such as deletions and translocations, play a crucial role in the development of plasma cell dyscrasias. These alterations are often linked to altered expression levels of miRNAs in MGUS and MM compared with normal plasma cells. This has been unveiled through studies utilizing gene expression profiling and high-resolution microarray analysis.[60,61]

Deletion of chromosome 13q14, which is implicated in CLL, is a commonly occurring genetic alteration in MM, seen in almost 50% of these patients. Its deletion correlates with reduced expression of miR-15 and miR-16. These miRNAs function to impede cell proliferation by suppressing the expression of cyclin D1 and cyclin D2, targeting the antiapoptotic gene *Bcl-2*, and inhibiting the NF-κB and AKT3 pathways. There is a notable underexpression of these miRNAs in MM compared to normal plasma cells and MGUS. Given that miR-15 and miR-16 are associated with the inhibition of cell proliferation, their diminished expression may be linked to the progression of MM. Down regulation of miR-15 and 16 has also been found to be associated with increased angiogenesis in MM.[54,60-62]

miR-361-3p and miR-30e are implicated in increased growth and survival of cells in MM. These miRNAs are upregulated in MM with t(11;14) and act through the activation of IL-6 signaling pathway.[63] MM with t(4;14) shows down regulation of miR-146a and miR-135b, which is related to increased proliferation through the IL-1 pathway by involvement of two IL-1 receptor-associated kinase genes, *PELI2* and *IRAK1*.[61] In addition, the expression of miR-99b and miR-125a-5p is upregulated with t(4;14). Translocations t(14;16) and t(14;20) are poor prognostic markers in MM, and are frequently

TABLE 2: Cytogenetic abnormalities with associated miRNA dysregulation in MM.		
Cytogenetic abnormalities	Dysregulated miRNAs	Expression
Del 13q14	miR-15 and miR-16	Decreased
t (11;14)	miR-361-3p and miR-30e	Increased
t (4;14)	miRNA-146a and miR-135	Decreased
	miR-99b and miR-125a-5p	Increased
t(14;16) and t(14;20)	miR-1, miR-133a, and miR-133b	Increased
del 17p13	miR-192, miR-194, and miR-215	Decreased
(MM: multiple myeloma; miRNA: microRNA)		

associated with upregulation of miR-1, miR-133a, and miR-133b.[64] The deletion at 17p13 leads to reduced expression of miR-192, miR-194, and miR-215, pivotal players in myelomagenesis by elevating levels of MDM-2—an inhibitor of the p53 tumor suppressor gene.[65]

Table 2 shows the cytogenetic abnormalities with their associated miRNA dysregulation in MM.

Epigenetic phenomena play a crucial role in governing the expression of miRNAs. Dysregulation of miRNAs in plasma cell dyscrasias can arise from epigenetic abnormalities, manifesting as either hypermethylation or histone modification. miR-34, miR-194, miR-192, and miR-215 are down regulated by methylation in MM. Similarly, miR-26 appears to be downregulated in MM with t(4;14) due to heterochromatin modification.[56,66-68]

Modulation of Bone Marrow Microenvironment by MicroRNAs in Plasma Cell Dyscrasias

As already discussed in the previous section, growth and survival of clonal plasma cells requires a favorable and supportive microenvironment in the BM. The BM microenvironment consists of BM stromal cells, osteoclasts, and a variety of immune cells. The clonal plasma cells interact with BM stromal cells and ECM components and cause reprogramming of certain miRNAs expressed on these cells. This may be responsible for the pathogenetic effects of miRNAs in the form of growth and survival advantage, decreased apoptosis, increased angiogenesis, and drug resistance.[69] miR-27b-3p and miR-214-3p expressed by BM fibroblasts are upregulated by interaction with clonal PCs and they mark the transition from MGUS to MM.[70] In MM, BM stromal cells overexpress miR-10a which increases cell proliferation. NOVA-1 is another miRNA which is overexpressed in MM cells and causes decreased apoptosis.

The clonal plasma cells also contribute to the elevation of secretion and activation of specific cytokines and growth factors by BM stromal cells. In MM, there is a diminished expression of miR-199a-5p, which serves as a negative regulator of hypoxia-inducible factor-1alpha (HIF-1α).[25,69] This causes overexpression of HIF-α responsible for angiogenesis and disease progression. MM cells decrease secretion of Osteoprotegerin by BM stromal cells and osteoblasts through the upregulation of miR-21. This impaired Osteoprotegerin secretion is responsible for interaction with the RANKl and development of osteolytic lesions in MM. BM T-lymphocytes undergo polarization toward the Th17 subtype because of the secretion of IL-6 and TGF-β by malignant plasma cells in MM. The IL-17 generated by Th17 cells plays a crucial role in disease progression by activating osteoclasts and forming lytic bone lesions. The overexpression of miR-21 in MM fosters the differentiation of Th17 cells.[71,72]

MicroRNA and Angiogenesis in Plasma Cell Dyscrasias

Angiogenesis plays a crucial role as a pathogenic mechanism in the initiation and advancement of MM. In fact, MM is one of the first malignancies in which the role of angiogenesis and antiangiogenic drugs was first established. Clonal plasma cells in plasma cell dyscrasias cause overexpression of HIF-1α with resultant increased angiogenesis via angiogenic factors such as VEGF, b-FGF, HGF, and IL-8.[69] The secretion of these growth factors and cytokines increases as we move forward through the spectrum of plasma cell dyscrasias from MGUS to smouldering MM to MM. A study on VEGF expression in MM postulated that its expression is even more in the aggressive forms of MM, such as plasmablastic myeloma.[73]

As already highlighted above, downregulation of miR-199-5p causes increased HIF-1α in MM. Studies have demonstrated the usefulness of synthetic miR-199a-5p mimetics in reducing HIF-1 expression, increased adhesion and decreased migration of the MM plasma cells.[74] In addition, down regulation of miR-15/16 also increases VEGF expression.[75] miR-145 is another anti-angiogenic miRNA that is downregulated in MM. Certain proangiogenic miRNAs that are upregulated in MM include members of the let-7 family and miR-92a. These miRNAs increase angiogenesis by targeting antiangiogenic molecules, HIF-3α and angiopoietin-like protein-1 (ANGPT-1), respectively.[69]

MicroRNA and Drug-resistance in Multiple Myeloma

Despite significant progress and the introduction of novel therapies for managing MM, a considerable number of patients still encounter refractory disease due to the emergence of drug resistance. miRNAs might play a pivotal role in governing the response of malignant plasma cells to therapies involving bortezomib, melphalan, and dexamethasone. The potential mechanisms linked to the involvement of miRNAs in drug resistance encompass the modulation of apoptotic, anti-apoptotic, and cell-cycle signaling pathways.[76] Interestingly, "miRNA pharmacogenomics" is an emerging field of study to determine the influence of miRNA on efficacy of chemotherapeutic drugs.

Reduced expression of miR-451 in MM leads to the heightened expression of the oncogene MDR1, a contributor to drug resistance. Certain studies propose that the downregulation of miR-15a, miR-16-5p, miR-20a-5p, and miR-17-5p is linked to resistance against bortezomib in MM. Additionally, miR-21 has been identified as upregulated in cases of MM exhibiting resistance to melphalan. Overexpression of miR-221/222 with resultant inhibition of the tumor suppressor gene, PUMA is linked to melphalan resistance. It also causes resistance to dexamethasone due to suppression of the autophagy-related gene-12 and m-TOR pathway. These miRNAs may serve as potential targets for drug therapy in MM.[25,77,78]

The emergence of MM cancer stem cells (CSCs) may cause the disease to become highly drug resistant due to the overexpression of ABC transporters and ATP-binding cassette transporters, which result in drug efflux. Few studies have found miR-451 to be expressed differently in CSCs as compared with non-CSCs, and demonstrated induction of responsiveness to bortezomib and melphalan therapy by inhibition of miR-451 by triggering apoptosis. Upregulation of miR-125b causes inactivation of p53 and resistance to dexamethasone.[79]

CONCLUSION

MicroRNAs affect almost all the phenomena that are involved in the initiation and progression of plasma cell dyscrasias. An understanding of the biology of miRNAs is critical for comprehension of their role in the pathogenesis of these neoplasms. The exploitation of this knowledge for the development of potential miRNA therapeutic targets in MM holds a promising future.

REFERENCES

1. Kyle RA, Rajkumar SV. Multiple myeloma. N Engl J Med. 2004;351:1860-73.
2. Rajkumar SV. Multiple myeloma: 2022 update on diagnosis, risk stratification, and management. Am J Hematol. 2022;97:1086-107.
3. Kyle RA, Rajkumar SV. Epidemiology of the plasma-cell disorders. Best Pract Res Clin Haematol. 2007;4:637-64.
4. Kyle RA, Therneau TM, Rajkumar SV, Larson DR, Plevak MF, Offord JR, et al. Prevalence of monoclonal gammopathy of undetermined significance. N Engl J Med. 2006;354:1362-9.
5. Turesson I, Kovalchik SA, Pfeiffer RM, Kristinsson SY, Goldin LR, Drayson MT, et al. Monoclonal gammopathy of undetermined significance and risk of lymphoid and myeloid malignancies: 728 cases followed up to 30 years in Sweden. Blood. 2014;123: 338-45.
6. Fend F, Dogan A, Cook JR. Plasma cell neoplasms and related entities—evolution in diagnosis and classification. Virchows Arch. 2023;482:163-77.
7. McKenna RW, Kyle RD, Kuehl WM, Harris NL, Coupland R, Fend F. Plasma cell neoplasms. In: Swerdlow SH, Campo E, Harris NL, Jaffe ES, Pileri S, Stein H, et al. (Eds). WHO Classification of Tumours of Hematopoietic and Lymphoid Tissues. Lyon: IARC; 2017. pp. 241-53.

8. Ríos-Tamayo R, Paiva B, Lahuerta JJ, López JM, Duarte RF. Monoclonal gammopathies of clinical significance: A critical appraisal. Cancers. 2022;14:5247.
9. Alaggio R, Amador C, Anagnostopoulos I, Attygalle AD, de Oliveira Araujo IB, Berti E, et al. The 5th edition of the World Health Organization Classification of Haematolymphoid Tumours: Lymphoid Neoplasms. Leukemia. 2022;36:1720-48.
10. Campo E, Jaffe ES, Cook JR, Quintanilla-Martinez L, Swerdlow SH, Anderson KC, et al. The International consensus classification of mature lymphoid neoplasms: A report from the clinical advisory committee. Blood. 2022;140:1229-53.
11. Barwick BG, Gupta VA, Vertino PM, Boise LH. Cell of origin and genetic alterations in the pathogenesis of multiple myeloma. Front Immunol. 2019;10:1121.
12. Heider M, Nickel K, Högner M, Bassermann F. Multiple myeloma: Molecular pathogenesis and disease evolution. Oncol Res Treat. 2021;44:672-81.
13. Flores-Montero J, de Tute R, Paiva B, Perez JJ, Böttcher S, Wind H, et al. Immunophenotype of normal vs. myeloma plasma cells: Toward antibody panel specifications for MRD detection in multiple myeloma. Cytometry B Clin Cytom. 2016;90:61-72.
14. Raja KR, Kovarova L, Hajek R. Review of phenotypic markers used in flow cytometric analysis of MGUS and MM, and applicability of flow cytometry in other plasma cell disorders. Br J Haematol. 2010;149:334-51.
15. Soliman AM, Lin TS, Mahakkanukrauh P, Das S. Role of microRNAs in diagnosis, prognosis and management of multiple myeloma. Int J Mol Sci. 2020;21:7539.
16. Bergsagel PL, Stewart AK, Russell SJ, Fonseca R. Molecular genetic aspects of plasma cell disorders. In: John PG, Daniel AA, Bertil G, List AF, Means RT, Paraskevas F, et al. (Eds). Wintrobe's Clinical Hematology, 13th edition. Philadelphia: Wolters Kluwer, Lippincott Williams & Wilkins Health; 2014. pp. 2022-7.
17. Prideaux SM, Conway O'Brien E, Chevassut TJ. The genetic architecture of multiple myeloma. Adv Hematol. 2014;2014:864058.
18. Abdallah N, Rajkumar SV, Greipp P, Kapoor P, Gertz MA, Dispenzieri A, et al. Cytogenetic abnormalities in multiple myeloma: Association with disease characteristics and treatment response. Blood Cancer J. 2020;10(8):82.
19. Kumar S, Fonseca R, Ketterling RP, Dispenzieri A, Lacy MQ, Gertz MA, et al. Trisomies in multiple myeloma: Impact on survival in patients with high-risk cytogenetics. Blood. 2012;119:2100-5.
20. Kumar SK, Rajkumar SV. The multiple myelomas - current concepts in cytogenetic classification and therapy. Nat Rev Clin Oncol. 2018;15:409-21.
21. Quail DF, Joyce JA. Microenvironmental regulation of tumor progression and metastasis. Nat Med. 2013;19:1423-37.
22. Hideshima T, Mitsiades C, Tonon G, Richardson PG, Anderson KC. Understanding multiple myeloma pathogenesis in the bone marrow to identify new therapeutic targets. Nat Rev Cancer. 2007;7:585-98.
23. Giuliani N, Rizzoli V. Myeloma cells and bone marrow osteoblast interactions: Role in the development of osteolytic lesions in multiple myeloma. Leuk Lymphoma. 2007;48:2323-9.
24. Kumar V, Abbas AK, Aster JC (Eds). Robbins Basic Pathology, 10th edition. Philadelphia: Elsevier; 2018.
25. Handa H, Murakami Y, Ishihara R, Kimura-Masuda K, Masuda Y. The role and function of microRNA in the pathogenesis of multiple myeloma. Cancers (Basel). 2019;11:1738.
26. Caprio C, Sacco A, Giustini V, Roccaro AM. Epigenetic aberrations in multiple myeloma. Cancers (Basel). 2020;12:2996.
27. Walker BA, Wardell CP, Chiecchio L, Smith EM, Boyd KD, Neri A, et al. Aberrant global methylation patterns affect the molecular pathogenesis and prognosis of multiple myeloma. Blood. 2011;117:553-62.

28. Singh S, Jain K, Sharma R, Singh J, Paul D. Epigenetic modifications in myeloma: Focused review of current data and potential therapeutic applications. Indian J Med Paediatr Oncol. 2021;42:395-405.
29. Xie Z, Bi C, Chooi JY, Chan ZL, Mustafa N, Chng WJ. MMSET regulates expression of IRF4 in t(4;14) myeloma and its silencing potentiates the effect of bortezomib. Leukemia. 2015;29:2347-54.
30. Bartel DP. MicroRNAs: Target recognition and regulatory functions. Cell. 2009;136: 215-33.
31. Peng Y, Croce CM. The role of MicroRNAs in human cancer. Signal Transduct Target. 2016;1:15004.
32. Calin GA, Ferracin M, Cimmino A, Leva GD, Shimizu M, Wojcik SE, et al. A MicroRNA signature associated with prognosis and progression in chronic lymphocytic leukemia. N Engl J Med. 2005;353:1793-801.
33. Svoronos AA, Engelman DM, Slack FJ. OncomiR or tumor suppressor? The duplicity of microRNAs in cancer. Cancer Res. 2016;76:3666-70.
34. Visone R, Croce CM. MiRNAs and cancer. Am J Pathol. 2009;174:1131-8.
35. Al-Masri A, Price-Troska T, Chesi M, Chung TH. MicroRNA expression analysis in multiple myeloma. Blood. 2005;106:1554.
36. Chen D, Yang X, Liu M, Zhang Z, Xing E. Roles of miRNA dysregulation in the pathogenesis of multiple myeloma. Cancer Gene Ther. 2021;28:1256-68.
37. Calvo KR, Landgren O, Roccaro AM, Ghobrial IM. Role of microRNAs from monoclonal gammopathy of undetermined significance to multiple myeloma. Semin Hematol. 2011;48:39-45.
38. Xiao C, Srinivasan L, Calado DP, Patterson HC, Zhang B, Wang J, et al. Lymphoproliferative disease and autoimmunity in mice with increased miR-17-92 expression in lymphocytes. Nat Immunol. 2008;9:405-14.
39. Ventura A, Young AG, Winslow MM, Lintault L, Meissner A, Erkeland SJ, et al. Targeted deletion reveals essential and overlapping functions of the miR-17 through 92 family of miRNA clusters. Cell. 2008;132:875-86.
40. Chen CZ, Li L, Lodish HF, Bartel DP. MicroRNAs modulate hematopoietic lineage differentiation. Science. 2004;303:83-6.
41. Jima DD, Zhang J, Jacobs C, Richards KL, Dunphy CH, Choi WWL, et al. Deep sequencing of the small RNA transcriptome of normal and malignant human B cells identifies hundreds of novel microRNAs. Blood. 2010;116:e118-27.
42. Zhang J, Jima DD, Jacobs C, Fischer R, Gottwein E, Huang G, et al. Patterns of microRNA expression characterize stages of human B-cell differentiation. Blood. 2009;113: 4586-94.
43. Martins G, Calame K. Regulation and functions of Blimp-1 in T and B lymphocytes. Annu Rev Immunol. 2008;26:133-69.
44. Zhu B, Ju S, Chu H, Shen X, Zhang Y, Luo X, et al. The potential function of microRNAs as biomarkers and therapeutic targets in multiple myeloma. Oncol Lett. 2018;15: 6094-106.
45. Szudy-Szczyrek A, Ahern S, Krawczyk J, Szczyrek M, Hus M. MiRNA as a potential target for multiple myeloma therapy-current knowledge and perspectives. J Pers Med. 2022;12:1428.
46. Loffler D, Brocke-Heidrich K, Pfeifer G, Stocsits C, Hackermüller J, Kretzschmar AK, et al. Interleukin-6 dependent survival of multiple myeloma cells involves the Stat3-mediated induction of microRNA-21 through a highly conserved enhancer. Blood. 2007;110(4):1330-3.
47. Pichiorri F, Suh SS, Ladetto M, Kuehl M, Palumbo T, Drandi D, et al. MicroRNAs regulate critical genes associated with multiple myeloma pathogenesis. Proc Natl Acad Sci U S A. 2008;105:12885-90.

48. Leone E, Morelli E, Di Martino MT, Amodio N, Foresta U, Gullà A, et al. Targeting miR-21 inhibits in vitro and in vivo multiple myeloma cell growth. Clin Can Res. 2013;19:2096-106.
49. Wang K, Li PF. Foxo3a regulates apoptosis by negatively targeting miR-21. J Biol Chem. 2010;285:16958-66.
50. Novotny GW, Sonne SB, Nielsen JE, Hansen MA, Skakkebaek NE, Meyts ER, et al. Translational repression of E2F1 mRNA in carcinoma in situ and normal testis correlates with expression of the miR-17-92 cluster. Cell Death Differ. 2007;14:879-82.
51. Di Martino MT, Gullà A, Cantafio ME, Lionetti M, Leone E, Amodio N, et al. In vitro and in vivo anti-tumor activity of miR-221/222 inhibitors in multiple myeloma. Oncotarget. 2013;4:242-55.
52. Zhao JJ, Chu ZB, Hu Y, Lin J, Wang Z, Jiang M, et al. Targeting the miR-221-222/ PUMA/ BAK/BAX pathway abrogates dexamethasone resistance in multiple myeloma. Cancer Res. 2015;75:4384-97.
53. Qu XY, Zhang SS, Wu S, Hong M, Li JY, Chen LJ, et al. Expression level of microRNA-92a and its clinical significance in multiple myeloma patients. Chin J Hematol. 2013;34: 332-6.
54. Roccaro AM, Sacco A, Thompson B, Leleu X, Azab AK, Azab F, et al. *MicroRNAs* 15a and 16 regulate tumor proliferation in multiple myeloma. Blood. 2009;113:6669-80.
55. Wong KY, Huang X, Chim CS. DNA methylation of microRNA genes in multiple myeloma. Carcinogenesis. 2012;33:1629-38.
56. Zhang W, Wang YE, Zhang Y, Leleu X, Reagan M, Zhang Y, et al. Global epigenetic regulation of microRNAs in multiple myeloma. PLoS ONE. 2014;9:e110973.
57. Okada N, Lin CP, Ribeiro MC, Biton A, Lai G, He X, et al. A positive feedback between p53 and miR-34 miRNAs mediates tumor suppression. Genes Dev. 2014;28:438-50.
58. Amodio N, Stamato MA, Gullà AM, Morelli E, Romeo E, Raimondi L, et al. Therapeutic Targeting of miR-29b/HDAC4 epigenetic loop in multiple myeloma. Mol Cancer Ther. 2016;15:1364-75.
59. Amodio N, Leotta M, Bellizzi D, Di Martino MT, D'Aquila P, Lionetti M, et al. DNA-demethylating and anti-tumor activity of synthetic miR-29b mimics in multiple myeloma. Oncotarget. 2012;3:1246-58.
60. Saki N, Abroun S, Hajizamani S, Rahim F, Shahjahani M. Association of chromosomal translocation and miRNA expression with the pathogenesis of multiple myeloma. Cell J. 2014;16:99-110.
61. Gutiérrez NC, Sarasquete ME, Misiewicz-Krzeminska I, Delgado M, De Las Rivas J, Ticona FV, et al. Deregulation of microRNA expression in the different genetic subtypes of multiple myeloma and correlation with gene expression profiling. Leukemia. 2010;24:629-37.
62. Gatt ME, Zhao JJ, Ebert MS, Zhang Y, Chu Z, Mani M, et al. MicroRNAs 15a/16-1 function as tumor suppressor genes in multiple myeloma. Blood. 2011;117:7188.
63. Lionetti M, Biasiolo M, Agnelli L, Todoerti K, Mosca L, Fabris S, et al. Identification of microRNA expression patterns and definition of a microRNA/mRNA regulatory network in distinct molecular groups of multiple myeloma. Blood. 2009;114(25):e20-6.
64. Pichiorri F, DeLuca L, Aqeilan RI. MicroRNAs: New players in multiple myeloma. Front Genet. 2011;2:22.
65. Pichiorri F, Suh SS, Rocci A, De Luca L, Taccioli C, Santhanam R, et al. Downregulation of p53-inducible microRNAs 192, 194, and 215 impairs the p53/MDM2 autoregulatory loop in multiple myeloma development. Cancer Cell. 2010;18(4):367-81.
66. Chim CS, Wong KY, Qi Y, Loong F, Lam WL, Wong LG, et al. Epigenetic inactivation of the miR-34a in hematological malignancies. Carcinogenesis. 2010;31(4):745-50.
67. Kimura K, Kuroda Y, Masuda Y, Yamane A, Hattori H, Tahara K, et al. Loop regulation between microRNAs and epigenetics underlie microRNA dysregulation in multiple myeloma and is associated with the disease progression. Blood. 2015;126:3013.

68. Wong KY, Huang X, Chim CS. DNA methylation of microRNA genes in multiple myeloma. Carcinogenesis. 2012;33:1629-38.
69. Raimondi L, De Luca A, Morelli E, Giavaresi G, Tagliaferri P, Tassone P, et al. MicroRNAs: Novel crossroads between myeloma cells and the bone marrow microenvironment. Biomed Res Int. 2016;2016:6504593.
70. Frassanito MA, Desantis V, Di Marzo L, Craparotta I, Beltrame L, Marchini S, et al. Bone marrow fibroblasts overexpress miR-27b and miR-214 in step with multiple myeloma progression, dependent on tumour cell-derived exosomes. J Pathol. 2019;247(2):241-53.
71. Pitari MR, Rossi M, Amodio N, Botta C, Morelli E, Federico C, et al. Inhibition of miR-21 restores RANKL/OPG ratio in multiple myeloma-derived bone marrow stromal cells and impairs the resorbing activity of mature osteoclasts. Oncotarget 2015;6(29):27343-58.
72. Papanota AM, Karousi P, Kontos CK, Ntanasis-Stathopoulos I, Scorilas A, Terpos E. Multiple myeloma bone disease: Implication of microRNAs in its molecular background. Int J Mol Sci. 2021;22(5):2375.
73. Palta A, Kaur M, Tahlan A, Dimri K. Evaluation of angiogenesis in multiple myeloma by VEGF immunoexpression and microvessel density. J Lab Physicians. 2020;12(1):38-43.
74. Raimondi L, Amodio N, Di Martino MT, Altomare E, Leotta M, Caracciolo D, et al. Targeting of multiple myeloma-related angiogenesis by miR-199a-5p mimics: In vitro and in vivo anti-tumor activity. Oncotarget. 2014;5(10):3039-54.
75. Sun C, She X, Qin Y, Chu ZB, Chen L, Ai LS, et al. miR-15a and miR-16 affect the angiogenesis of multiple myeloma by targeting VEGF. Carcinogenesis. 2013;34(2):426-35.
76. Solimando AG, Malerba E, Leone P, Prete M, Terragna C, Cavo M, et al. Drug resistance in multiple myeloma: Soldiers and weapons in the bone marrow niche. Front Oncol. 2022;12:973836.
77. Hao M, Zhang L, An G, Sui W, Yu Z, Zou D, et al. Suppressing miRNA-15a/-16 expression by interleukin-6 enhances drug-resistance in myeloma cells. J Hematol Oncol. 2011;4:37.
78. Zhao JJ, Chu ZB, Hu Y, Lin J, Wang Z, Jiang M, et al. Targeting the miR-221/222/PUMA/BAK/BAX pathway abrogates dexamethasone resistance in multiple myeloma. Cancer Res. 2015;75(20):4384-97.
79. Ghosh N, Matsui W. Cancer stem cells in multiple myeloma. Cancer Lett. 2009;277(1):1-7.

CHAPTER 10

Genomic Profiling for Clinical Decision-making in Hematological Malignancies

Harish Chandra

■ INTRODUCTION

Hematology is one of the dynamic sections of medical science receiving eruption of new knowledge day by day. The genomics explosion changes the scenario very much, and after the new 5th Edition of the WHO[1] where various new subclasses are added based on the genomic profiling of disease; it turns the table now toward a new therapeutic approach called precision medicine.

The basis of precision medicine lies in the concept of right patient, right time, and right drug, with the help of genomic profile of the disease in any patient, we can decide the best-suited targeted therapy for that individual and hence, the concept of "One size fit for all" is obsolete nowadays.[2]

Why precision oncology is gaining attention nowadays? It is just because of reduced toxicity due to chemotherapy in conventional therapy, it is economical to save money, also improves patient's outcome and reduces time and money on futile treatment.

Although morphology is an important tool to diagnose hematological malignancies (HM), but as the sub-classifications of HM are very common now and their responses to treatment also differ, it creates a need for further exploration required beyond morphology. Chromosomal analysis, fluorescence in situ hybridization (FISH), polymerase chain reaction (PCR), reverse transcription-PCR (RT-PCR), and microarray are continuously helping scientist and clinicians to explore further the understanding of pathobiology of the disease and accordingly that modifications are being done in therapeutics. However, with the recent development in genomics which include next-generation sequencing, its make the life more challenging.

Next-generation sequencing (NGS) information is critical for HM as it provides vital information for the diagnosis, risk assessment, therapeutic decisions, measurable residual disease (MRD) monitoring, progression of disease, and response to treatment **(Fig. 1)**.

Genomic profiling plays an important role in clinical decision-making for the management of various HM like acute leukemia, lymphomas and

CHAPTER 10: Genomic Profiling for Clinical Decision-making...

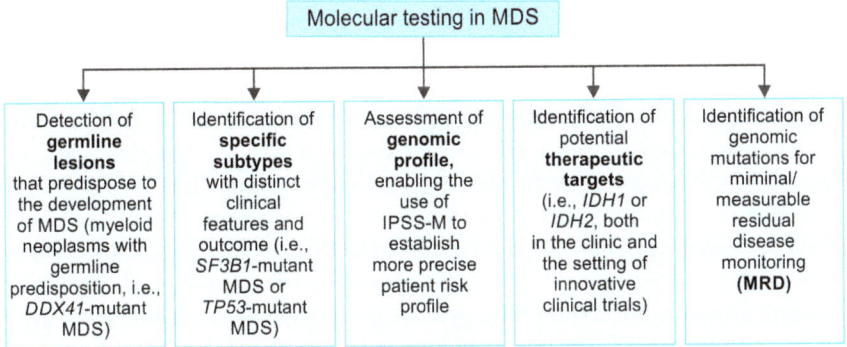

FIG. 1: How molecular profiling can inform clinical decision-making in MDS.
(IPSS-M: Molecular International Prognostic Scoring System; MDS: myelodysplastic syndrome; MRD: minimal/measurable residual disease)
Source: Professional illustration by Patrick Lane, ScEYEnce Studios.[4]

multiple myeloma. Most of the HM are characterized by genetic and molecular heterogeneity, which makes individual neoplasm-specific and plays an important role in the diagnosis, sub-classification, prognosis and management of these neoplasms. It signifies the importance of genomic changes seen in the HM and provides management as per the specific tumor. Clinical molecular pathology analysis or genomic profiling has therefore become an indispensable laboratory tool that can be used to characterize tumor biology and to drive therapeutic decisions. Molecular studies with chromosome banding analysis enhances the diagnostic capabilities of clinical genetics, allowing for a more comprehensive understanding of genetic disorders and abnormalities. The combination of traditional and molecular techniques contributes to a more accurate and detailed characterization of the genome.

In this chapter, we will discuss the role of genomics in day-to-day practice to the management of HM. First, we will discuss about the routine conventional molecular and immunophenotypic measures by which we can diagnose and categorized these entities followed by HM individually.

■ CONVENTIONAL MOLECULAR METHODS

Chromosomal Banding Analysis (Cytogenetics)

We know that this is the most conventional method to know about chromosomal numbers, losses, translocations, deletions, and amplifications. The limitations of CG (cytogenetics) is that the requirement of live cells (metaphase arrest) for better resolutions, as well as the resolution is low (5–10 Mb only) with low sensitivity (10^{-1}). This whole process is also time-consuming and mostly takes 2–3 weeks time.

FISH

Fluorescence in situ hybridization (FISH) is a powerful tool and helps to identify various translocations, deletions, and amplifications in various HM. The main advantages is that we do not need to culture cell or required any live tissue/cells. We can perform it on even tissue sections or on interface nuclei. The FISH probes are specifically designed for particular target regions, so its sensitivity is much more than routine CG/Karyotyping. With the help of FISH, we can detect 100–200 kb changes in DNA/Chromosome. It can detect abnormalities even up to 1–5% of affected cells with an analytical sensitivity of approximately 10^{-2}. The entire process generally will not take much time as compared with CG, results available usually between 1–3 days. It is very helpful in detecting cytogenetically cryptic changes.

Chromosomal Microarrays

Chromosomal microarrays (CMAs) are used to identify small unbalanced abnormalities or cryptic copy number alterations (CNA) but do not able to detect balanced rearrangements. CMA includes single-nucleotide polymorphism (SNP) probes to identify loss of heterozygosity (LOH) helping in the determination of chromosomal ploidy. It can detect abnormalities across the whole genome and did not required live cells. CMA can detect small abnormalities (20-100 kb) present in 20-30% of tumor cells. The analytical sensitivity of CMA is $>10^{-1}$.[3] Turnaround time in CMA ranges from 3–14 days.

Optical Genome Mapping

This method uses enzymatic digestion of high molecular weight DNA and is used to identify structural variants, such as translocations, inversions, and CNAs. It is not widely used nowadays in clinical practice.

Polymerase Chain Reaction

The PCR method is widely used to detect mutations in a gene of interest. In HM, this technique is used to detect single-gene mutations (e.g., JAK2 p.V617F, and KIT p.D816V) and distinct fusions (e.g., BCR::ABL1) for diagnosis and disease monitoring. Turnaround time in PCR generally ranges between 2 and 5 days. With the help of PCR, we can detect one mutation at a time. Variations in the form of qPCR (quantitative real-time PCR) and digital PCR are also available. The sensitivity of droplet digital PCR (ddPCR) is 10^{-4} which means that it can detect one mutation in 10,000 normal cells. This method can be widely used in MRD analysis.

Sanger Sequencing

With the help of Sanger sequencing, we can detect even a single base pair change in DNA (PCR product). Here, with the help of electrophoresis individual DNA bases identified by random incorporation of fluorescently labeled chain terminating dideoxynucleotide by DNA polymerase. It is generally used to detect gene mutations confined to single exons (e.g., *CEBPA*, and *CALR*) and has a relatively low analytic sensitivity of approximately 20% ($>10^{-1}$). It has an advantage over NGS because of its short turnaround time and easy data interpretation.

NGS-BASED MOLECULAR METHODS

Background

Next-generation sequencing also known as high throughput sequencing designed to know the sequences of nucleotide in a genomic sample. Here, we use millions or billions of parallel sequencing reactions to identify genomic abnormalities. NGS has significantly advanced our ability to understanding of genomic and genetics. NGS used to identify full range of genomic variation, including single nucleotide variant (SNV), small insertion/deletions, CNAs, chromosomal translocations/gene fusions, gene expression, and DNA methylation, and can be used in initial diagnosis as well as during monitoring. NGS has various key features, which makes it unique among all molecular and genomic technologies.

Key Features

High Throughput

Next-generation sequencing allows simultaneous sequencing of millions and billions of DNA fragments in a single run. This high throughput has greatly reduced the cost and time required for the large-scale sequencing projects.

Speed

Next-generation sequencing sequencing is faster than traditional Sanger sequencing. This speed is essential for applications where rapid sequencing is crucial such as in clinical diagnostics and studying time-sensitive biological processes.

Parallel Sequencing

Next-generation sequencing platform performs sequencing in massively parallel fashion. They generate millions of short DNA sequences in parallel, which are then computationally reconstructed to obtain the complete genome or target region sequence.

Clinical Applications

Genomic Sequencing

Next-generation sequencing has been used to sequence entire genome, not only human being but also applicable to other species. It has facilitated large-scale genome project like Human Genome Project.

Transcriptomics
This method is used to study transcriptome, which, involves sequencing of the entire RNA molecule in a cell or tissue. This enriches our experience in gene expression, alternative splicing, and many more.

Epigenetics
Next-generation sequencing allows for the study of epigenetic modifications, such as DNA methylation and histone modifications, which play a crucial role in gene regulation.

Metagenomics
Next-generation sequencing is used to sequence DNA from a complex mixture of microorganisms, like those of human microbiome.

Cancer Genomics
Next-generation sequencing is a valuable tool in understanding the genetic mutations and alterations that drive cancer. It is used for identifying potential therapeutic targets and personalized medicine approaches.

Cancer Diagnostics
Next-generation sequencing is increasingly used in clinical settings for the diagnosis of cancer by identifying mutations and monitoring MRD in various cancer patients.

Short Reads versus Long Reads
Next-generation sequencing platform can produce both short and long reads. Short reads are typically less expensive and have high accuracy, while long reads are helpful in resolving complex genomic regions and structural variations.

Table 1 depicts the advantages, limitations, and clinical applications of various genomic methods used in clinical practice.

Which molecular test will be appropriate depends upon the clinical scenario or disease category. The genes to be tested as per clinical conditions is given in **Table 2**.[4]

Now, we will discuss the role of genomic testing in various HM and premalignant conditions where it will help in accurate diagnosis, which further helps in subcategorization of disease category. Apart from this, these mutations detected by genomic testing will be helpful in prognosis and choosing appropriate therapy. A set of gene mutations for different hematological malignancies or premalignant conditions which can be used in diagnosis, prognosis MRD assay and risk stratifications is given in **Table 3**.

ROLE OF GENOMICS IN PATIENTS WITH CYTOPENIA AND SUSPICION OF MYELODYSPLASTIC SYNDROME

Persistent cytopenias are matter of concern to the hematologists, as this might be a spectrum of underlying MDS (myelodysplastic syndrome).

TABLE 1: General advantages, limitations, and clinical applications of comprehensive genomic methods.[4]

Technique	CG	FISH	CMA	OGM	Targeted	Exome	WGS	RNA-seq
Viable cells	yes	No	No	No	No	No	No	No
Resolution	~5 Mb	100–200 kb	20–100 kb	5–50 kb	1 bp	1 bp	1 bp	1 bp
Coverage	Genome	Targeted	Genome	Genome	Targeted	Exome	Genome	Genome
Alterations	CNV, SV	CNV, SV	Genome	CNV, SV	← SNV, Indel, CNV, SV, LOH →			Gene expression, SV
Sensitivity (VAF)	5–10%	1–5%	30%	5%	2%	5–10%	10%	5%
TAT (days)*	2–21	1–3	3–14	4–7	5–14	5–14	3–14	5–14
Cost*	$	$	$$	$$$	$$-$$$	$$$	$$$$	$$-$$$
Worldwide use*	High	High	Low	Low	Medium	Low	Low	Low
Used in								
MDS and MDS/MPN	D, FU	D, FU	D, R	D, R	D, MRD†	D	D, ND	
MPN	D	D	D	D	D, MRD†	D	D	ND
AML	D, R	D	D	D, R	D, MRD†	D	D	D
ALL	D, R	D	D, R	D, R	D	D	D	D

*TATs, cost, and use approximated. Actual TATs, cost, and use vary significantly by region and laboratory.
†When used in conjunction with high coverage sequencing and error correction methods for increased sensitivity/specificity for low-abundance mutation.
(ALL: acute lymphoblastic leukemia; AML: acute myeloid leukemia; CG: cytogenetics; CMA: chromosomal microarray; CNV: copy number variations; D: diagnosis; ES: exome sequencing; FISH: fluorescence in situ hybridization; FU: follow-up; Indel, small insertion/deletions; LOH: loss of heterozygosity; MPN: myeloproliferative neoplasm; ND: not done; OGM: optical genome mapping; R: relapse; SNV: single-nucleotide variant; SV: structural variant; TAT: turnaround time; $: cost in USD)

TABLE 2: Gene mutations in myeloid neoplasms and leukemia indicated for clinical testing.[4]

Indication	Single-gene mutations	Structural variants
MDS, MDS/MPN, cytopenia	ASXL1, BCOR, BCORL1, CBL, CEBPA, CSF3R, DDX41, DMNT3A, ETV6, ETNK1, EZH2, FLT3-ITD, FLT3-TKD, GATA2, GNB1, IDH1, IDH2, JAK2, KIT, KRAS, KMT2A-PTD, NF1, NPM1, NRAS, PHF6, PPM1D, PRPF8, PTPN11, RAD21, RUNX1, SAMD9[†], SAMD9L[†], SETBP1, SF3B1, SRSF2, STAG2, TET2, TP53, U2AF1, UBA1, WT1, ZRSR2	
MPN and mastocytosis[‡]	ASXL1, CALR, CBL, CSF3R, DNMT3A, EZH2, IDH1, IDH2 JAK2§, KIT, KRAS, MPL, NRAS, PTPN11, RUNX1, SETBP1, SF3B1, SH2B3, SRSF2, TET2, U2AF1, ZRSR2	BCR::ABL1[§]
Eosinophilia	ASXL1, CBL, DNMT3A, EZH2, KRAS, NRAS, RUNX1, SF3B1, SRSF2, STAT5B, TET2, U2AF1	BCR::ABL1[§], FGFR1::R, FLT3::R, JAK2::R, PDGFRA::R, PDGFRB::R
AML	*Genes required for diagnosis and risk stratification:* ASXL1, BCOR, CEBPA, DDX41, EZH2, FLT3-ITD[§], FLT3- TKD[§], IDH1[§], IDH2[§], NPM1, RUNX1, SF3B1, SRSF2, STAG2, TP53, U2AF1, ZRSR2 *Additional genes recommended to test for at diagnosis and for use in disease monitoring:* ANKRD26, BCORL1, BRAF, CBL, CSF3R, DNMT3A, ETV6, GATA2, JAK2, KIT, KRAS, NRAS, NF1, PHF6, PPM1D, PTPN11, RAD21, SETBP1, TET2, WT1	BCR::ABL1[§], CBFB::MYH11, DEK::NUP214 MECOM::R, KMT2A::R, NUP98::R, RUNX1::RUNX1T1, PML::RARA[§]
B-ALL	CREBBP, CRLF2, FLT3, IDH1, IDH2, IKZF1, IL7R, JAK1, JAK2, JAK3, KMT2D, KRAS, NF1, NRAS, PAX5, PTPN11, SETD2, SH2B3, TP53	ABL1::R[§], ABL2::R, CRLF2::R, CSF1R::R, DUX4::R, EPOR::R, ETV6::R, JAK2::R, KMT2A::R, MEF2D::R, NUTM1::R, PAX5::R, PDGFRA::R, PDGFRB::R, TCF3::R, ZNF384::R
T-ALL	DNMT3A, ETV6, EZH2, FBXW7, FLT3, IDH1, IDH2, IL7R, JAK1, JAK3, KRAS, MSH2, NOTCH1, NRAS, PHF6, PTEN, U2AF1, WT1	BCL11B::R, LMO2::R, MYB::R, NUP::ABL1, NUP214::R, STIL::R, TAL::R, TLX1::R, TLX3::R

*Conventional karyotype should be performed on all cases at diagnosis. Specific FISH, RT-PCR, or gene fusion NGS assays (targeted DNA/RNA or WGS) may be included depending on clinical context and results of other clinical studies.

[†]Pediatric patients.

[‡]Mast cell disease with suspicion of associated hematologic neoplasm.

[§]Food and Drug Administration–approved targeted therapy.

(ALL: acute lymphoblastic leukemia; AML: acute myeloid leukemia; MDS/MPN: myelodysplastic/myeloproliferative neoplasms)

TABLE 3: Features of CHIP, ICUS, CCUS, and MDS.[4]

	Cytopenia/ Dysplasia	VAF Cutoff	Commonly mutated driver genes	Higher risk features
CHIP	No/Minimal (<10%) to none	>2%	*DNMT3A, TET2, ASXL1, PPM1D, JAK2, ZBTB33, ZNF318, TP53, CBL, GNB1, SF3B1, SRSF2*, loss of Y chromosome	Mutations in TP53, ASXL1, JAK2, SF3B1, SRSF2, U2AF1, or IDH1/IDH2; >1 driver mutations; VAF > 10%
ICUS	Yes/Minimal (<10%) to none	None	None	None
CCUS	Yes/Minimal (<10%) to none	>2%	*TET2, DNMT3A, ASXL1, SRSF2, ZRSR2, SF3B1, U2AF1, IDH1/2, RUNX1, EZH2, JAK2, CBL, KRAS, CUX1, TP53*	Spliceosome gene mutations *DNMT3A, ASXL1, TET2* in commutational patterns (RUNX1, EZH2, CBL, BCOR, CUX1, TP53, or IDH1/IDH2 most specific), >1 driver mutation; VAF > 10%
MDS	Yes/Yes	None	See in MDS	See in MDS

(CCUS: clonal cytopenia of undetermined significance; CHIP: clonal hematopoiesis of indeterminate potential; ICUS: idiopathic cytopenia of undetermined significance; MDS: myelodysplastic syndrome)

Conventional cytogenetics plays an important role in classification and risk stratification in MDS, e.g., del(5q), del(7q), and complex cytogenetic patterns. Genomic testing especially for driver mutations is crucial for further identification of subclasses. If driver mutations are absent in a background of persistent cytopenias, we will consider it as idiopathic cytopenias of undetermined significance (ICUS) on the other hand, if driver mutations are present in the same scenario, then it will be considered as clonal cytopenias of undetermined significance (CCUS). However, in some cases, particularly in elderly persons sometimes, these driver mutations are present without having any cytopenias or dysplasia in hematopoietic cells, this situation is considered as clonal hematopoiesis of undetermined significance (CHIP) **(Table 3)**.

These CHIP-positive populations are at the risk of developing hematological[5] or cardiovascular disorders.[6] In clinical practice, we will not directly go into search for driver mutation by NGS in elderly; routinely, we follow it in clinical context, followed by basic lab investigations and then if required, we will advise the patients to these high-end tests if it will not be explained by routine lab investigations.

Cytopenias are defined as hemoglobin <10 gm/dL, absolute neurtophil count <1800/mm^3 and platelets <10,000/mm^3. Although 6 months of unexplained cytopenias establish their chronicity for some MDS subtypes,[7] here the gene panel sequencing is suggested to further confirm the diagnosis and its subtyping.

There is a high concordance of mutation detection seen in between peripheral blood (PB) and bone marrow samples. An idea emerged that can we avoid more invasive, painful, and costly bone marrow (BM) investigation once we have mutational panel available with peripheral blood. However, to rule out MDS, where BM morphology is important and simultaneously this will help us to differentiate it from CCUS. Although, in subsequent follow-up of the disease, PB mutational analysis will be a good choice to monitor the progress of the disease.[8]

In CCUS, patients with driver mutations with higher variant allele frequency is indicative of malignant transformation. If VAF of the driver mutation is reported 10%, it is predictive of disease progression.[9] Mutations in spliceosome genes and/or co-mutation patterns of epigenetic genes *DNMT3A, TET2,* and *ASXL1* are highly predictive of progression to a myeloid malignancy with co-occurring mutations in *RUNX1, EZH2, CBL, BCOR, CUX1, TP53,* or *IDH1/IDH2* being most specific for progression to a myeloid neoplasm with MDS.[10]

ROLE OF GENOMIC IN MDS AND MDS/MPN

Currently, there is a proposed classification of MDS [Molecular International Prognostic Scoring System (IPSS-M)] based on mutations, which predicts overall survival, leukemia-free survival and AML transformation. The advantages of applying genomic information in treatment like IDH inhibitors, sub-classification, for example MDS with mutated SF3B1, MDS, and MDS/AML with mutated TP53, and MDS/myeloproliferative neoplasms (MPNs) with thrombocytosis and SF3B1 mutation, all these carry poor prognosis.[11] NGS data (mutated TP53) can play an important role in management of intermediate-risk MDS as per International Prognostic Scoring System-Revised (IPSS-R), who underwent allogeneic hematopoietic stem cell transplantation (allo-HSCT).

In MDS/MPN entity, CMML has shown a driver mutations in >90% of cases which include combination of *TET2* (biallelic variant) and *SF3B1*. This also acts as a diagnostic tool and will be helpful in cases where monocytosis is not evident on morphology (clonal monocytosis of undetermined significance, CMUS). Sometimes, it is also useful to exclude possibility of MDS and MDS/MPN through genomic profiling, if BCR:ABL1 is positive, it excludes any possibility of MDS and MDS/MPNs.

In CMML, somatic mutations play an important role in prognostication also, for this, the gene panel also included analysis of *ASXL1, NRAS, RUNX1,* and *SETBP1*.[12] These patients are eligible for transplantation. Somatic mutations in TP53 also show therapeutic advantages in MDS and MDS/MPNs entities, those who harbor this mutation shows good response to hypomethylating agents (HMAs).[13]

With the help of somatic mutations seen in genomic analysis, we can analyze response to therapy in MDS and MDS/MPNs during follow-up. If after transplantation, still these mutations seen or appearances of newer one, suggests poor outcome or progressive disease.[14] However, still these genomic testing are not in use in clinical practice, it requires further large studies and clinical trials.

In recent clinical trials, many new compounds targeted toward proteins or disrupted signaling pathways because of recurrently mutated genes.[15] One of the best example is lenalidomide in MDS with 5q deletion.

Copy neutral loss of heterozygosity (CN-LOH) detection through SNP array is an important tool to capture multihit TP53 lesions in MDS or MDS/MPN, which carry a poor prognosis.[16]

Although, there are multiple somatic mutations seen in MDS and MDS/MPN, but TP53, FLT3, MLL, and SF3B1 are most clinically relevant.

GENOMICS IN MPNS, MAST CELL NEOPLASMS, AND EOSINOPHILIC NEOPLASM

Classical Myeloproliferative Neoplasms

In routine clinical setting, generally, we screen MPNs for JAK2, CALR, and MPN for establishing the diagnosis. However, in some cases, where these driver mutations are not seen, the NGS panel will look for additional mutations like indel in JAK2 exon 12. In some MPNs mimics (hereditary thrombocytosis or erythrocytosis), NGS panel can differentiate it with MPNs that carry germline variants in JAK2/MPL. A measurement of the VAF of JAKP.V617.F from a PB DNA sample can be helpful in estimating the treatment response or if there is a gradual increasing trend seen in VAF, this is suggestive of progressive disease[17] or resistance to therapy. A base line VAF at the time of diagnosis is recommended for this purpose. NGS testing for other myeloid-related genes also has prognostic value, such as *ASXL1, EZH2, SRSF2, IDH1, IDH2,* and *U2AF1*, these are considered as "high molecular risk" mutations in primary myelofibrosis.[18]

At present, there is still no clear consensus regarding how extensive this NGS panel should be for MPNs, but the inclusion of TP53, NRAS/KRAS, and RUNX1 suggested that it has an impact on prognosis and resistance to therapy.[19] According to some studies, CSF3R mutations also have some role in the treatment response especially toward dasatinib.[20]

If mutations associated with MPNs continue to exist after 3–6 months post-allo-HSCT, this signifies relapse. For this purpose, a PCR test for JAK2P.V617F is highly recommended.[21] Although the confirmation of molecular remission in post-allo-HSCT is confirmed, monitoring of variants is not in clinical practice; however, it may be useful for follow-up in cases of suspected relapse.[4]

Chronic Neutrophilic Leukemia

Among 60–80% of the patients are tested positive for variants in CSF3R In cases of CNL; however, it is not specific to CNL only. This mutation also has also been reported in cases of aCML and CMML. Therapeutic sensitivity of Ruxolitinib also depends on the presence of p.T618I mutation, which shows favorable response to therapy.

Systemic Mastocytosis

In >90% of the cases of systemic mastocytosis (SM), KITp.D816V mutation was identified at the time of diagnosis. Over NGS, here allele-specific PCR or dPCR is preferred for the identification of this mutation. This mutation (KITp.D816V) is reported in terms of VAF, is easily calculated from DNA. In follow-up after initiating therapy with KIT inhibitors (midostaurin, avapritinib), we can assess VAF from PB, which is indicative of response to therapy; although, it is still not used in current clinical practice.[22] Detection of additional somatic mutations by NGS, such as SRSF-2, ASXL1, or RUNX1 carry poor prognosis.[23] In therapy-resistant cases of SM, additional new mutations were seen along with previous one such as KRAS/NRAS and TP53. Cytogenetics carry importance at the time of diagnosis as well as in follow-up (poor prognosis seen in -5,-7, and complex cytogenetics).[24]

Neoplasms with Eosinophilia

The two most common mutations reported in these cases, the first one is FIP1L1::PDGFRA (detected by reverse transcriptase PCR, FISH and NGS assay). The second one KITp.D618V is suggestive of SM as the cause for eosinophilia.[25] BM cytogenetic analysis reveals myeloid/lymphoid neoplasm with eosinophilia MLN—eos (PDGFRA (4q12), PDGFRB (5q31-33), FGFR1 (8p11), FLT3 (13q12), and JAK2 (9p24) and TK gene fusion. Clonality of eosinophilia can be ascertained by the presence of somatic mutations as well as chromosomal deletions, monosomies, and complex karyotyping. FISH is an ideal test for *TK* gene rearrangement; however, NGS is best for the detection of cryptic fusions. During follow-up, FISH (for PDGFRA rearrangement) and RT-PCR (fusion transcripts) are used when patient is on TKIs.[4]

Clonal T cells (checked by PCR or NGS) can be seen in reactive as well as in clonal eosinophilia suggestive of lymphocytic hypereosinophilic syndrome variant.

Chronic Myeloid Leukemia

Chronic myeloid leukemia is one of the most commonly used HM where genomic studies are extensively applied. The detection of BCR::ABL1 translocation with the help of FISH or RT-PCR is the mainstay at the time of diagnosis. However, follow-up after TKIs quantitative estimation of BCR-ABL is indicative of therapeutic response. Rise in copy number of BCR::ABL1 suggests the resistance or relapse of disease. The resistance to therapy is due to ABL1 Kinase domain mutations in approximately 50% of the cases. However, NGS panel studies suggests that other myeloid neoplasm-related mutations also appears in rest of the therapy-resistance cases.[26] These include RUNX1 and ASXL1 mutations, and IKZF1 deletions. NCCN guidelines suggest cases of CML in lymphoid blast crisis or accelerated phase and those CML cases which are negative for kinase domain mutations should be searched for myeloid mutation panel. Although, myeloid mutation panel is not seen among cases of lymphoid blast crisis.

GENOMIC TESTING IN ACUTE MYELOID LEUKEMIA

In a newly reported case of acute myeloid leukemia (AML), before going to costly genomic testing, we have to narrow down the diagnosis with the help of morphology, Cytogenetics, FISH, RT-PCR, and multicolor flow cytometry (MFC). However, as there is recent development in molecular sub-classification of AML by WHO[27], it is required that each and every AML should have genomic testing for common myeloid mutations. It is suggested that we can wait for at least 5 days till the reports of mutational analysis available through NGS panel[28] before starting of therapy.

With the help of NGS panel, we can further sub-classify AML (risk stratification) and design a targeted therapy, such as adverse risk AML (AML with MDS-related mutations), intermediate risk (AML with FLT3-ITD) and favorable (AML with CEBPA mutations). NGS panel should also include the IDH1, IDH2, FLT-ITD, and FLT3-TKD. So targeted therapy can be planned accordingly. The last two mutations are usually detected separately through PCR and capillary electrophoresis.

Immunohistochemistry also advised in resource-limited conditions, for which protein expression of NPM1 can detected on formalin-fixed paraffin embedded samples or cell block. Similarly, IDH1 and IDH2 also demonstrated. Mutation in p53 expressed as accumulation of null protein, on IHC and suggestive of AML with TP53 mutation.[29]

As recurrent genetic abnormalities are quite common in AML, "Myeloid FISH Panels" is suggested especially where metaphase cytogenetics facilities are not available.[30] However, above all, if facilities are available for NGS, it is highly recommended to go for whole genome sequencing (WGS). It will answer all queries related to indel, SNV, CNV, SV (structural variant), and LOH (loss of heterozygosity). However, currently in India, this facility is not easily available at every tertiary care center or medical institutes.

Another aspect of NGS is the monitoring of AML in follow-up after chemotherapy. This MRD assay can be done by qPCR, dPCR (digital droplet PCR) and MFC also. By MRD assay, we can identify the impending response of therapy, and it will help us to modify the treatment if required. In the case of favorable AML category, we can plan for all-HSCT after consolidation phase where MRD is still positive. On the basis of MRD, a 5-year overall survival can also be predicted as it was confirmed through a meta-analysis of >10,000 patients, where significant differences were reported among MRD-positive and MRD-negative groups (34% vs. 68%).[31]

MRD monitoring is done using MFC as well as by RT-PCR, but if mutation is seen in *NPM1* gene and core-binding factor (CBF), MRD evaluation best done using RT-PCR technique. Estimation of tumor load should be performed at the time of diagnosis as well, so the kinetics of disease can be understood.[32]

NGS has upper edge over RT-PCR and MFC. It can detect newer mutations that appear during the course of treatment, which were not present at the time of diagnosis. Which MRD detection method will work best depends on the type of mutations present and the phenotype of the disease.[33] Driver mutations, such as RUNX1::RUNX1T1 and CBFB::MYH11, which are typically present on initial clonal cells are also seen in MRD analysis; although, the quantitation may change. But the mutations of signaling genes such as FLT3-ITD, NRAS/KRAS are often sub-clonal and may not be present on each and every clone over time. Hence, we cannot use it for MRD evaluation. Similarly, we should not take epigenetic mutations as an indicator of relapse, especially "DTA" (DNMT3A, TET2, ASXL1); they represent the preleukemic clone and do not indicate a relapse.[34]

The importance of MRD in AML was confirmed in a meta-analysis of >80 publications with >10,000 patients; the estimated 5-year overall survival was 68% versus 34% in patients in AML remission with MRD$^-$ versus MRD$^+$ status.[31] Although proven interventions to eradicate MRD are currently lacking, the detection of persistent MRD after completion of consolidation, or MRD "relapse," correlates with inferior outcomes including increased risk of relapse and decreased overall survival. Current guidelines recommend MRD assessments after two cycles of standard therapy at the end of treatment, and then evaluation every 3 months (if BM) or every 4–6 weeks (if PB) for 24 months.[35]

In cases of AML, MRD estimation by molecular methods versus MFC, the results are equivalent. However, in cases where RT-qPCR assay (e.g., NPM1, CBF fusion) is available, it can be the preferred method for MRD over NGS, and it should be done at diagnostic sample as well as on MRD to understand dynamics of disease and evaluate response to therapy.[32] Diagnostic sensitivity of bone marrow sample is definitely above the peripheral blood.

Apart from the RT-qPCR, NGS is considered as an alternative method for MRD assay, it can provide a detailed information about the dynamics of underlying malignancies over time, appearances of new mutations along with previous one over a time scale. FCM and NGS both can be used for MRD assay depending upon the mutations present and the phenotype. The results of both of these techniques are mutually agreeable.[33] Note that the sensitivity of most routine NGS panels is ~2% VAF; however, the ELN recommends error-corrected NGS with a minimum sensitivity of ~0.1% VAF[35] Caution must be taken in the interpretation of residual epigenetic mutations, including "DTA" (DNMT3A, TET2, ASXL1), which represent pre leukemic clones and are not predictive of relapse.[34] Residual SRSF2 and IDH1/2 mutations may be similarly non-informative for MRD assessment.[36]

ACUTE LYMPHOBLASTIC LEUKEMIA

Genomic studies have significantly expand our knowledge of cute lymphoblastic leukemia (ALL) and have led to the discovery of new entities within this disease allowing, for more precise diagnosis, prognosis, and treatment strategies. This represent a more personalized and targeted approach to manage ALL.

Sequencing-based approaches in ALL play a critical role in MRD-based risk-adapted therapy by providing a comprehensive and dynamic view of the ALL's genetic features. This enable more precise individualized treatment decisions, ultimately improving the prognosis and outcome for ALL patients. The choice of diagnostic approaches in genomic testing in ALL is a multifaceted decision that takes into account the purpose of the diagnosis, the available tools and the broader clinical and operational context. We can further divide these investigations into three categories and will discuss their advantages as well as limitations in context of ALL.

Routine Diagnostic Approaches

Chromosomal banding analysis and FISH are indispensible tools in the diagnosis and management of ALL. They enable the precise identification of aneuploidy, subtype defining chromosomal alterations, translocations, and gene fusions (e.g., BCR::ABL1, ETV6::RUNX1, KMT2A::AFF1, TCF3::PBX1, and iAMP21). This in turn informs the risk assessment and selection of targeted therapies, leading to more personalized and effective treatment strategies for ALL. Limitations of FISH seen during identification of focal insertion of EPOR into immunoglobulin loci, and sequence mutations in JAK signaling genes, FISH not able to pick it up. However, PCR easily get all these sequence mutations.

The role of quantitative RT-PCR in BCR::ABL1 is Like ALL, where it provides valuable information about the gene expression profile; however, it may not be able to identify all the driver kinase activation alteration. That is why subsequent testing is required in the form of FISH and sequencing. Limitations of RT-PCR are that it will not provide information about the underlying DNA sequences or any structural abnormalities in gene. However, RT-PCR can identify deregulated gene expression which is specific to recently recognized ALL subtypes (DUX4, EPOR, NUTM1, and CDX2/UBTF).[37]

The MCF can be useful to identify subclasses of ALL, which has a rearrangement of *DUX4* gene, this type of ALL is showing the expression of CD371. MCF detects CD371 in these ALL cells and can helpful in identifying these rare types of ALL which have specific prognosis and response to therapy. Similarly, there is another subtype of B-ALL (CRFL2 rearranged ALL) where leukemic cells show the expression of thymic stromal lymphopoietin receptor (TSLPR). MFC can easily identify these antigens on leukemic cells and help in further sub-classification of ALL.

Capture-based Sequencing Approaches

Capture-based or amplicon-based sequencing are advanced techniques used in genomics to identify alteration including chimeric fusion (primarily focused on entronic regions) in various HM including ALL also. These methods are highly effective in identifying many common chimeric fusions, for example, BCR::ABL1 like B-ALL.

However, there are certain limitations to these capture-based or amplicon-based methods also. These methods are unable to identify complex rearrangements such as insertion of *EPOR* gene into immunoglobulin loci, which can involve intricate structural changes that are challenging to be captured using these methods.

Apart from this, another limitations of capture-based techniques is that it cannot identify intronic breakpoints, because their primary focus is on exonic region breakpoints. To address this limitation, long-read sequencing or whole genome sequencing may be used.

Multiplex ligation-dependent probe amplification (MLPA) is a valuable molecular biology technique used to identify specific DNA CNAs in a single gene or genomic regions. In B-ALL, this technique is used to detect IKZF1^{plus} composite genotype. It includes deletion of IKZF1 co-occurring with other genes, such as CDKN2A/B, PAX5 or the pseudoautosomal region 1 (PAR1). Altogether, this deletion carries poor prognosis.

The MLPA has certain limitations, for instance, it may not be able to identify all relevant alterations associated with a specific gene arrangement in ALL. It can detect only few cases of CRFL2 – ALL (where PAR1 deletion is detected) rest become undetected like IGH::CRFL2. Similarly, ERG deletions are associated with only 50% of the cases of ALL with DUX4 subtype; it means the rest 50% of the cases will remain undetected by MLPA.

To compensate this deficiency, other molecular testing should be used in conjunction with FISH, qRT-PCR, and NGS to overcome the limitations of individual test. Together, all these tests can provide a more detailed information about specific genetic rearrangements, breakpoints and fusion genes. Combining multiple diagnostic methods can enhance the accuracy of subtype classification and risk assessment in ALL, giving appropriate treatment strategies for the affected individual.

Transcriptomic and Genomic Sequencing

Transcriptome sequencing often referred to WTS or RNA sequencing, is a powerful tool that provides a comprehensive view of transcriptome, allowing for the characterization of gene expression, identification of fusion transcript chimeras, mutant allele expression and ploidy.[38] It can identify different subgroups and phenocopies within a disease like, BCR::ABL1 like ALL, ETV6::RUNX1 like ALL, KMT2A like ZNF 384/362.

WTS is a valuable tool for studying gene expression, it may face challenges in detection of rearrangement that involves complex and repetitive regions of the genome, such as antigen receptor loci or DUX4.[39] Whole genome sequencing (WGS) is often employed to complement WTS, providing a more comprehensive analysis of the entire genome, especially in cases where detailed information about structural variations or noncoding regions is crucial. WTS is less effective in detecting sequence variants that are not expressed or that result in nonsense-mediated decay. It means, variants are present in DNA but are not actively transcribed.

To address the limitations of WTS, WGS is often used. WGS provides a broader view of the entire genome including complex and repetitive regions and can detect non-expressed variants. It can be particularly valuable in cases where WTS falls short.

T-ALL subgroup can be defined as the deregulation of T-lineage transcription factor and their downstream target genes. These transcription factors play a critical role in normal T-cell development, and their dysregulation can lead to leukemia. The gene involved and the specific genomic drivers of dysregulation can vary widely from one T-ALL cases to another. Diversity of gene and genomic drivers involved in T-ALL, NGS-based methods can analyze the genetic alteration and identify specified deregulated genes and pathways.

In deregulation of T-lineage transcription factor, it is important to note that they are not continuously associated with clinical outcome. In some cases, the specific subtype of T-ALL may not have significant impact on prognosis and treatment response. Therefore, T-ALL subgroup may not be rationally included in the current diagnostic workflow aimed at risk assessment or treatment stratification. WGS can detect diverse genomic alteration in T-ALL which includes intergenic regions (e.g., TLX3, T-cell receptor gene loci) that deregulate oncogenes, and noncoding sequence mutations that generate neo-enhancers (e.g., TAL1 and LMO1/2).[40]

Early T-cell precursor ALL (ETP-ALL) is an interesting entity of clinical relevance and represents a high-risk subset of T-Lineage leukemia. It is characterized by specific immunophenotypic (CD7$^+$, Cyto CD3$^+$, CD2$^+$, CD1a$^-$, CD8$^-$, MPO$^-$ but positive for at least one stem cell marker CD34/CD117)[39] features, which make it distinct from other types of T-ALL. It carries poor prognosis. Apart from distinctive immunophenotype, it also shows specific genetic abnormalities, which include mutations in gene like *DNMT2A* and *FLT3*. This T-ALL requires more aggressive chemotherapy and HSCT as treatment. Presence of structural variants affecting BCL11B in ETP-ALL highlights the genetic complexity of this leukemia subtype. A distinct immunophenotype suggests the possibility of BCL11B (CD117/CD34$^+$, cyto CD3$^+$, always CD2$^+$, always CD5$^-$, always CD8$^-$, variable for MPO and other myeloid markers). An interesting feature seen in BCL11B subtype is that it shows activating mutations in *FLT3* gene (identified in 80.1% samples) which draw the attention for targeted therapy with gilteritinib. Venetoclax (anti-BCL2) also shows promising results in ETP-ALL cases. With the help of NGS and FISH, we can easily detect that structural variants deregulate BCL11B locus **(Table 4)**.[41,42]

Molecular Quantitation of Measurable Residual Disease

Monitoring MRD during and after the induction and consolidation phase of leukemia therapy is of paramount importance for assessing a patient's response to treatment and predicting their prognosis. It also plays a critical role in tailoring therapeutic strategies. The following are common methods for evaluating MRD:

Multicolor Flow Cytometry

It can detect the antigen expressed on the cell surface as well as in cytoplasm. It is a widely used method for MRD assessment in cases of leukemia. It has the sensitivity of around $\leq 10^{-4}$, which makes it relevant in many cases.

Allele-specific PCR for IG/TCR Gene Rearrangement

A-PCR technique is used to identify as well as quantify specific gene arrangement in leukemic cells. The sensitivity of this method is around 10^{-4}.

High-throughput Next Generation Sequencing

It involves the sequencing of DNA of leukemic cells, specially targeting the *IG* and *TCR* gene. Its sensitivity reaches up to 10^{-6} and makes it capable of detecting extremely low levels of MRD.

The choice of MRD methods depends on various factors including the clinical context, the patient's specific disease characteristics and the available resources. NGS with its high sensitivity is increasingly being used in clinical practice and research because it can detect very low level of MRD that might otherwise missed. This is particularly beneficial to risk assessment and early interventions in high-risk cases.

■ GENERAL CONCLUSIONS AND FUTURE DIRECTIONS

Hematological neoplasms are characterized by a complex and dynamic interplay of multiple clones of abnormal cells that evolve over time. This complexity is often referred to as clonal heterogeneity. The coexistence of multiple evolving clones is a hallmark of HM (myeloid neoplasms and acute leukemia). The complexity highlights the need for personalized treatment strategies that takes into account the genetic heterogeneity and dynamic changes within the disease ultimately improving the management of these conditions.

Recent advancements in single-cell level studies have provided unique insight into the clonal architecture of disease including HM. These studies reveal the intricate interactions and relationship between different clones shedding lights on how the presence of distinct clones can influence each other growth and fitness. These interactions have a profound impact on the behavior and progression of disease. This information can influence treatment strategies and potentially leads to more effective therapeutic interventions.

As our understanding of genomics and molecular basis of HM improves, there is a growing emphasis on precision medicine. This approach tailored

TABLE 4: Food and Drug Administration (FDA) approved targeted therapies for tumors that have an associated biomarker.[43]

Preferred name	Direct drug target	Company	FDA approved indication—disease(s)	FDA approved indication—biomarker(s)
Bosutinib	ABL1, BCR-ABL1, SRC	Pfizer	Chronic myelogenous leukemia	BCR-ABL1
Dasatinib	ABL1, KIT, BRAF, BCR-ABL1, ABL2, PDGFRA, PDGFRB, SRC, DDR1, DDR2, EPHA3 Amplification, EPHA2, FYN, LCK, LYN, YES1	Bristol-Myers Squibb	Chronic myelogenous leukemia	BCR-ABL1
			Acute lymphoblastic leukemia	BCR-ABL1
Enasidenib	IDH2	Agios Pharmaceuticals	Acute myeloid leukemia	IDH2 mutation
Gemtuzumab ozogamicin	CD33	Pfizer	Acute myeloid leukemia	CD33$^+$
Imatinib	PDGFRA, KIT, BCR-ABL1, ABL1, PDGFRB	Novartis Pharmaceuticals	Gastrointestinal Stromal Tumors	KIT$^+$
			Chronic myeloid leukemia, Acute lymphoblastic leukemia	BCR-ABL1
			Myelodysplastic/Myeloproliferative diseases	PDGFRA fusion
			Chronic eosinophilic leukemia	FIP1L1-PDGFRA
Midostaurin	KDR, FLT3, PDGFRA, PDGFRB, SYK, AKT1, FLT1, AKT2, AKT3, KIT, SRC, PRKCA, PRKCB, PRKCG, CDK1, FGR, ETV6-NTRK3	Novartis Pharmaceuticals	Acute myeloid leukemia	FLT3 mutation
Nilotinib	BCR-ABL1	Novartis Pharmaceuticals	Chronic myelogenous leukemia	BCR-ABL1
Ponatinib	PDGFRA, KDR, SRC, ABL1, FGFR1, BCR-ABL1, KIT, RET	Ariad Pharmaceuticals	Acute lymphoblastic leukemia/lymphoblastic lymphoma, chronic myeloid leukemia	BCR-ABL1, T315I
			Chronic myeloid leukemia, acute lymphoblastic leukemia	BCR-ABL1
Venetoclax	BCL2	AbbVie	Chronic lymphocytic leukemia	c.CHR17p deletion
Rituximab	CD20	Genentech	Non-Hodgkin's lymphoma, chronic lymphocytic leukemia	CD20$^+$

TABLE 5: Targeted therapy and their efficacy in HM.[42]

Drug	Disease indication	Line of therapy	Aberrant gene	Number of studies*	Response rate (%)
Hematologic malignancies: Fusion target					
All trans-retinoic acid	APL	1+	PML-RARA	1	72
Bosutinib	CML	2+	BCR-ABL	2	31
Dasatinib	CML	1+	BCR-ABL	2	63
Imatinib	CML	1	BCR-ABL	1	73
Nilotinib	CML	1+	BCR-ABL	1	84
Ponatinib	CML	2+	BCR-ABL	1	46
Hematologic malignancies: Target non-fusion					
Enasidenib	AML	2+	IDH2	1	23
Gilteritinib	AML	2+	FLT3	1	21
Ivosidenib	AML	2+	IDH1	1	33
Vemurafenib	ECD	1+	BRAF	1	55

*Refers to the number of studies provided in the US Food and drug administration package insert; the response rate was per package insert. If >1 study was listed, the mean is shown.

treatment strategies to the individual genetic and molecular characteristics of patient and their disease. As more targeted therapy available, recommendations for testing and treatment are likely to become more personalized.

Recently (2018) Food and Drug Administration (FDA), USA approved targeted therapy for certain tumors that have an associated biomarker given in **Table 4**.

Although we are talking too much about targeted therapy but still there are other factors which also influence the outcome, which is still under experimental research (like microenvironment) that's why the efficacy of these magical drugs are limited to certain extent only **Table 5**.

Recommendations for testing and treatment in the field of HM as well as other areas of medicine are continually evolving. This evolution is driven by advances in our understanding of disease, changes in disease classification, and the development of new treatments and the ongoing refinement of genetic testing methods. Staying up to date with latest guidelines and participating in ongoing education and research are critical for health care professionals to provide the best care for patients.

REFERENCES

1. Alaggio R, Amador C, Anagnostopoulos I, Attygalle AD, Araujo IB de O, Berti E, et al. The 5th edition of the World Health Organization Classification of Haematolymphoid Tumours: Lymphoid Neoplasms. Leukemia. 2022;36(7):1720-48.

2. Warner JL. Giving up on precision oncology? Not so fast! Clin Transl Sci. 2017;10(3): 128-9.
3. Riehn M, Klopocki E, Molkentin M, Reinhardt R, Burmeister T. A BACH2-BCL2L1 fusion gene resulting from a lymphoma cell line BLUE-1. Cancer. 2011;396:389-96.
4. Duncavage EJ, Bagg A, Hasserjian RP, DiNardo CD, Godley LA, Iacobucci I, et al. Genomic profiling for clinical decision making in myeloid neoplasms and acute leukemia. Blood. 2022;140(21):2228-47.
5. Desai P, Mencia-Trinchant N, Savenkov O, Simon MS, Cheang G, Lee S, et al. Somatic mutations precede acute myeloid leukemia years before diagnosis. Nat Med [Internet]. 2018;24(7):1015-23.
6. Bick AG, Pirruccello JP, Griffin GK, Gupta N, Gabriel S, Saleheen D, et al. Genetic interleukin 6 signaling deficiency attenuates cardiovascular risk in clonal hematopoiesis. Circulation. 2020;141(2):124-31.
7. Arber DA, Orazi A, Hasserjian R, Thiele J, Borowitz MJ, Le Beau MM, et al. The 2016 revision to the World Health Organization classification of myeloid neoplasms and acute leukemia. Blood. 2016;127(20):2391-405.
8. Duncavage EJ, Uy GL, Petti AA, Miller CA, Lee YS, Tandon B, et al. Mutational landscape and response are conserved in peripheral blood of AML and MDS patients during decitabine therapy. Blood [Internet]. 2017;129(10):1397-401. Available from: http://dx.doi.org/10.1182/blood-2016-10-745273
9. Malcovati L, Gallì A, Travaglino E, Ambaglio I, Rizzo E, Molteni E, et al. Clinical significance of somatic mutation in unexplained blood cytopenia. Blood. 2017;129(25):3371-8.
10. Gallì A, Todisco G, Catamo E, Sala C, Elena C, Pozzi S, et al. Relationship between clone metrics and clinical outcome in clonal cytopenia. Blood. 2021;138(11):965-76.
11. Bernard E, Tuechler H, Greenberg PL, Hasserjian RP, Arango Ossa JE, Nannya Y, et al. Molecular international prognostic scoring system for myelodysplastic syndromes. NEJM Evid. 2022;1(7):1-14.
12. Elena C, Gallì A, Such E, Meggendorfer M, Germing U, Rizzo E, et al. Integrating clinical features and genetic lesions in the risk assessment of patients with chronic myelomonocytic leukemia. Blood. 2016;128(10):1408-17.
13. Welch JS, Petti AA, Miller CA, Fronick CC, O'Laughlin M, Fulton RS, et al. TP53 and Decitabine in Acute Myeloid Leukemia and Myelodysplastic Syndromes . N Engl J Med. 2016;375(21):2023-36.
14. Duncavage EJ, Jacoby MA, Chang GS, Miller CA, Edwin N, Shao J, et al. Mutation clearance after transplantation for myelodysplastic syndrome. N Engl J Med. 2018;379(11):1028-41.
15. Sallman DA, DeZern AE, Garcia-Manero G, Steensma DP, Roboz GJ, Sekeres MA, et al. Eprenetapopt (APR-246) and azacitidine in TP53-mutant myelodysplastic syndromes. J Clin Oncol. 2021;39(14):1584-94.
16. Yoshizato T, Nannya Y, Atsuta Y, Shiozawa Y, Iijima-Yamashita Y, Yoshida K, et al. Genetic abnormalities in myelodysplasia and secondary acute myeloid leukemia: impact on outcome of stem cell transplantation. Blood [Internet]. 2017;129(17):2347-58.
17. Loscocco GG, Guglielmelli P, Gangat N, Rossi E, Mannarelli C, Betti S, et al. Clinical and molecular predictors of fibrotic progression in essential thrombocythemia: a multicenter study involving 1607 patients. Am J Hematol. 2021;96(11):1472-80.
18. Vannucchi AM, Lasho TL, Guglielmelli P, Biamonte F, Pardanani A, Pereira A, et al. Mutations and prognosis in primary myelofibrosis. Leukemia [Internet]. 2013;27(9):1861-9.
19. Coltro G, Rotunno G, Mannelli L, Mannarelli C, Fiaccabrino S, Romagnoli S, et al. RAS/CBL mutations predict resistance to JAK inhibitors in myelofibrosis and are associated with poor prognostic features. Blood Adv. 2020;4(15):3677-87.

20. Schwartz MS, Wieduwilt MJ. CSF3R truncation mutations in a patient with B-cell acute lymphoblastic leukemia and a favorable response to chemotherapy plus dasatinib. Leuk Res Reports [Internet]. 2020;14:100208.
21. Wolschke C, Badbaran A, Zabelina T, Christopeit M, Ayuk F, Triviai I, et al. Impact of molecular residual disease post allografting in myelofibrosis patients. Bone Marrow Transplant [Internet]. 2017;52(11):1526-9.
22. Gotlib J, Reiter A, Radia DH, Deininger MW, George TI, Panse J, et al. Efficacy and safety of avapritinib in advanced systemic mastocytosis: interim analysis of the phase 2 PATHFINDER trial. Nat Med. 2021;27(12):2192-9.
23. Jawhar M, Schwaab J, Schnittger S, Meggendorfer M, Pfirrmann M, Sotlar K, et al. Additional mutations in SRSF2, ASXL1 and/or RUNX1 identify a high-risk group of patients with KIT D816V+ advanced systemic mastocytosis. Leukemia [Internet]. 2016;30(1):136-43.
24. Jaiswal S, Ebert BL. Clonal hematopoiesis in human aging and disease. Science (80-). 2019;366(6465):eaan4673.
25. Kluin-Nelemans HC, Reiter A, Illerhaus A, van Anrooij B, Hartmann K, Span LFR, et al. Prognostic impact of eosinophils in mastocytosis: analysis of 2350 patients collected in the ECNM Registry. Leukemia [Internet]. 2020;34(4):1090-101.
26. Branford S, Kim DDH, Apperley JF, Eide CA, Mustjoki S, Ong ST, et al. Laying the foundation for genomically-based risk assessment in chronic myeloid leukemia. Leukemia [Internet]. 2019;33(8):1835-50.
27. Khoury JD, Solary E, Abla O, Akkari Y, Alaggio R, Apperley JF, et al. The 5th edition of the World Health Organization Classification of Haematolymphoid Tumours: Myeloid and Histiocytic/Dendritic Neoplasms. Leukemia. 2022;36(7):1703-19.
28. Röllig C, Kramer M, Schliemann C, Mikesch JH, Steffen B, Krämer A, et al. Does time from diagnosis to treatment affect the prognosis of patients with newly diagnosed acute myeloid leukemia? Blood. 2020;136(7):823-30.
29. Tashakori M, Kadia T, Loghavi S, Daver N, Kanagal-Shamanna R, Pierce S, et al. TP53 copy number and protein expression inform mutation status across risk categories in acute myeloid leukemia. Blood [Internet]. 2022;140(1):58-72.
30. Nelson ND, McMahon CM, El-Sharkawy Navarro F, Freyer CW, Roth JJ, Luger SM, et al. Rapid fluorescence in situ hybridisation optimises induction therapy for acute myeloid leukaemia. Br J Haematol. 2020;191(5):935-8.
31. Short NJ, Zhou S, Fu C, Berry DA, Walter RB, Freeman SD, et al. Association of measurable residual disease with survival outcomes in patients with acute myeloid leukemia: a systematic review and meta-analysis. JAMA Oncol. 2020;6(12):1890-9.
32. Gorello P, Cazzaniga G, Alberti F, Dell'Oro MG, Gottardi E, Specchia G, et al. Quantitative assessment of minimal residual disease in acute myeloid leukemia carrying nucleophosmin (NPM1) gene mutations. Leukemia. 2006;20(6):1103-8.
33. Jongen-Lavrencic M, Grob T, Hanekamp D, Kavelaars FG, al Hinai A, Zeilemaker A, et al. Molecular minimal residual disease in acute myeloid leukemia. N Engl J Med. 2018;378(13):1189-99.
34. Tanaka T, Morita K, Loghavi S, Wang F, Furudate K, Sasaki Y, et al. Clonal dynamics and clinical implications of postremission clonal hematopoiesis in acute myeloid leukemia. Blood [Internet]. 2021;138(18):1733-9.
35. Heuser M, Freeman SD, Ossenkoppele GJ, Buccisano F, Hourigan CS, Ngai LL, et al. 2021 Update on MRD in acute myeloid leukemia: a consensus document from the European LeukemiaNet MRD working party. Blood. 2021;138(26):2753-67.
36. Cappelli LV, Meggendorfer M, Baer C, Nadarajah N, Hutter S, Jeromin S, et al. Indeterminate and oncogenic potential: CHIP vs CHOP mutations in AML with NPM1 alteration. Leukemia. 2022;36(2):394-402.

37. Kimura S, Montefiori L, Iacobucci I, Zhao Y, Gao Q, Paietta EM, et al. Enhancer retargeting of CDX2 and UBTF::ATXN7L3 define a subtype of high-risk B-progenitor acute lymphoblastic leukemia. Blood. 2022;139(24):3519-31.
38. Montefiori LE, Bendig S, Gu Z, Chen X, Pölönen P, Ma X, et al. Enhancer hijacking drives oncogenic bcl11b expression in lineage-ambiguous stem cell leukemia. Cancer Discov. 2021;11(11):284-67.
39. Coustan-Smith E, Mullighan CG, Onciu M, Behm FG, Raimondi SC, Pei D, Cheng C, Su X, Rubnitz JE, Basso G, Biondi A, Pui CH, Downing JR, Campana D. Early T-cell precursor leukaemia: a subtype of very high-risk acute lymphoblastic leukaemia. Lancet Oncol. 2009;10(2):147-56.
40. Iacobucci I, Kimura S, Mullighan CG. Biologic and therapeutic implications of genomic alterations in acute lymphoblastic leukemia. J Clin Med. 2021;10(17):3792.
41. Montefiori LE, Mullighan CG. Redefining the biological basis of lineage-ambiguous leukemia through genomics: BCL11B deregulation in acute leukemias of ambiguous lineage. Best Pract Res Clin Haematol. 2021;34(4):101329.
42. Nikanjam M, Okamura R, Barkauskas DA, Kurzrock R. Targeting fusions for improved outcomes in oncology treatment. Cancer. 2020;126(6):1315-21.
43. Kurnit KC, Dumbrava EE, Litzenburger B, Khotskaya YB, Johnson AM, Yap TA, et al. Precision oncology decision support: current approaches and strategies for the future. Clin Cancer Res. 2018;24(12):2719-31.

CHAPTER 11

Hereditary Hemorrhagic Telangiectasia/Osler–Weber–Rendu Syndrome

Nuzhat Samoon, Ambreen Beigh

■ INTRODUCTION

Hereditary hemorrhagic telangiectasia (HHT) synonymous with Osler–Weber–Rendu syndrome is an inherited vascular disorder that causes abnormal vascular connections, called arteriovenous malformations (AVMs), to develop between small vessels. This disease is named after the physicians William Osler, Frederick Parkes Weber, and Henri Jules Louis Marie Rendu.[1]

It often poses a diagnostic dilemma due to variable clinical presentations including mucocutaneous telangiectasia, epistaxis, gastrointestinal (GI) bleeding, and deficiency anemias.[2-4] Its severity can vary greatly from patient to patient.

Hereditary hemorrhagic telangiectasia is a multisystemic disorder commonly occurring in the pulmonary, hepatic, and cerebral circulations, which may manifest as pulmonary hypertension, hepatic failure, cardiac failure, and cerebrovascular events.

All individuals are susceptible from any racial and ethnic class for HHT. HHT if diagnosed early, effective treatments are available. However, there is no cure for HHT.

■ EPIDEMIOLOGY

Hereditary hemorrhagic telangiectasia affects nearly 1 in 5,000 individuals in North America.[5] The prevalence is highest in the Afro-Caribbean regions of the Dutch Antilles and France.[6]

Individuals with HHT have a reduced life expectancy, highly depending on the severity of condition. Patients without internal organ manifestations (such as hepatic, cerebral, or pulmonary AVMs) are expected to have a normal or near-normal lifespan, but approximately 10% of patients may become debilitated or scum to death from HHT-related complications.[7]

Pathogenesis

It is an autosomal disorder characterized by vascular malformations including AVMs and telangiectasias. AVMs may be composed of small (1-3 cm), micro (< 1 cm) AVMs, or direct high flow connections.[8] The diagnosis of HHT is clinical, based on Curacao criteria **(Table 1)**.

Gene Mutations

Hereditary hemorrhagic telangiectasia is suspected to be haploinsufficiency where two wild-type copies of a gene for a normal phenotype is required and one functional gene copy cannot produce enough protein to preserve function of the cell.[9]

In 97% of individuals with HHT diagnosis, a causative mutation is identified in one of the genes: *Endoglin, activin A receptor-like type 1* (*ACVRL1*), and *SMAD4*.[10]

Classification and Genetics of Most Common Hereditary Hemorrhagic Telangiectasia Subtypes (Table 2)

HHT1

HHT1 originates from mutations in the gene *Endoglin*, located on chromosome 9q34 encoding protein endoglin (CD105).[11] This was the first gene to be identified showing implication in the HHT pathogenesis.

Endoglin, a cell surface glycoprotein and part of the transforming growth factor-beta (TGF-β) receptor complex is needed for vascular modeling and its integrity.

TABLE 1: Curacao criteria for the diagnosis of HHT.	
Epistaxis	Spontaneous or recurrent nose bleeds
Telangiectasia	Multiple at characteristic sites (lips, oral cavity, nose, and fingers)
Visceral arteriovenous malformations/ telangiectasias	Any of the following: • Cerebral AVM • Spinal AVM • Pulmonary AVM • Hepatic AVM • Gastrointestinal telangiectasias
Family history	A first degree relative with HHT according to these criteria: • Definite HHT: 3–4 criteria present • Possible/suspected HHT: 2 criteria present • Unlikely HHT: 0–1 criteria are present

(AVM: arteriovenous malformation; HHT: hereditary hemorrhagic telangiectasia)

TABLE 2: Classification and genetics of most common HHT subtypes.

HHT	Genetic mutation	Visceral manifestations	Function of gene product involved
Type 1	Endoglin-ENG (9q34.11)	• Pulmonary AVMs • Brain AVMs	Membrane glycoprotein receptor on endothelial cells, part of the transforming growth factor-beta receptor pathway
Type 2	Activin receptor-like kinase 1 (ALK1)-ACVRL1	• Hepatic AVMs • Spinal AVMs • Pulmonary AVMs	ALK1, a cell surface serine/threonine-protein kinase receptor
Type 3: JP-HHT (associated with juvenile polyposis)	MADH4 (SMAD4)	• Gastrointestinal polyps • Pulmonary hypertension	MADH4 encodes SMAD4 (a mediator in the TGF-β signaling pathway)

(AVM: arteriovenous malformation; HHT: hereditary hemorrhagic telangiectasia)

HHT2

HHT2 condition results from mutations in *ACVRL1* gene on chromosome 12q13 encoding protein activin receptor-like kinase 1 (ALK1).[12] Activin receptor-like kinase 1 a type 1 cell-surface receptor functions as a part of TGF-β signaling complex and plays a role in the regulation of angiogenesis.[13]

HHT3: Associated with Juvenile Polyposis (JPHT or JP-HHT)

HHT3 arises from the mutation in the gene mothers against decapentaplegic homolog 4 (*MADH4*) that encodes SMAD4, a transcription factor which is a critical downstream effector of TGF-β signaling pathway.[14] The mutation types including nonsense, missense, frameshift, and de novo in HHT3 are located on the last four exons of SMAD4.[15]

All the three identified genes *Endoglin*, *ALK1*, and *SMAD4* involved in implication of HHT interfere in normal cellular functions via TGF-β/BMP signaling pathway, which play a key role in cell growth, differentiation, apoptosis, and angiogenesis. TGF-β signaling occurs through phosphorylation of TGF-β receptor 1 by TGF-β receptor 2 which activates downstream signaling by phosphorylation of SMADs on the membrane of the cells. SMAD4 (specific SMAD protein) transfers this information to the nucleus and regulates transcription of the target genes.

In healthy affected individuals, ligands such as TGF-β, activins, and BMPs in extracellular space bind to serine/threonine receptors of the cell membrane. TGF-β1/2/3 ligand binds to the type II receptor of the TGF-β signaling cascade (TGFβRII) that becomes phosphorylated and recruits the TGF-β type I receptors ALK1 or ALK5.[16]

HISTOPATHOLOGY

Histological changes show dilated different calibre walled vessels lined by flattened endothelial cells and abrupt changes in thickness of medial and elastic layers of vessels.

Clinical Manifestations

It is characterized by presence of multiple AVMs. Smaller ones are known as telangiectasis and the larger ones (few millimeters to several centimeters in diameter) are referred to as AVMs.

Common AVM manifestations include epistaxis, telangiectasis, neurological changes, GI bleeding, iron deficiency anemia, pulmonary hypertension, heart failure, and hepatic failure.

Epistaxis

Minor trauma to the nasal mucosa results in recurrent episodes of nasal bleed. Around 90% individuals have onset before the attainment of adulthood.

The episodes of epistaxis increases with age as has been reported that 95% of all HHT patients eventually develop recurrent epistaxis.[17]

However, many do not have nose bleeds that are severe enough to call for medical attention and have been graded as mild, moderate, and severe depending on the episodes and treatment required.
- Grade 1—a few episodes of epistaxis per week without requirement of transfusion
- Grade 2—one or two episodes of epistaxis per day, with <10 transfusions required
- Grade 3—frequent episodes lasting longer than half an hour, with >10 transfusions required

Telangiectasis

Telangiectasias is defined as lesions on mucocutaneous surfaces, such as skin, aerodigestive tract, and lower gut mucosa. About 30% of affected patients report telangiectasis appearing first before the age of 40 years.[18]

Neurologic Symptoms

Central nervous system AVMs are present at birth occurring in 10% of affected individuals.[19] Brain abscess and cerebrovascular accidents are more commonly encountered in HHT patients than in normal healthy individuals. The loss of normal filtering function of the pulmonary vasculature is a cause in pulmonary AVM patients. These AVMs lead to thrombotic and septic emboli reach to brain leading to brain abscesses and cerebrovascular accidents. Among them, untreated patients have a 2% risk of stroke and a 1% risk of brain abscess per year. These are commonly located in the superficial layers of the brain parenchyma, primarily in the parietal lobe parenchyma where micro infarcts and septic emboli can occur.[20]

Gastrointestinal and Hepatic Symptoms

Recurrent GI bleeding which affects about less than 50% of patients, usually does not occur until the fourth decade of life.[21] Affected individuals usually complain of passage of black tarry stools (melena). Liver vascular malformations are seen in 75% of individuals of HHT. Most of the patients remain asymptomatic. Symptomatic individuals present with right-upper-outer quadrant pain, jaundice, and bleeding from esophageal varices. Sometimes, patients with HHT may present with cirrhosis and liver failure.

Anemias

Gastrointestinal bleeding can be often mild, intermittent, and chronic with few noticeable symptoms until it leads to anemia. Anemia results in chest pain, fatigue, and shortness of breath. Patients with severe epistaxis or GI bleed are advised to undergo a GI endoscopy for diagnosis and treatment of GI AVMs.

GENETIC TESTING

Genetic mutation testing has been advised and recommended in all the affected patients meeting 1-2 of the Curacao criteria or children and family members with family history of HHT.[22] Screening tests for the three most common mutations, *Endoglin*, *ALK1*, and *SMAD4*, should be done and should also be done in first degree family members of affected patients. Around 10-15% of HHT patients do not show any of these gene mutations.

Screening should be done meticulously, regardless of a patient's clinical symptoms, due to the danger of undiagnosed silent AVMs.

Assessment and Management

The significant AVMs can be identified by following ways: (1) skin examination: (2) ENT assessment; (3) brain magnetic resonance imaging (MRI)/magnetic resonance angiography; (4) transthoracic echocardiogram with bubble study; (5) colonoscopy; (6) endoscopy/video capsule endoscopy; (7) abdominal Doppler ultrasound, computed tomographic scan, MRI of the liver. Hematologic evaluation must also include complete blood count (CBC), erythrocyte sedimentation rate (ESR), reticulocyte count, total iron-binding capacity, and ferritin. Ferritin levels may be increased due to inflammation associated in the many patients of HHT. So ferritin alone may not accurately reflect iron stores.

Treatment options are always patient-specific and the best approach should be stepwise approach based on local versus systemic measures. There are no standard medical therapies for HHT but does include supportive care, local lesion-specific therapy, and systemic treatment.

Preventative measures of epistaxis include the local measures and systemic measures like use of topical moisturizers, emollients, nasal saline washes, local hygiene maintained with humidifiers, and avoidance blood thinners, and local triggering factors like trauma, dryness, and congestion.[22,23] During active episodes of nasal bleed, bleed can be managed conservatively by using topical decongestant spray, both anterior and posterior absorbable nasal packings, manual pressure, and/or chemical cauterization using silver nitrate.[24] We should avoid nondissolvable nasal packing due to the risk of increased mucosal trauma with the procedure-related effects on insertion and removal of the packing. Refractory episodes can be managed by surgical interventions.[22]

Iron deficiency anemia requires iron replacement, either orally or intravenously (IV). For refractory and severe anemia, blood transfusions and IV iron infusions may be required regularly. Blood transfusions should be considered in severe cases. Newer therapies like hormonal, bevacizumab, and thalidomide have also shown promising results but require further evaluation for their long-term use.[25]

Gastrointestinal AVM management requires endoscopic cauterization and an adjunct therapy may be used to prevent ongoing bleeding in the form of hormones or antifibrinolytic therapy.[26]

Pulmonary AVMs being of high medical concern should be treated with transcatheter embolization using embolic materials such as metallic coils and Amplatzer vascular plugs.[27-29]

An association between oral microorganisms and pulmonary AVM-associated brain abscesses have been documented.[30] Thus, recommendation is to use prophylactic treatment with antibiotics for any procedure that carries a risk of infection, commonly seen with dental procedures.

Hepatic AVMs are managed based on the symptoms and complications. HHT patients with hepatic AVMs may suffer from high-output cardiac failure, portal hypertension, and/or cirrhosis, managed medically. Blood transfusions for anemia, salt and fluid restriction, beta-blockers, and diuretics are used as treatment in high cardiac output. Liver transplantation is reserved for refractory cases failed to respond medical management.[31]

Symptomatic cardiac AVM patients or with risk factors, such as a family history of cerebral hemorrhage/infarct, treatment options are embolization, microsurgery, stereotactic radiation, or a combination of these treatment options. Spetzler–Martin grading scale has been used in estimating the risk of open surgery for cerebral AVMs.[32]

CONCLUSION

Hereditary hemorrhagic telangiectasia, also known as Osler–Weber–Rendu disease, is an autosomal dominant disorder characterized by vascular dysplasia, leading to malformations in various blood vessels. This condition has the potential to cause bleeding and blood shunting. HHT is frequently underdiagnosed, and affected families may be unaware of available screening and treatment options, which can result in life-threatening events.

The initial manifestation of HHT often involves chronic nosebleeds. Malformations in blood vessels can lead to abnormalities affecting the lungs, brain, spinal cord, and liver. To address the diverse features of HHT and enhance the quality of life while preventing life-threatening complications, a range of treatments is available.

Appropriate interventions can significantly improve the prognosis for individuals with HHT, allowing them to achieve a near-normal life expectancy. It is crucial to raise awareness of the condition, promote early diagnosis, and facilitate access to the various treatments available for managing this autosomal dominant disorder.

REFERENCES

1. Kritharis A, Al-Samkari H, Kuter DJ. Hereditary hemorrhagic telangiectasia: Diagnosis and management from the hematologist's perspective. Haematologica. 2018;103(9):1433-43.
2. Jackson SB, Villano NP, Benhammou JN, Lewis M, Pisegna JR, Padua D. Gastrointestinal manifestations of hereditary hemorrhagic telangiectasia (HHT): A systematic review of the literature. Dig Dis Sci. 2017;62(10):2623-30.
3. Morgan T, McDonald J, Anderson C, Ismail M, Miller F, Mao R, et al. Intracranial hemorrhage in infants and children with hereditary hemorrhagic telangiectasia (Osler-Weber-Rendu syndrome). Pediatrics. 2002;109(1):E12.
4. Shovlin CL, Guttmacher AE, Buscarini E, Faughnan ME, Hyland RH, Westermann CJ, et al. Diagnostic criteria for hereditary hemorrhagic telangiectasia (Rendu-Osler-Weber syndrome). Am J Med Genet. 2000;91(1):66-7.
5. Marchuk DA. Genetic abnormalities in hereditary hemorrhagic telangiectasia. Curr Opin Hematol. 1998;5(5):332-8.
6. Westermann CJ, Rosina AF, de Vries V, de Coteau PA. The prevalence and manifestations of hereditary hemorrhagic telangiectasia in the Afro Caribbean population of the Netherlands Antilles: A family screening. Am J of Med Genet. 2003;116(4):324-8.
7. Golzarian J, Sun S, Sharafuddin M. Springerlink (Online Service. Vascular Embolotherapy: A Comprehensive Approach, Volume 1: General Principles, Chest, Abdomen, and Great Vessels. Berlin, Heidelberg: Springer Berlin Heidelberg; 2006.
8. Kritharis A, Al-Samkari H, Kuter DJ. Hereditary hemorrhagic telangiectasia: Diagnosis and management from the hematologist's perspective. Haematologica. 2018;103(9):1433-43.
9. Halderman AA, Ryan MW, Clark C, Sindwani R, Reh DD, Poetker DM, et al. Medical treatment of epistaxis in hereditary hemorrhagic telangiectasia: An evidence-based review. Int Forum Allergy Rhinol. 2018;8(6):713-28.
10. McDonald J, Wooderchak-Donahue W, VanSant Webb C, Whitehead K, Stevenson DA, Bayrak-Toydemir P. Hereditary hemorrhagic telangiectasia: Genetics and molecular diagnostics in a new era. Front Genet. 2015;6:1.
11. McAllister KA, Grogg KM, Johnson DW, Gallione CJ, Baldwin MA, Jackson CE, et al. Endoglin, a TGF-beta binding protein of endothelial cells, is the gene for hereditary haemorrhagic telangiectasia type 1. Nat Genet. 1994;8(4):345-51.
12. Johnson DW, Berg JN, Baldwin MA, Gallione CJ, Marondel I, Yoon SJ, et al. Mutations in the activin receptor-like kinase 1 gene in hereditary haemorrhagic telangiectasia type 2. Nat Genet. 1996;13(2):189-95.
13. Azuma H. Genetic and molecular pathogenesis of hereditary hemorrhagic telangiectasia. J Med Invest. 2000;47(3-4):81-90.

14. Gallione CJ, Repetto GM, Legius E, Rustgi AK, Schelley SL, Tejpar S, et al. A combined syndrome of juvenile polyposis and hereditary haemorrhagic telangiectasia associated with mutations in MADH4 (SMAD4). Lancet. 2004;363(9412):852-9.
15. Govani FS, Shovlin CL. Hereditary haemorrhagic telangiectasia: A clinical and scientific review. Eur J Hum Genet. 2009;17(7):860-71.
16. Fernández-L A, Sanz-Rodriguez F, Blanco FJ, Bernabéu C, Botella LM. Hereditary hemorrhagic telangiectasia, a vascular dysplasia affecting the TGF-signaling pathway. Clin Med Res. 2006;4(1):66-78.
17. AAssar OS, Friedman CM, White RI, Jr. The natural history of epistaxis in hereditary hemorrhagic telangiectasia. Laryngoscope. 1991;101(9):977-80.
18. Berg J, Porteous M, Reinhardt D, Gallione C, Holloway S, Umasunthar T, et al. Hereditary haemorrhagic telangiectasia: A questionnaire based study to delineate the different phenotypes caused by endoglin and ALK1 mutations. J Med Genet. 2003;40(8):585-90.
19. Brinjikji W, Iyer VN, Wood CP, Lanzino G. Prevalence and characteristics of brain arteriovenous malformations in hereditary hemorrhagic telangiectasia: A systematic review and meta-analysis. J Neurosurg. 2017;127(2):302-10.
20. McDonald MJ, Brophy BP, Kneebone C. Rendu-Osler-Weber syndrome: a current perspective on cerebral manifestations. J Clin Neurosci. 1998;5(3):345-50.
21. Goodenberger DM. Visceral manifestations of hereditary hemorrhagic telangiectasia. Trans Am Clin Climatol Assoc. 2004;115:185-99.
22. Grigg C, Anderson D, Earnshaw J. Diagnosis and treatment of hereditary hemorrhagic telangiectasia. Ochsner J. 2017;17(2):157-61.
23. Tunkel DE, Anne S, Payne SC, Ishman SL, Rosenfeld RM, Abramson PJ, et al. Clinical practice guideline: Nosebleed (epistaxis). Otolaryngol Head Neck Surg. 2020;162(1_suppl):S1-S38.
24. Sautter NB, Smith TL. Treatment of hereditary hemorrhagic telangiectasia-related epistaxis. Otolaryngol Clin North Am. 2016;49(3):639-54.
25. Shovlin CL. Hereditary haemorrhagic telangiectasia: Pathophysiology, diagnosis and treatment. Blood Rev. 2010;24(6):203-19.
26. Faughnan ME, Palda VA, Garcia-Tsao G, Geisthoff UW, McDonald J, Proctor DD, et al. HHT Foundation International - Guidelines Working Group. International guidelines for the diagnosis and management of hereditary haemorrhagic telangiectasia. J Med Genet. 2011;48(2):73-87.
27. Garg N, Khunger M, Gupta A, Kumar N. Optimal management of hereditary hemorrhagic telangiectasia. J Blood Med. 2014;5:191-206.
28. Faughnan ME, Mager JJ, Hetts SW, Palda VA, Lang-Robertson K, Buscarini E, et al. Second international guidelines for the diagnosis and management of hereditary hemorrhagic telangiectasia. Ann Intern Med. 2020;173(12):989-1001.
29. Faughnan ME, Palda VA, Garcia-Tsao G, Geisthoff UW, McDonald J, Proctor DD, et al. HHT Foundation International - Guidelines Working Group. International guidelines for the diagnosis and management of hereditary haemorrhagic telangiectasia. J Med Genet. 2011;48(2):73-87.
30. Shovlin C, Bamford K, Wray D. Post-NICE 2008: Antibiotic prophylaxis prior to dental procedures for patients with pulmonary arteriovenous malformations (PAVMs) and hereditary haemorrhagic telangiectasia. Br Dent J. 2008;205(10):531-3.
31. Lerut J, Orlando G, Adam R, Sabbà C, Pfitzmann R, Klempnauer J, et al. European Liver Transplant Association. Liver transplantation for hereditary hemorrhagic telangiectasia: Report of the European liver transplant registry. Ann Surg. 2006;244(6):854-62; discussion 862-4.
32. Spetzler RF, Martin NA. A proposed grading system for arteriovenous malformations. J Neurosurg. 1986;65(4):476-83.

CHAPTER 12

Pathogenesis of Chemotherapy and Cancer-induced Anemia: Recent Updates

Snigdha Petwal, Sana Umar

INTRODUCTION

Cancer patients, especially those undergoing chemotherapy, frequently experience anemia. The emergence of anemia related to cancer (referred to as cancer-induced anemia or CIA) is a multifaceted and intricate process.[1] Gastrointestinal, genitourinary, and gynecological cancers can cause blood loss, while lymphoma and chronic lymphocytic leukemia often lead to hemolysis. Chemotherapy and radiotherapy can suppress red blood cell (RBC) production.[2] Some chemotherapeutic agents can cause nephrotoxicity, affecting erythropoietin (EPO) production. Anemia of chronic illness, possibly influenced by cytokines like interferon-γ and interleukin (IL)-1, is observed in cancer patients with no identifiable cause.[2,3] Other factors causing anemia in cancer patients include surgery-related blood loss, tumor infiltration into the bone marrow, loss of appetite, and nutritional deficiencies.[4]

Cancer-induced anemia is typically normochromic and normocytic. It is often hypoproliferative, indicated by low reticulocyte count and reticulocyte index value. Serum iron concentrations are normal-to-low, while ferritin levels may be elevated, suggesting functional iron deficiency. CIA is marked by low levels of circulating EPO despite preserved kidney function.[5-8]

PREVALENCE OF CANCER-INDUCED ANEMIA

A significant proportion of cancer patients, exceeding 30% even at the point of diagnosis, grapple with CIA. This prevalence surges further during treatment, reaching approximately 67%.[9-11] The stage of the disease influences the prevalence of CIA especially in advanced cancer patients not receiving chemotherapy, where high percentages of men (77%) and women (68%) show anemia[12] attaining an advanced age during diagnosis could potentially augment the likelihood of an increased occurrence of anemia.[4] The frequency of CIA displays significant variation across different types of cancer, with higher percentages observed in lung cancer, as well as in gynecologic, genitourinary, and gastrointestinal tumors.[4,10,13] A large observational study found that 63% of cancer patients had CIA at diagnosis, increasing with advanced cancer staging and decreased performance status. It was found that lung and ovarian cancer patients had the highest incidence of CIA (73.5% and 67.9%, respectively), and greater anemia severity was observed in these cases.[14]

PATHOGENESIS OF CANCER-INDUCED ANEMIA

Cancer-induced anemia emerges without any signs of bleeding, neoplastic bone marrow involvement, hemolysis, or dysfunction in the kidneys or liver. Its origin is rooted mainly in persistent inflammation associated with advanced-stage cancer, driven by the production of proinflammatory cytokines from both immune cells and cancer cells.[15]

The chief pathogenetic mechanisms through which inflammation causes anemia include reduced erythrocyte survival and increased erythrocyte destruction, suppression of erythropoiesis in the bone marrow, effects on EPO production, iron metabolism alteration mediated by hepcidin increase.[6]

Proinflammatory stimuli activate macrophages, increase RBC destruction. This, combined with iron restriction and cytokine inhibition of erythropoietic progenitors, leads to inadequate erythropoiesis and reduced RBC production. In chronic inflammatory diseases like cancer, reduced EPO synthesis results in insufficient circulating EPO levels to maintain hemoglobin (Hb) levels, independent of renal function.[16]

Tumor necrosis factor (TNF)-α, IL-6, and IL-1 are the proinflammatory cytokines that affect iron balance, erythropoiesis, EPO synthesis and activity, RBC lifespan, and energy metabolism **(Table 1)**.[17] IL-1 and TNF-α negatively regulate HIF1 expression through GATA2 and nuclear factor-κ B.[5] IL-6 induces hepcidin synthesis, disrupting iron homeostasis, and affecting erythropoiesis by reducing iron absorption and release via ferroportin 1 degradation.[18] Chronic inflammation increases ROS levels, contributing to the EPO deficit.[19] ROS inhibit EPO synthesis by generating false oxygen signals, leading to oxidative stress that affects erythrocyte fragility, maturation, and survival.[20-23] Proinflammatory cytokines also inhibit erythroid precursor proliferation through ROS.[24]

ROLE OF PROINFLAMMATORY CYTOKINES

Interleukin-1 exercises its impact by directly and precisely hindering the progression and maturation of erythroid precursors (BFU-E and CFU-E), reducing the abundance of EPO receptors, and prompting a disturbance in the production of EPO. Moreover, IL-1 also causes activation of macrophages for erythrophagocytosis and thus leading to premature destruction and reduced survival of erythrocytes.[25,26] IL-1 also influences energy metabolism and nutritional well-being, leading to appetite loss and decreased food consumption.[27] It hampers the release of neuropeptide Y, indirectly elevating levels of corticotropin-releasing factor, which in turn reduces

TABLE 1: Role of proinflammatory cytokines in cancer-induced anemia.	
Proinflammatory cytokines	**Role in cancer-induced anemia**
IL-1	• Suppresses maturation of erythroid precursors • Reduces expression of erythropoietin (EPO) receptor, and impairs EPO synthesis • Activates macrophages for erythrophagocytosis, induces premature destruction • Influences energy metabolism • Inhibits neuropeptide Y release • Increases corticotropin-releasing factor levels, reduces GH production and IGF-1 levels • Contributes to insulin resistance • Negatively affects erythropoiesis and glucose metabolism
IL-6	• Interferes iron homeostasis and inhibits erythroid progenitor proliferation and their response to EPO • Alters hepcidin synthesis • Inhibits hemoglobin synthesis
TNF-α	• Causes impairment of erythropoiesis • Increases apoptosis of immature erythroblast • Decreases apoptosis of mature erythroblast • Reduces responsiveness of erythroid progenitors to EPO • Affects lipid metabolism leading to lipoatrophy and reduced erythroid progenitor maturation

(GH: growth hormone; IGF: insulin-like growth factor; IL: interleukin; TNF: tumor necrosis factor)

the production of growth hormone (GH) and insulin-like growth factor-1 (IGF-1). This cascade subsequently contributes to the decline in muscle mass seen in advanced cancer patients.[28-30] IL-1-modulated pathways in the central nervous system have been linked to anemia. Replacing GH leads to increased Hb, hematocrit, and RBC count.[31] IGF promotes erythroid progenitor proliferation and differentiation.[32-34] Low IGF levels have been associated with anemia.[35] IL-1 also restrains the synthesis of insulin, resulting in an elevation of insulin levels and resistance to its effects, a condition known as hyperinsulinemia and insulin resistance. These factors could potentially play a role in the development of CIA.[30] Moreover, the presence of elevated glucose levels and insulin resistance has adverse implications for the process of erythropoiesis.[36] Glucose metabolism plays a crucial role in erythroid cell differentiation.[37,38] IL-1 exerts a range of effects on the process of erythropoiesis, contributing to the emergence of CIA. Its influence extends to immune and metabolic changes within individuals with advanced cancer.

Interleukin-6 plays a significant role in the progression of CIA by disturbing iron balance within the body and hindering the growth of erythroid progenitors, as well as their capacity to adequately react to EPO.[29] It also alters hepcidin synthesis and liver gene expression.[6] IL-6 can independently inhibit Hb synthesis by impairing mitochondrial function in maturing erythroid cells.[39] Furthermore, IL-6 also induces immune and metabolic alterations, like cachexia, commonly observed in advanced cancer, contributing to CIA.[40] Hepcidin stimulation can result from cross-talk between the IL-6/JAK2-STAT3 pathway and another inflammatory pathway involving activin B and its Smad signaling mechanism.[41,42] In advanced cancer patients, IL-6 is a crucial determinant of muscle mass. The activation of IL-6/STAT3 signaling and the regulation of the PI3K/AkT-mTOR pathway, along with highly increased degradation and reduction in availability of amino acids, contribute to defective erythropoiesis. Anorexia and insulin resistance further inhibit the mTOR pathway. Anemia, which reduces the efficiency of oxygen transport to the peripheral tissues, can cause inhibition of mTOR signaling, primarily due to impairment of oxidative phosphorylation and reduced ATP synthesis.[43,44]

Tumor necrosis factor-α impairs erythropoiesis and differentiation, leading to increase in immature erythroblast apoptosis, decrease in mature erythroblast apoptosis, and reduction in erythroid progenitor responsiveness to EPO.[45] It also induces metabolic changes, including lipid metabolism alterations, insulin resistance and cancer cachexia typical in advanced cancer patients.[46] TNF-α negatively affects lipoprotein lipase activity, free fatty acids (FFA) transporters, and lipogenesis enzymes, inducing lipolysis.[47] TNF-α's signaling impacts peroxisome proliferator-activated receptor gamma (PPAR-γ), affecting lipid metabolism leading to lipoatrophy and reduced erythroid progenitor maturation.[48-50] EPO deficit explains the increase in ROS ($O°$, H_2O_2, and $OH-$) concentrations linked to chronic inflammation.[51,52] ROS can inhibit EPO synthesis, causing increased erythrocyte fragility, decreased maturation, and reduced survival of red cells. It also mediates the inhibitory effect of proinflammatory cytokines on erythroid precursor proliferation.[20-24] Sustained oxidative stress-induced hepcidin expression in the liver may contribute to cancer-related anemia (CRA).[53]

■ IRON HOMEOSTASIS AND CHANGES IN CANCER-INDUCED ANEMIA

The equilibrium of iron within the body is governed by hepcidin, an endocrine hormone responsible for overseeing iron levels in the bloodstream. Hepcidin regulates the processes of iron absorption, storage, and release. Most circulating iron comes from recycled RBCs, while a small portion comes from the diet. Iron is bound to Hb in RBCs and stored in hepatocytes and macrophages. Transferrin transports iron to the bone marrow for RBC production and is stored in a complex with ferritin in cells of the reticuloendothelial system.[18]

Reduced transferrin-bound iron can inhibit erythropoiesis, but other processes are generally unaffected by mild iron depletion unless it becomes severe. Iron from the diet is taken up by duodenal enterocytes and subsequently released into the bloodstream via ferroportin, a transporter that facilitates the transfer of iron from storage sites to the blood circulation. Macrophages play a critical role in recycling of iron from senescent RBCs by erythrophagocytosis. Hepcidin produced by the liver and macrophages, controls iron recycling, storage, and export by regulating ferroportin. The production of hepcidin is regulated by positive feedback mechanisms based on high plasma iron levels and negatively by hypoxia and increased erythropoiesis.[18] Erythroferrone, generated by erythroblasts in reaction to EPO, functions to suppress hepcidin. This inhibition facilitates the export of intracellular iron, the absorption of iron in the intestines, and ultimately supports the process of erythropoiesis.[54]

Both CIA and anemia in association with chronic inflammatory diseases disrupt iron homeostasis. They lead to increase in iron storage in the macrophages and limited iron availability for RBC production, causing decreased erythropoiesis. Elevated intracellular iron levels hinder erythropoiesis by degrading HIF1α and inhibiting EPO synthesis.[54-56] This "functional iron deficiency" state is characterized by normal or elevated reserves of iron in the bone marrow, increased levels of ferritin, increased iron-binding capacity, and normal or decreased levels of serum iron.[57] Elevated hepcidin production, driven by inflammatory cytokines like IL-6, redirects the movement of iron by obstructing the absorption of iron in the duodenum and the release of iron from precursor macrophages.[58,59]

In advanced cancer and chronic inflammatory diseases, high IL-6 levels induce increased hepatic hepcidin production, degrading cellular ferroportin. This blockage in iron excretion, leading to increased iron storage in hepatocytes, enterocytes, and macrophages, limiting iron delivery to plasma transferrin. Consequently, heme synthesis is impaired, affecting erythroid replication and maturation.[60]

Macrophages, particularly M1 macrophages, play a vital role in iron metabolism and immune responses, consuming iron through phagocytosis of senescent or injured cells.[61] M1 macrophages retain iron, exhibiting proinflammatory activity, and promoting antimicrobial and antitumoral effects. They are characterized by high expression of hepcidin and ferritin, low transferrin receptor and ferroportin levels, and increased iron storage.[62]

A strong correlation exists between M1 polarized tumor-associated macrophages (TAMs) and CRA in ovarian cancer patients. TAM M1 polarization is associated with elevated hepcidin and IL-6 levels, and altered iron metabolism pathways with increased ferritin and decreased free iron levels.[63] In advanced cancer patients, hepcidin values negatively correlate with Hb levels and positively associate with IL-6 and ferritin levels, while negatively correlating with serum iron and transferrin saturation values.[64,65]

ASSOCIATION BETWEEN NUTRITIONAL STATUS AND CANCER-INDUCED ANEMIA

The progression of cancer often leads compromise in the patients nutritional status, resulting in symptoms such as weight loss, reduced muscle mass, increased energy expenditure, anorexia, nausea, and vomiting. Loss of weight along with body mass index (BMI) has been identified as unfavorable predictive marker in cancer patients, independent of tumor characteristics such as site, stage, and performance status. Even a minor reduction in body weight (>2.4%) upon diagnosis is linked to elevated risks of morbidity.[66] This weight loss is a hallmark of cancer cachexia, an inflammatory-driven syndrome that commonly occurs in advanced stages of the disease.[67] However, the loss of body weight in cachectic cancer patients cannot be solely attributed to reduced nutrient intake caused by anorexia. Changes in energy metabolism, resulting in increased resting metabolic expenditure, substantially contribute to loss of weight.[68]

Chronic inflammation associated with cancer contributes to alterations in energy metabolism pathways, including glucose metabolism, lipoprotein lipase activity, and protein synthesis and degradation. These alterations result in a decline in the lean body mass. There is a drop in the production of muscle protein and an uptick in proteolysis due to heightened enzymatic proteolytic activity among the cancer patients. In contrast, the metabolic dynamics in the liver exhibit distinct characteristics. In spite of stable or reduced albumin synthesis, the production of other proteins is elevated in the liver, particularly acute phase inflammation proteins (CRP, hepcidin, and fibrinogen).[69] These metabolic changes, along with inflammation, also contribute to reduced albumin levels, which are associated with a deteriorated Glasgow prognostic score (GPS)—an inflammatory/nutritional status-based score, strongly associated with the deterioration of CIA.[14]

Malnutrition, weight loss, and reduced food intake are consistently correlated with anemia in chronic inflammatory disease.[70] In advanced cancer, anemia associated with chronic inflammation is typically linked to weight loss and altered energy metabolism caused by the cancer itself.

Leptin, a marker of nutritional and metabolic status, is associated with anemia.[71-73] Lower levels of leptin in ovarian cancer patients are correlated with lower Hb levels. A large prospective study in different cancer types showed a positive correlation between leptin, albumin, cholesterol, BMI, and Hb levels[14] Leptin, IL-6, and cancer stage were predictive variables for Hb levels. Leptin also influences erythropoiesis and stimulates human erythroid progenitors in vitro.[74] As in patients of cancer anemia is influenced by nutritional factors affecting iron and micronutrient levels necessary for erythropoiesis, leptin serves as a sensitive nutritional marker that correlates with Hb levels.[1]

CHEMOTHERAPY-INDUCED ANEMIA

As a result of myelosuppressive chemotherapy, anemia is a common complication in cancer patients, impacting functional capacity and quality of life.[75,76] Its severity is influenced by disease extent, treatment intensity, and cumulative effects **(Table 2)**. The incidence and severity of chemotherapy-related anemia vary based on treatment factors and patient characteristics, with symptom severity linked to anemia degree, underlying malignancy, and pulmonary/cardiovascular function.[75] Elderly cancer patients may experience anemia-related symptoms at higher Hb levels compared to noncancer anemic patients. Assessing lower-grade toxic effects, including mild anemia, is crucial as they significantly affect patients' energy levels and quality of life.[76,77]

Small-cell Lung Cancer

Cisplatin along with etoposide is a preferred regimen for the treatment of small-cell lung cancer. Grade 3 or 4 anemia is commonly associated with this regimen, occurring in 16–55% of the patients undergoing treatment.[78-80]

Non-small-cell Lung Cancer

In advanced non-small-cell lung cancer (NSCLC) platinum-based combination chemotherapy is the first-line of treatment. Patients with this cancer commonly experience clinically significant decrease in Hb as a side effect of platinum.[81]

Breast Cancer

The combination of cyclophosphamide-doxorubicin-5-FU commonly causes grade 1 or 2 anemia in 55% and grade 3 or 4 anemia in 11% of patients

TABLE 2: Chemotherapeutic drugs and degree of anemia in various cancer types.		
Cancer type	**Chemotherapeutic drugs**	**Degree of anemia**
Small-cell lung cancer	• Cisplatin • Etoposide	Grade 3 or 4
Non-small cell cancer	Platinum	Grade 3
Ovarian cancer	• Paclitexal • Topotecan	• Grade 3 or 4 • Grade 1 or 2
Breast cancer	Cyclophosphamide–doxorubicin–5-FU	Grade 1 or 2
Lymphoma	Procarbazine–methotrezate–leucovorin–doxorubicin–cyclophosphamide–etoposide	Grade 1 or 2
Head and neck cancer	• 5-FU • Irinotecan	• Grade 1 or 2 • Grade 1 or 2

treated for metastatic breast cancer. Newer agents like paclitaxel, docetaxel, and vinorelbine also show high response in metastatic breast cancer cause higher incidence of grade 1 or 2 anemia. For instance, paclitaxel causes grade 1 or 2 anemia in 36-51% of previously treated patients with metastatic breast cancer.[82,83]

Ovarian Cancer

Paclitaxel and topotecan are the treatment of choice in advanced ovarian cancer. Administering higher doses and prolonging the infusion duration of paclitaxel is linked to heightened myelosuppression, including a higher occurrence of grade 3 or 4 anemia. Topotecan causes a high incidence of grade 1 or 2 anemia and a higher incidence of grade 3 or 4 anemia than paclitaxel in previously treated patients.[84,85]

Lymphoma

Treatment regimens involving combinations of procarbazine-methotrexate-leucovorin-doxorubicin-cyclophosphamide-etoposide, mechlorethamine-vincristine-procarbazine-prednisone (MOPP), and methotrexate-leucovorin-doxorubicin-cyclophosphamide-vincristine-prednisone-bleomycin resulted in grade 1 or 2 anemia in 63% and 55% of NHL patients, respectively. Additionally, grade 3 or 4 anemia occurred in 9% and 10% of the patients in each group, respectively.[86]

Colorectal Cancer

5-FU, is a cornerstone of chemotherapy for advanced colorectal cancer, induces grade 1 or 2 anemia in approximately 50% of previously untreated patients, while grade 3 or 4 anemia affects 5-8% of them.[87,88] On the other hand, irinotecan, a recently introduced treatment for advanced colorectal cancer, is associated with a high occurrence of grade 1 or 2 anemia (49-60%), with grade 3 or 4 anemia affecting 8-10% of patients.[89]

Head and Neck Cancer

In head and neck cancer, single-agent therapies using bleomycin, cisplatin, methotrexate, carboplatin, 5-FU, docetaxel, paclitaxel, and gemcitabine exhibit high rates of grade 1 or 2 anemia and low rates of grade 3 or 4 anemia. Among previously untreated patients with advanced disease, single-agent paclitaxel resulted in grade 1 or 2 anemia in 39% and grade 3 anemia in 13%. Conversely, single-agent methotrexate led to grade 1 or 2 anemia in 25% and grade 3 anemia in 3%.[90,91]

■ MANAGEMENT OF CHEMOTHERAPY-INDUCED ANEMIA

The management of anemia resulting from chemotherapy depends upon the severity of anemia. Multiple treatment options used include crystalloid and hematinic treatment, RBC transfusion, and epoetin alfa administration.

TRANSFUSION OF CONCENTRATED ERYTHROCYTES

Red blood cell transfusions serve as a swift and efficacious therapeutic approach to elevate Hb levels and enhance the capacity for oxygen transport in cancer patients experiencing severe symptomatic anemia (Hb <7–8 g/dL).[92,93]

TREATMENT WITH RECOMBINANT HUEPO

Recombinant HuEPO (rHuEPO) was first approved for anemia in chronic kidney failure and later for cancer patients.[94] Both short- and long-acting formulations, such as rHuEPOα, rHuEPOβ, and darbepoetin α, are accessible. Among these, rHuEPO exhibits an extended half-life after subcutaneous administration compared to natural EPO, spanning around 24 hours for rHuEPOα and 20.5 hours for rHuEPOβ.[94] On the other hand, darbepoetin α, an altered hyperglycosylated epoetin, presents an even lengthier half-life after subcutaneous administration, approximately 49 hours. This prolonged duration between doses facilitates less frequent administration while maintaining the desired Hb levels.[95] Many other biosimilar EPOs have been formulated and incorporated in clinical practice (e.g., biosimilar epoetin alfa and epoetin zeta), highly similar to reference drugs in structure and mechanism of action.[96]

IRON SUPPLEMENTATION

Cancer-induced anemia is characterized by impaired iron incorporation into developing RBCs and EPO deficiency. Treatment options for CIA may involve treatment options involving both erythropoiesis-stimulating agents (ESAs) and supplementation with iron. Iron can be delivered either through oral or parenteral routes, offering cancer patients a range of formulations to choose from. These options include low-molecular-weight iron dextran, ferric gluconate, and iron sucrose. The amalgamation of iron with ESAs has been substantiated by meta-analyses to enhance hematopoietic response, reduce transfusion rates, and increase Hb levels. When combined with ESAs, intravenous iron supplementation has demonstrated greater effectiveness compared with oral iron, resulting in improved Hb response and reduced transfusion needs. Lactoferrin, an iron-binding protein, has demonstrated comparable efficacy to intravenous iron in increasing Hb levels. Therefore, iron supplementation is recommended for CIA patients, especially when they do not respond adequately to erythropoietic agents alone.[97-99]

SUMMARY

Cancer-induced anemia is a complex disorder stemming from the interplay between cytokines, resulting from intricate interactions between tumor cells and the immune system. The overproduction of inflammatory cytokines leads to a shortened lifespan of RBCs, the suppression of erythroid progenitor cells, compromised iron utilization, and inadequate EPO production. Macrophages play a pivotal role in this process, with their activation being the primary driver of increased RBC destruction. Moreover, both radiotherapy and chemotherapy have the potential to compromise the immune system and bone marrow, consequently impeding erythropoiesis. However, the severity of anemia can vary based on the specific treatment approach adopted.

CONCLUSION

Cancer-induced anemia is a multifaceted condition resulting from a complex interaction between various factors within the body which is primarily influenced by the interplay of cytokines, the immune system, and tumor cells. Inflammatory cytokines, produced in excess due to this interaction, contribute to the shortened lifespan of RBCs, hinder the production of EPO, suppress erythroid progenitor cells, and impair iron utilization. Macrophages, particularly when activated, significantly contribute to the destruction of RBCs in this process. Additionally, treatments like radiotherapy and chemotherapy, while targeting cancer cells, have the unintended consequence of compromising the immune system and bone marrow, thereby affecting the production of RBCs.

In essence, CIA emerges from a complex web of interactions involving inflammatory cytokines, immune responses, tumor cells, and the impact of cancer treatments on the body's ability to produce RBCs. The understanding of these interactions is crucial for devising effective strategies to manage and treat cancer-induced anemia.

REFERENCES

1. Abdel-Razeq H, Hashem H. Recent update in the pathogenesis and treatment of chemotherapy and cancer induced anemia. Crit Rev Oncol Hematol. 2020;145:102837.
2. Cullis J. Anaemia of chronic disease. Clin Med (Northfield Il). 2013;13(2):193-6.
3. Nemeth E, Rivera S, Gabayan V, Keller C, Taudorf S, Pedersen BK, et al. IL-6 mediates hypoferremia of inflammation by inducing the synthesis of the iron regulatory hormone hepcidin. J Clin Invest. 2004;113(9):1271-6.
4. Schwartz RN. Anemia in patients with cancer: incidence, causes, impact, management, and use of treatment guidelines and protocols. Am J Health-Syst Pharmacy. 2007;64(3_Supplement_2):S5-13.
5. Spivak JL. The anaemia of cancer: Death by a thousand cuts. Nature Rev Cancer 2005;5(7):543-55.
6. Adamson JW. The anemia of inflammation/malignancy: Mechanisms and management. ASH Educ Program. 2008:159-65.
7. Rodgers GM, Gilreath JA, Achebe MM, Alwan L, Arcasoy M, Ali Beth S, et al. NCCN. Cancer and chemotherapy-induced anemia, version 2. 2017.
8. Wish JB. Assessing iron status: Beyond serum ferritin and transferrin saturation. Clin J Am Soc Nephrol. 2006;1(Suppl. 1):S4-8.
9. Ludwig H, Van Belle S, Barrett-Lee P, Birgegård G, Bokemeyer C, Gascón P, et al. The European Cancer Anaemia Survey (ECAS): A large, multinational, prospective survey

defining the prevalence, incidence, and treatment of anaemia in cancer patients. Eur J Cancer. 2004;40(15):2293-306.
10. Birgegård G, Aapro MS, Bokemeyer C, Dicato M, Drings P, Hornedo J, et al. Cancer-related anemia: Pathogenesis, prevalence and treatment. Oncology. 2005;68 (Suppl. 1):3-11.
11. Caro JJ, Salas M, Ward A, Goss G. Anemia as an independent prognostic factor for survival in patients with cancer: A systematic, quantitative review. Cancer. 2001;91(12):2214-21.
12. Dunn A, Carter J, Carter H. Anemia at the end of life: prevalence, significance, and causes in patients receiving palliative care. J Pain Sympt Manage. 2003;26(6):1132-9.
13. Knight K, Wade S, Balducci L. Prevalence and outcomes of anemia in cancer: A systematic review of the literature. Am J Med. 2004;116(7):11-26.
14. Madeddu C, Gramignano G, Astara G, Demontis R, Sanna E, Atzeni V, et al. Pathogenesis and treatment options of cancer related anemia: Perspective for a targeted mechanism-based approach. Front Physiol. 2018;9:1294.
15. Weiss G, Goodnough LT. Anemia of chronic disease. New Engl J Med. 2005;352(10):1011-23.
16. Spivak JL. The blood in systemic disorders. Lancet. 2000;355(9216):1707-12.
17. Means Jr RT. Pathogenesis of the anemia of chronic disease: A cytokine-mediated anemia. Stem Cells. 1995;13(1):32-7.
18. Ganz T, Nemeth E. Iron homeostasis in host defence and inflammation. Nature Rev Immunol. 2015;15(8):500-10.
19. Means Jr RT. Recent developments in the anemia of chronic disease. Curr Hematol Report. 2003;2(2):116-21.
20. Sailaja YR, Baskar R, Saralakumari D. The antioxidant status during maturation of reticulocytes to erythrocytes in type 2 diabetics. Free Radic Biol Med. 2003;35(2):133-9.
21. Olszewska M, Wiatrow J, Bober J, Stachowska E, Gołembiewska E, Jakubowska K, et al. Oxidative stress modulates the organization of erythrocyte membrane cytoskeleton. Adv Hyg Exp Med. 2012;66:534-42.
22. Lang F, Abed M, Lang E, Föller M. Oxidative stress and suicidal erythrocyte death. Antioxid Redox Signal. 2014;21(1):138-53.
23. Bukowska B, Sicińska P, Pająk A, Koceva-Chyla A, Pietras T, Pszczółkowska A, et al. Oxidative stress and damage to erythrocytes in patients with chronic obstructive pulmonary disease—changes in ATPase and acetylcholinesterase activity. Biochem Cell Biol. 2015;93(6):574-80.
24. Prince OD, Langdon JM, Layman AJ, Prince IC, Sabogal M, Mak HH, et al. Late stage erythroid precursor production is impaired in mice with chronic inflammation. Haematologica. 2012;97(11):1648.
25. Faquin WC, Schneider TJ, Goldberg MA. Effect of inflammatory cytokines on hypoxia-induced erythropoietin production. Blood. 1992;79(8):1987-94.
26. Jelkmann W, Pagel H, Wolff M, Fandrey J. Monokines inhibiting erythropoietin production in human hepatoma cultures and in isolated perfused rat kidneys. Life Sci. 1992;50(4):301-8.
27. Patra SK, Arora S. Integrative role of neuropeptides and cytokines in cancer anorexia–cachexia syndrome. Clin Chim Acta. 2012;413(13-14):1025-34.
28. Gautron L, Layé S. Neurobiology of inflammation-associated anorexia. Front Neurosci. 2010;3:1147.
29. Saini A, Nasser AS, Stewart CE. Waste management—cytokines, growth factors and cachexia. Cytokine Growth Factor Rev. 2006;17(6):475-86.
30. Burke SJ, Stadler K, Lu D, Gleason E, Han A, Donohoe DR. IL-1β reciprocally regulates chemokine and insulin secretion in pancreatic β-cells via NF-κB. Am J Physiol Endocrinol Metabol. 2015;309(8):E715-26.

31. Christ ER, Cummings MH, Westwood NB, Sawyer BM, Pearson TC, Sönksen PH, et al. The importance of growth hormone in the regulation of erythropoiesis, red cell mass, and plasma volume in adults with growth hormone deficiency. J Clin Endocrinol Metab. 1997;82(9):2985-90.
32. Iglesias P, Diez JJ, Fernandez-Reyes MJ, Aguilera A, Burgués S, Martínez-Ara J, et al. Recombinant human growth hormone therapy in malnourished dialysis patients: A randomized controlled study. Am J Kidney Dis. 1998;32(3):454-63.
33. Nilsson-Ehle H, Bengtsson BÅ, Lindstedt G, Mellström D. Insulin-like growth factor-1 is a predictor of blood haemoglobin concentration in 70-yr-old subjects. Eur J Haematol. 2005;74(2):111-6.
34. Succurro E, Arturi F, Caruso V, Rudi S, Sciacqua A, Andreozzi F, et al. Low insulin-like growth factor-1 levels are associated with anaemia in adult non-diabetic subjects. Thromb Haemost. 2011;105(02):365-70.
35. Marini MA, Mannino GC, Fiorentino TV, Andreozzi F, Perticone F, Sesti G. A polymorphism at IGF1 locus is associated with anemia. Oncotarget. 2017;8(20):32398.
36. Oburoglu L, Romano M, Taylor N, Kinet S. Metabolic regulation of hematopoietic stem cell commitment and erythroid differentiation. Curr Opin Hematol. 2016;23(3):198-205.
37. Vander Heiden MG, Cantley LC, Thompson CB. Understanding the Warburg effect: The metabolic requirements of cell proliferation. Science. 2009;324(5930):1029-33.
38. Montel-Hagen A, Sitbon M, Taylor N. Erythroid glucose transporters. Curr Opin Hematol. 2009;16(3):165-72.
39. McCranor BJ, Kim MJ, Cruz NM, Xue QL, Berger AE, Walston JD, et al. Interleukin-6 directly impairs the erythroid development of human TF-1 erythroleukemic cells. Blood Cells Mol Dis. 2014;52(2-3):126-33.
40. Strassmann G, Fong M, Kenney JS, Jacob CO. Evidence for the involvement of interleukin 6 in experimental cancer cachexia. J Clin Invest. 1992;89(5):1681-4.
41. Babitt JL, Huang FW, Xia Y, Sidis Y, Andrews NC, Lin HY. Modulation of bone morphogenetic protein signaling in vivo regulates systemic iron balance. J Clin Invest. 2007;117(7):1933-9.
42. Besson-Fournier C, Latour C, Kautz L, Ganz T, Roth MP, Coppin H. Induction of activin B by inflammatory stimuli up-regulates expression of the iron-regulatory peptide hepcidin through Smad1/5/8 signaling. Blood. 2012;120(2):431-9.
43. Chung J, Bauer DE, Ghamari A, Nizzi CP, Deck KM, Kingsley PD, et al. The mTORC1/4E-BP pathway coordinates hemoglobin production with L-leucine availability. Sci Signal. 2015;8(372):ra34.
44. Nathan DG. Amino acid uptake in erythropoiesis. Sci Signal. 2015;8(372):fs9.
45. Buck I, Morceau F, Grigorakaki C, Dicato M, Diederich M. Linking anemia to inflammation and cancer: The crucial role of TNFα. Biochem Pharmacol. 2009;77(10):1572-9.
46. Patel HJ, Patel BM. TNF-α and cancer cachexia: Molecular insights and clinical implications. Life Sci. 2017;170:56-63.
47. Carbó N, Costelli P, Tessitore L, Bagby GJ, López-Soriano FJ, Baccino FM, et al. Anti-tumour necrosis factor-α treatment interferes with changes in lipid metabolism in a tumour cachexia model. Clin Sci. 1994;87(3):349-55.
48. Cawthorn WP, Sethi JK. TNF-α and adipocyte biology. FEBS Letters. 2008;582(1):117-31.
49. Bing C, Russell S, Becket E, Pope M, Tisdale MJ, Trayhurn P, et al. Adipose atrophy in cancer cachexia: Morphologic and molecular analysis of adipose tissue in tumour-bearing mice. Brit J Cancer. 2006;95(8):1028-37.
50. Nagasawa E, Abe Y, Nishimura J, Yanase T, Nawata H, Muta K. Pivotal role of peroxisome proliferator–activated receptor γ (PPARγ) in regulation of erythroid progenitor cell proliferation and differentiation. Exp Hematol. 2005;33(8):857-64.

51. Macciò A, Madeddu C, Gramignano G, Mulas C, Tanca L, Cherchi MC, et al. The role of inflammation, iron, and nutritional status in cancer-related anemia: Results of a large, prospective, observational study. Haematologica. 2015;100(1):124.
52. Maccio A, Madeddu C, Massa D, Mudu MC, Lusso MR, Gramignano G, et al. Hemoglobin levels correlate with interleukin-6 levels in patients with advanced untreated epithelial ovarian cancer: Role of inflammation in cancer-related anemia. Blood. 2005;106(1):362-7.
53. Millonig G, Ganzleben I, Peccerella T, Casanovas G, Brodziak-Jarosz L, Breitkopf-Heinlein K, et al. Sustained submicromolar H_2O_2 levels induce hepcidin via signal transducer and activator of transcription 3 (STAT3). J Biol Chem. 2012;287(44):37472-82.
54. Rodgers GM, Gilreath JA. The role of intravenous iron in the treatment of anemia associated with cancer and chemotherapy. Acta Haematol. 2019;142(1):13-20.
55. Kautz L, Jung G, Valore EV, Rivella S, Nemeth E, Ganz T. Identification of erythroferrone as an erythroid regulator of iron metabolism. Nat Genet. 2014;46(7):678-84.
56. Kling PJ, Dragsten PR, Roberts RA, Santos BD, Brooks DJ, Hedlund BE, et al. Iron deprivation increases erythropoietin production in vitro, in normal subjects and patients with malignancy. Brit J Haematol. 1996;95(2):241-8.
57. Bron D, Meuleman N, Mascaux C. Biological basis of anemia. Seminars in Oncology. WB Saunders; 2001, vol. 28, pp. 1-6.
58. Alvarez-Hernandez X, Liceaga J, McKay IC, Brock JH. Induction of hypoferremia and modulation of macrophage iron metabolism by tumor necrosis factor. Lab Invest. 1989;61(3):319-22.
59. Torti FM, Torti SV. Regulation of ferritin genes and protein. Blood. 2002;99(10):3505-16.
60. Ludwiczek S, Aigner E, Theurl I, Weiss G. Cytokine-mediated regulation of iron transport in human monocytic cells. Blood. 2003;101(10):4148-54.
61. Schmidt PJ. Regulation of iron metabolism by hepcidin under conditions of inflammation. J Biol Chem. 2015;290(31):18975-83.
62. Recalcati S, Locati M, Gammella E, Invernizzi P, Cairo G. Iron levels in polarized macrophages: Regulation of immunity and autoimmunity. Autoimmun Rev. 2012;11(12):883-9.
63. Madeddu C, Mantovani G, Gramignano G, Astara G, Macciò A. Muscle wasting as main evidence of energy impairment in cancer cachexia: Future therapeutic approaches. Future Oncol. 2015;11(19):2697-710.
64. Basseri RJ, Nemeth E, Vassilaki ME, Basseri B, Enayati P, Shaye O, et al. Hepcidin is a key mediator of anemia of inflammation in Crohn's disease. J Crohns Colitis. 2013;7(8): e286-91.
65. Shu T, Jing C, Lv Z, Xie Y, Xu J, Wu J. Hepcidin in tumor-related iron deficiency anemia and tumor-related anemia of chronic disease: Pathogenic mechanisms and diagnosis. Eur J Haematol. 2015;94(1):67-73.
66. Martin L, Senesse P, Gioulbasanis I, Antoun S, Bozzetti F, Deans C, et al. Diagnostic criteria for the classification of cancer-associated weight loss. J Clin Oncol. 2015;33(1):90-9.
67. Fearon K, Strasser F, Anker SD, Bosaeus I, Bruera E, Fainsinger RL, et al. Definition and classification of cancer cachexia: An international consensus. Lancet Oncol. 2011;12(5):489-95.
68. Friesen DE, Baracos VE, Tuszynski JA. Modeling the energetic cost of cancer as a result of altered energy metabolism: implications for cachexia. Theoret Biol Med Model. 2015;12:1-8.
69. Porporato PE. Understanding cachexia as a cancer metabolism syndrome. Oncogenesis. 2016;5(2):e200.
70. Hung SC, Tung TY, Yang CS, Tarng DC. High-calorie supplementation increases serum leptin levels and improves response to rHuEPO in long-term hemodialysis patients. Am J Kidney Dis. 2005;45(6):1073-83.

71. Abella V, Scotece M, Conde J, Pino J, Gonzalez-Gay MA, Gómez-Reino JJ, et al. Leptin in the interplay of inflammation, metabolism and immune system disorders. Nat Rev Rheumatol. 2017;13(2):100-9.
72. Mantovani G, Macciò A, Mura L, Massa E, Mudu MC, Mulas C, et al. Serum levels of leptin and proinflammatory cytokines in patients with advanced-stage cancer at different sites. J Mol Med. 2000;78:554-61.
73. Macciò A, Madeddu C, Massa D, Astara G, Farci D, Melis GB, et al. Interleukin-6 and leptin as markers of energy metabolicchanges in advanced ovarian cancer patients. J Cell Mol Med. 2009;13(9b):3951-9.
74. Umemoto Y, Tsuji K, Yang FC, Ebihara Y, Kaneko A, Furukawa S, et al. Leptin stimulates the proliferation of murine myelocytic and primitive hematopoietic progenitor cells. Blood, J Am Soc Hematol. 1997;90(9):3438-43.
75. Ludwig H, Strasser K. Symptomatology of anemia. Seminars in oncology. WB Saunders; 2001, vol. 28, pp. 7-14.
76. Groopman JE, Itri LM. Chemotherapy-induced anemia in adults: Incidence and treatment. J Nat Cancer Instit. 1999;91(19):1616-34.
77. Oburoglu L, Romano M, Taylor N, Kinet S. Metabolic regulation of hematopoietic stem cell commitment and erythroid differentiation. Curr Opin Hematol. 2016;23(3):198-205.
78. Hainsworth JD, Levitan N, Wampler GL, Belani CP, Seyedsadr MS, Randolph J, et al. Phase II randomized study of cisplatin plus etoposide phosphate or etoposide in the treatment of small-cell lung cancer. J Clin Oncol. 1995;13(6):1436-42.
79. Loehrer Sr PJ, Ansari R, Gonin R, Monaco F, Fisher W, Sandler A, et al. Cisplatin plus etoposide with and without ifosfamide in extensive small-cell lung cancer: A Hoosier Oncology Group study. J Clin Oncol. 1995;13(10):2594-9.
80. Nowrousian MR. Prevalence, pathophysiology, predictive factors, and prognostic significance of anemia in cancer chemotherapy. In: Nowrousian MR (Ed). Recombinant Human Erythropoietin (rhEPO) in Clinical Oncology: Scientific and Clinical Aspects of Anemia in Cancer. Springer Vienna. 2012; pp. 63-100.
81. Schiller JH. Current standards of care in small-cell and non-small-cell lung cancer. Oncology. 2001;61(Suppl. 1):3-13.
82. Nabholtz JM, Gelmon K, Bontenbal M, Spielmann M, Catimel G, Conte P, et al. Multicenter, randomized comparative study of two doses of paclitaxel in patients with metastatic breast cancer. J Clin Oncol. 1996;14(6):1858-67.
83. Dieras V, Marty M, Tubiana. Net al Phase II randomized study of paclitaxel versus mitomycin in advanced breast cancer. Semin Oncol. 1995;22(4 Suppl 8):33-9.
84. Bokkel Huinink W ten, Gore M, Carmichael J, Gordon A, Malfetano J, Hudson I, et al. Topotecan versus paclitaxel for the treatment of recurrent epithelial ovarian cancer. J Clin Oncol. 1997;15(6):2183-93.
85. Creemers GJ, Bolis G, Gore M, Scarfone G, Lacave AJ, Guastalla JP, et al. Topotecan, an active drug in the second-line treatment of epithelial ovarian cancer: Results of a large European phase II study. J Clin Oncol. 1996;14:3056-61.
86. Sertoli MR, Santini G, Chisesi T, Congiu AM, Rubagotti A, Contu A, et al. MACOP-B versus ProMACE-MOPP in the treatment of advanced diffuse non-Hodgkin's lymphoma: Results of a prospective randomized trial by the non-Hodgkin's Lymphoma Cooperative Study Group. J Clin Oncol. 1994;12(7):1366-74.
87. Hill M, Norman A, Cunningham D, Findlay M, Watson M, Nicolson V, et al. Impact of protracted venous infusion fluorouracil with or without interferon alfa-2b on tumor response, survival, and quality of life in advanced colorectal cancer. J Clin Oncol. 1995;13(9):2317-23.
88. Petrelli N, Douglass HO Jr, Herrera L, Russell D, Stablein DM, Bruckner HW, et al. The modulation of fluorouracil with leucovorin in metastatic colorectal carcinoma: A

prospective randomized phase III trial. Gastrointestinal Tumor Study Group [published erratum appears in J Clin Oncol 1990;8:185]. J Clin Oncol. 1989;7:1419-26.
89. Rougier P, Bugat R, Douillard JY, Culine S, Suc E, Brunet P, et al. Phase II study of irinotecan in the treatment of advanced colorectal cancer in chemotherapy-naive patients and patients pretreated with fluorouracil-based chemotherapy. J Clin Oncol. 1997;15(1):251-60.
90. Forastiere AA, Neuberg D, Taylor S, DeConti R, Adams G. Phase II evaluation of Taxol in advanced head and neck cancer: An Eastern Cooperative Oncology group trial. J Nat Cancer Instit Monogr. 1993;(15):181-4.
91. Forastiere AA, Metch B, Schuller DE, Ensley JF, Hutchins LF, Triozzi P, et al. Randomized comparison of cisplatin plus fluorouracil and carboplatin plus fluorouracil versus methotrexate in advanced squamous-cell carcinoma of the head and neck: A Southwest Oncology Group study. J Clin Oncol. 1992;10(8):1245-51.
92. Koeller JM. Clinical guidelines for the treatment of cancer-related anemia. Pharmacotherapy. 1998;18(1):156-69.
93. Ganz T, Nemeth E. Iron balance and the role of hepcidin in chronic kidney disease. Seminars in Nephrology. WB Saunders; 2016;36(2):87-93.
94. Storring PL, Tiplady RJ, Das REG, Stenning BE, Lamikanra A, Rafferty B, et al. Epoetin alfa and beta differ in their erythropoietin isoform compositions and biological properties. Brit J Haematol. 1998;100(1):79-89.
95. Bohlius J, Weingart O, Trelle S, Engert A. Cancer-related anemia and recombinant human erythropoietin—an updated overview. Nat Clin Pract Oncol. 2006;3(3):152-64.
96. Haag-Weber M, Eckardt KU, Hürl WH, Roger SD, Vetter A, Roth K. Safety, immunogenicity and efficacy of subcutaneous biosimilar epoetin-α (HX575) in non-dialysis patients with renal anemia: A multi-center, randomized, double-blind study. Clin Nephrol. 2012;77(1):8-17.
97. Mhaskar R, Wao H, Miladinovic B, Kumar A, Djulbegovic B. The role of iron in the management of chemotherapy-induced anemia in cancer patients receiving erythropoiesis-stimulating agents. Cochrane Database Syst Rev. 2016;2(2):CD009624.
98. Fishbane S, Kowalski EA. The comparative safety of intravenous iron dextran, iron saccharate, and sodium ferric gluconate. In: Seminars in Dialysis; Boston, MA: Blackwell Science Inc. 2000;13(6):381-4.
99. Auerbach M, Ballard H, Trout JR, McIlwain M, Ackerman A, Bahrain H, et al. Intravenous iron optimizes the response to recombinant human erythropoietin in cancer patients with chemotherapy-related anemia: A multicenter, open-label, randomized trial. J Clin Oncol. 2004;22(7):1301-7.

CHAPTER 13

Anemia in CKD—Pathophysiology and Recent Updates in Treatment Strategy

Brijesh Thakur

INTRODUCTION

The general pathologic causes of normocytic anemia include endocrine deficiency, renal insufficiency, hemolytic or post-hemorrhagic anemia, anemia of chronic disorder or hypersplenism. The common manifestation of chronic kidney disease (CKD) is anemia possibly related to erythropoietin (EPO) deficiency (major factor), chronic stage, reduced red blood cells (RBCs) life span, underlying iron deficiency, or blood loss particularly in hemodialysis. Presence as well as severity of anemia may worsen the quality of life and survival. Anemia in CKD is associated with significant increase in morbidity and mortality either independently or other coexisting disorders in CKD patients. Major complications of anemia in CKD are superadded inflammation, progressive left ventricular hypertrophy, more risk of myocardial infarction and worse cardiac outcomes. Approximately, 90% of patients having glomerular filtration rate (GFR) <30 mL/min are found to be anemic.[1] Variable prevalence rates of anemia up to 60% have been reported in studies focused on nondialysis-dependent CKD.[2]

Although pathogenesis of anemia in CKD is multifactorial, the predominant cause is reduced production of endogenous EPO which may be absolute and/or functional deficiency. Implication of recombinant human EPO in 1989 was a therapeutic landmark in the treatment of anemia in CKD; however, disappointing results with use of erythropoiesis-stimulating agents (ESAs) to increase hemoglobin (Hb) to range of normal levels have been found in some of the trials.[1] Globally, variable recommendations for the management of anemia in CKD have been considered. The iron therapy and the use of ESAs have caused significant betterment of patients with anemia of CKD. Few newer therapeutic trials are under assessment as well which have been discussed later.[3]

EVALUATION OF ANEMIA IN CHRONIC KIDNEY DISEASE
Stages of Chronic Kidney Disease
- *Stage 1*: Kidney damage with normal or increased GFR (equal/more than 90 mL/min/1.73 m^2)
- *Stage 2*: Kidney damage with mild decreased GFR (60-89 mL/min/1.73 m^2)
- *Stage 3*: Moderate decreased GFR (30-59 mL/min/1.73 m^2)
- *Stage 4*: Severe decreased GFR (15-29 mL/min/1.73 m^2)
- *Stage 5*: Kidney failure (<15 mL/min/1.73 m^2 or dialysis)

Before labeling patients with anemia attributed to CKD, a thorough work up should be done to exclude other reversible processes or associated factors which may be the cause of decreased hemoglobin in CKD. Particularly, iron deficiency is significantly frequent in patients with renal insufficiency. Almost all dialysis patients reveal iron deficiency at some stage. Iron deficiency may be attributed to blood loss during dialysis or increased iron demand secondary to ESAs.

Anemia is defined as—in adults and children >15 years with CKD when the Hb concentration is <13.0 g/dL (or 130 g/L) in males and <12.0 g/dL (or 120 g/L) in females (KDIGO 2012 guidelines).[4] CKD should be considered as a possible cause of anemia when the GFR is <60 mL/min/1.73 m^2; even more likely if the GFR is <30 mL/min/1.73 m^2 (<45/min/1.73 m^2 in patients with diabetes) and no other specific cause of anemia is identified.[4,5]

Investigations must be performed for a thorough evaluation of anemia in CKD (regardless of age and CKD stage)—no definite supporting evidences for different guidelines for anemia evaluation in pediatric age group have been described till date.
- *Complete blood count (CBC) including:*
    - Hb concentration
    - Mean corpuscular hemoglobin (MCH)
    - Mean corpuscular volume (MCV)
    - Mean corpuscular hemoglobin concentration (MCHC)
    - White blood cell count and differential count
    - Platelet count
    - Absolute reticulocyte count to assess bone marrow responsiveness (if indicated).
- *Test to determine iron status*: Two important aspects for iron status evaluation include the presence or absence of iron stores and it's accessibility for erythropoiesis.
    - Percentage of hypochromic red blood cells (%HRC): A fresh sample is needed and processing of blood sample to be done within 6 hours of sample collection.
    - In case, fresh sample is not available: Equivalent tests like reticulocyte Hb equivalent or combination of transferrin saturation (TSAT) and serum ferritin may be done in case %HRC or reticulocyte Hb equivalent are not available or the patient has thalassemia or

CHAPTER 13: Anemia in CKD—Pathophysiology and Recent Updates...

thalassemia trait. At times, finding of a TSAT <20% coupled with a ferritin level greater than 500 µg/L may pose an interpretational difficulty for clinicians.

- ○ Serum ferritin to assess iron stores: Low serum ferritin is a useful marker to diagnose the absolute iron deficiency. Normal or high serum ferritin values (≥100 µg/L) do not exclude iron deficiency completely, which may be related to other causes, for example, infection or inflammation. Hence, ferritin values should be interpreted with caution in CKD patients.
- *Plasma/serum C-reactive protein (CRP):* To assess the inflammatory status of the patient.
- *Serum B12 and folate levels:* To rule out the coexisting deficiencies; although uncommon.
- Tests for hemolysis (plasma/serum levels of haptoglobin, lactate dehydrogenase, bilirubin, and Coomb's test).
- *Plasma/serum and/or urine protein electrophoresis:* Especially to rule out the presence of M-band.
- Hb electrophoresis
- Free light chains and bone marrow examination
- *EPO levels:* The EPO levels cannot be used to distinguish renal anemia from other causes of anemia. The measurement of EPO level is rarely helpful for the diagnosis or management of anemia in CKD patients. Even these patients may have EPO levels equal to or higher than that in normal non-anemic individuals.

MONITORING OF CHRONIC KIDNEY DISEASE PATIENTS FOR ANEMIA (NOT GRADED)[4]

- KDIGO 2012 guidelines suggest the measurement of Hb level at least annually in patients with CKD 3, at least twice per year in patients with CKD 4-5ND (nondialysis) and at least every 3 months in patients with CKD 5HD (hemodialysis) and CKD 5PD (peritoneal dialysis) in CKD patients without anemia
- In cases if Hb levels are <110 g/L (<105 g/L if younger than 2 years) or they develop symptoms attributable to anemia.
- In case of CKD patients with anemia and not treated with ESAs, measure Hb concentration at least every 3 months in patients with CKD 3-5ND and CKD 5PD and at least monthly in patients with CKD 5HD.
- Patients should also be monitored for Hb level response to previous iron therapy, iron status (at least every 3 months), ESA response, changes in parameters of various investigations or blood loss.
- *If patient is on iron therapy*: Iron repletion is usually defined as: %HRC <6%/CHr (mean cellular hemoglobin content of reticulocytes), >29 pg/ferritin and TSAT (>100 µg/L and >20%).

PATHOPHYSIOLOGY OF ANEMIA IN CHRONIC KIDNEY DISEASE[6-8]

Typically, the erythropoietic profile is characterized by normocytic, normochromic morphology, a normal MCV, a low reticulocyte count, and an absence of polychromasia on the peripheral blood smear. Renal anemia is accompanied by failure of the normal EPO response or progressive reduction of endogenous EPO levels which is a major factor in the pathogenesis of anemia in CKD. However, other contributing factors to anemia in CKD patients have been considered like reduced iron levels due to blood loss or impaired iron absorption, increased hepcidin levels leading to impaired use of iron stores, systemic inflammation and associated comorbidities, such as diabetes mellitus, hyporesponsive bone marrow to EPO due to uremic toxins, decreased RBCs life span, or other deficiency states such as vitamin B12 or folic acid. EPO is a glycoprotein (165 amino acids, 30.4 kDa) produced mainly by the interstitial peritubular cells of the kidney, and lesser amount (about 10–15%) by liver (80% by hepatocytes, 20% by Ito cells); depending upon the condition of tissue oxygen tension. However, kidney is much more sensitive to the low oxygen tension for EPO production as compared with liver. In humans, the plasma half-life of EPO produced by the kidney is 5–6 hours due to high levels of glycosylation.

Receptor for EPO is present on the surface of erythroid progenitor or precursor cells including burst forming unit erythroid (BFU-E) and colony forming unit erythroid (CFU-E). The primary target cells of EPO are CFU-E cells, which are responsive to small amounts of EPO as well, and stimulated for their proliferation as well as differentiation. The binding of EPO to its receptor autophosphorylates Janus kinase 2 (JAK2), leading to the inhibition of apoptosis of progenitor cells via the activation of multiple regulatory processes including signal transducer and activator of transcription (STAT) pathway, phosphatidylinositol 3-kinase (PI3K) and AKT pathway as well. The EPO receptor expression is controlled by the transcription factor, that is, GATA-1 which allows increasing erythropoiesis quickly as required during the erythroid cells differentiation.

The *EPO* gene is present on chromosome 7 (q11–q22) and its transcription is activated by hypoxia-induced factor 1 (HIF-1). Other hypoxia-induced genes like vascular endothelial growth factor (VEGF), platelet-derived growth factor (PDGF), glycolytic enzymes, such as aldolase A, enolase-1, lactate dehydrogenase A, phosphofructokinase-1, and phosphoglycerate kinase-1 are also activated by HIF1. HIF1 consists of two subunits, HIF1α and HIF1β. HIF1β is constitutively expressed whereas under normal oxygen tension, HIF1α is hydroxylated by specific HIF prolyl-hydroxylase enzymes (also known as prolylhydroxylase domain or PHD enzymes) in presence of cofactors as oxygen, iron, and 2-oxoglutarate. Then E3 ubiquitin ligase von Hippel-Lindau (pVHL) binds HIF1α, and is targeted for proteosomal degradation, hence, HIF1α is absent under normoxic condition.

In hypoxic condition, as the action of PHDs is prevented, HIF1α accumulates and translocates to the nucleus and binds to HIF1β. The HIF1α-β heterodimer binds to DNA sequences (hypoxia response elements or HRE), regulating the downregulation or upregulation of various hypoxia-sensitive genes. In addition to *EPO* gene, various genes encoding EPO receptor, transferrin, and transferrin receptor, VEGF, or endothelin-1 are also upregulated **(Fig. 1)**.

■ IRON DEFICIENCY IN CHRONIC KIDNEY DISEASE

Another important contributing factor to renal anemia is the limited availability of iron for erythropoiesis. In dialyzed patients, reduced iron level is mainly attributed to excessive blood loss, especially related to the residual amount of blood inside the dialyzer, dialysis sets and needles after each hemodialysis, bleeding at intravenous (IV) access sites, and repeated blood sampling for investigations. Hence, negative iron balance and reduced iron stores may develop easily if the patient is not taking iron therapy. In renal disease, the EPO deficiency and chronic inflammation result in reduced number of EPO-stimulated erythroblasts which are the source of erythroferrone (ERFE), main erythroid hormonal regulator of hepcidin which in turn controls plasma iron

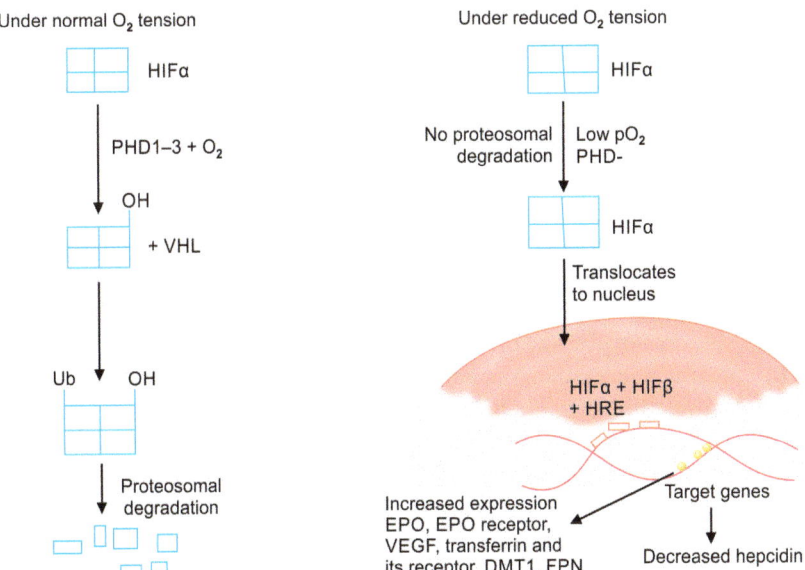

FIG. 1: Diagrammatic representation of role of HIF (hypoxia inducing factor) in the regulation of *EPO* gene expression and other erythropoiesis-related molecules and their receptors under normoxic as well as hypoxic conditions.

(DMT1: divalent metal transporter 1; EPO: erythropoietin; FPN: ferroportin; HRE: hypoxia response element; PHD: prolylhydroxylase domain; VEGF: vascular endothelial growth factor; VHL: von Hippel-Lindau)

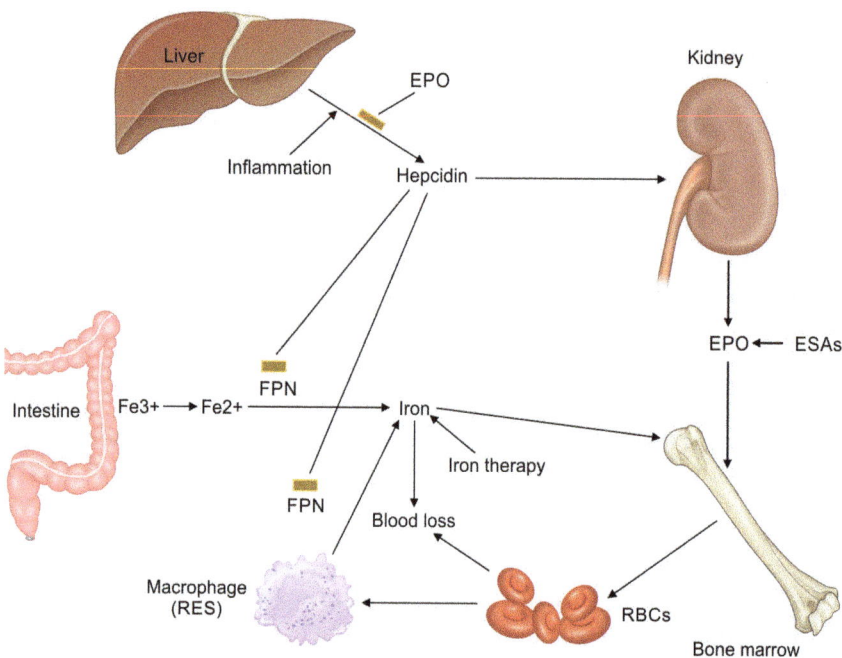

FIG. 2: Diagrammatic representation of regulation of iron balance by various factors.

levels and total body iron. Mobilization of stored and recycled iron as well as absorption of duodenal iron is increased by ERFE after bleeding or hemolysis **(Fig. 2)**.

Hepcidin, currently believed to be crucial in the regulation of iron metabolism, is inhibited by increased erythropoiesis or hypoxia while induced by excess iron levels or inflammation. Increased hepcidin levels decrease the level of iron by reducing dietary absorption and its release from iron stores as well. Although, routine measurement of hepcidin levels in the diagnosis of iron deficiency in dialyzed patients is not recommended. However, serum ferritin level is considered a relatively simple and reliable tool to confirm decreased iron stores. Other laboratory parameters, such as iron plasma concentrations (pFe), transferrin, and TSAT can be used to evaluate the functional iron deficiency. These tests may be complemented by the percentage of hypochromic RBCs, erythrocyte zinc protoporphyrin testing, or serum transferrin receptor levels, although the role of these parameters is not validated in CKD patients.

Absolute iron deficiency: It is defined as a serum ferritin concentration <100 ng/mL and TSAT <20%.

Functional iron deficiency: It is defined as TSAT <20% and normal/high ferritin levels. Despite normal or high iron stores, iron cannot be adequately mobilized from the reticuloendothelial system.

INFLAMMATION IN CHRONIC KIDNEY DISEASE

Systemic inflammation in renal failure may be attributed to autoimmune diseases, infections, diabetes mellitus, use of intravascular devices, and renal osteodystrophy leading to increased inflammatory cytokines which suppress EPO production and erythroid differentiation. Various cytokines, such as IL-6, TNF, interferon-γ (IFN-γ) and IL-1β play important role in these suppressive actions. Inflammation and infections also restrict iron supply to the bone marrow by inducing transcription of *HAMP* (which encodes hepcidin) via IL-6 signaling through the STAT3 pathway and activin B signaling through the BMP/Smad1/5/8 pathway.

OTHER CONTRIBUTING FACTORS TO RENAL ANEMIA

Other associated factors may contribute to the development of anemia or exacerbate renal anemia, for example, coincidental vitamin B12 and folate deficiency, drugs such as angiotensin converting enzyme (ACE) inhibitors, uremic toxins, secondary hyperparathyroidism, malnutrition, and tumors. Approximately, in 40% of the anemic kidney transplant cases, anemia is mainly due to impaired graft function. Immunosuppressive drugs also have a direct effect of bone marrow suppression. Cyclosporine A and mTOR inhibitors may cause hemolytic uremic syndrome and hemolysis in cases of renal transplants.

ERYTHROPOIETIN RESISTANCE

A proportion of CKD patients may have functional EPO deficiency or EPO resistance, indicating that bone marrow response to endogenous and exogenous EPO is not optimal. These patients present with low Hb even in the presence of normal EPO levels. EPO resistance is hypothesized to be attributed to various factors, such as proinflammatory cytokines release, enhanced hepcidin production, or selective hemolysis of young RBCs in patients on exogenous EPO.

UPDATES IN TREATMENT STRATEGY OF ANEMIA IN CHRONIC KIDNEY DISEASE[9,10]

There has been dramatic progress in the management of anemia in CKD, starting from the first oral iron supplements (ferrous sulfate) first introduced in 1830, the use of RBC transfusions along the 20th century, androgens as nontransfusional therapy to the approval of recombinant human EPO in 1989, followed by long-acting ESAs to the widespread use of IV iron therapy. Androgens can stimulate bone marrow as well as renal and/or liver EPO production which may lead to the improvement of anemia. Initially, the use of recombinant EPO was mainly done to prevent blood transfusion in anemic CKD patients but later studies revealed that ESAs have improved the quality of living, neurocognitive function, and major outcomes like regression of left ventricular hypertrophy. Currently, ESAs and IV iron therapy appear the key players of renal anemia treatment. Recently, pharmacologic activation of HIF response appears to have a great remedial effect, and seems to have better physiologic effect in renal anemia management rather than current approaches.

Four main randomized controlled trials were conducted to evaluate the effects in randomized patients to either higher "normal-range" hemoglobin targets or to lower target Hb levels [The NHCT (Normal Hematocrit Study), CHOIR (Correction of Hemoglobin and Outcomes in Renal Insufficiency) trial, CREATE (Cardiovascular Risk Reduction by Early Anemia Treatment) trial, TREAT (Trial to Reduce Cardiovascular Events With Aranesp Therapy)]. Their findings were not rewarding and only the CREATE trial was able to demonstrate an improved quality of life benefit for the high-target group.

Target Iron Levels

The guidelines recommend the following criteria for maintaining iron stores:

For adult patients with CKD who are not on dialysis, iron should be given to keep TSAT above 20% and ferritin level above 100 ng/mL. TSAT should not exceed 30%, and ferritin levels should not exceed 500 ng/mL.

For adult patients on dialysis, iron should be given to maintain TSAT above 30% and ferritin level above 200 ng/mL.

Some controversies occur about the optimal Hb and iron targets in different randomized controlled trials or guidelines.

Erythropoiesis-stimulating agents may be given to patients with anemia of CKD, to avoid blood transfusion; especially in patients who are considered suitable for transplantation. Various ESAs have different pharmacokinetic and pharmacodynamic properties, such as different half-lives and affinity for EPO receptor, allowing a less frequent dosing and ease of administration when long-acting ESAs are being used for nondialysis-dependent CKD patients. In the case of absolute iron deficiency (ferritin <100 μg/L), ESAs should not be started; however, they may be given if anemia persists even after correction of iron deficiency. If patients have functional iron deficiency, iron supplements should be initiated before or during initiation of ESA therapy. Common ESAs include Epoetin-alpha or beta, Darbepoetin and CERA (continuous EPO receptor activator).

Target or achievable Hb range between 10 and 12 g% in adults, young people, children aged 2 years and older; 9.5-11.5 g% in children younger than 2 years of age should be achieved. Determining factors for the first ESA dose include the patient's Hb level, body weight, clinical states (like history of thromboembolism, seizure, hypertension, or cardiovascular event), the target Hb level and the rate of increase in Hb level (recommended 1-2 g/dL/month). Subcutaneous (SC) route is the method of choice in nondialysis patients, while IV route is preferable in hemodialysis patients.

The SC route for short-acting ESA administration may reduce about 30% of the dose requirement for the same achievable Hb in comparison to IV access. ESA doses should ideally be reduced when a downward adjustment of desirable Hb level is needed. In patients with previous history of hypertension, stroke, or malignancy, ESAs should be prescribed or initiated with caution. ESA-dependent patients should not discontinue treatment in acute illness, surgical procedures or during hospitalization, unless it is contraindicated. ESAs should be ceased in patients developing ESA-induced pure red cell aplasia. Blood pressure should be monitored in all patients receiving ESAs, and hypertension should be treated by volume removal and/or antihypertensive drugs. Hyporesponsive patients with replenish iron stores should be evaluated to rule out other common causes of anemia.

Usually, oral iron may be enough to achieve target Hb in ESA-treated CKD patients not yet requiring dialysis and in those on peritoneal dialysis. For nondialysis-dependent CKD patients, the preferred method between oral versus parenteral iron is determined by the severity of iron deficiency, previous therapeutic response and side effects, venous attainability, and requirement for ESA therapy. For adults and young people, high-dose (HD), low-frequency (LF) IV iron should be considered preferential therapy. Parenteral iron therapy in patients with active infection should be avoided and serum ferritin should not exceed 800 µg/L in patients who are on iron therapy. Regular monitoring of iron status (every 1-3 months) in patients should be done to avoid toxicity or overload.

The CHOIR trial proposed that elevated or soaring doses of epoetin-alpha, rather than target Hb per se, were found to be linked with increased risk of death, myocardial infarction, congestive heart failure or stroke compared with lower epoetin doses. The CREATE study correlated that early correction of anemia to normal Hb did not reduce the risk of cardiovascular events. Indeed, the hazards ratio for primary endpoints of death from any cause or death from cardiovascular disease consistently (but not significantly) favored the lower Hb target group. Although important subgroups of patients, such as young adults, patients returning to dialysis after failed renal transplant, or patients with chronic lung disease were not enrolled or evaluated in any of these trials.

Inadequate response ("resistance") to ESA therapy is defined as inability to attain the target or desirable Hb level. The exploration for new therapeutic alternatives is relevant in this scenario. In this context, some molecules of the HIF system have already been studied as new targets for anemia treatment to increase the endogenous EPO production and to improve the utilization of iron stores. The uncovering of PHDs as oxygen sensors allowed a structural basis for the evolvement of HIF activating compounds, called PHD inhibitors (PHIs). These compounds inhibit PHD catalytic activity by binding to the ferrous iron-containing active site, thereby blocking the entry of the co-substrate 2 oxoglutarate (2OG). These HIF stabilizers have advantages as being considerable convenient, compliant, less expensive compared with

ESAs, nonimmunogenic, effective independent of iron repletion status or inflammation status of patients. However, these inhibitors may cause potential downstream harmful effects like pro-angiogenic effects or PHI-induced hypoxia responses or acceleration of proliferative retinopathy in diabetic patients. HIF stabilizers are still in clinical trials, no validated guideline for their use till date is recommended. One trial suggested that HIF-PHIs, such as daprodustat may be a better alternative to conventional ESAs.

CONCLUSION

- Anemia in CKD patients is a frequent manifestation with multifactorial pathophysiology and predominantly attributed to decrease in endogenous EPO production.
- Renal anemia may be a contributing factor for poor outcome, such as increased risk of left ventricular hypertrophy, myocardial infarction, and heart failure.
- Before starting ESAs, a thorough evaluation is needed to rule out associated conditions such as iron or vitamin deficiencies.
- ESAs have their different pharmacological properties and variable outcomes in CKD patients with ESA therapy and still it remains to be elucidated.
- PHIs are newer alternatives under clinical assessment. The available data proposed that these are safer options for the treatment of renal anemia in nondialyzed and dialysis-dependent CKD patients as compared with ESAs. However, added elucidated data is needed to validate these conclusions and to formulate new additional recommendations for better outcome of patients.

REFERENCES

1. Nakhoul G, Simon JF. Anemia of chronic kidney disease: Treat it, but not too aggressively. Cleve Clin J Med. 2016;83:613-24.
2. Portolés J, Martín L, Broseta JJ, Cases A. Anemia in Chronic Kidney Disease: From Pathophysiology and Current Treatments, to Future Agents. Front Med (Lausanne). 2021;8:642296.
3. Mikhail A, Brown C, Williams JA, Mathrani V, Shrivastava R, Evans J, et al. Renal association clinical practice guideline on Anaemia of Chronic Kidney Disease. BMC Nephrol. 2017;18:345.
4. KDIGO Clinical Practice for Anemia in Chronic Kidney Disease. Kidney Int. 2012;2(Suppl 4):279-366.
5. Locatelli F, Bárány P, Covic A, De Francisco A, Del Vecchio L, Goldsmith D, et al. Kidney Disease: Improving Global Outcomes guidelines on anaemia management in chronic kidney disease: a European Renal Best Practice position statement. Nephrol Dial Transplant. 2013;28:1346-59.
6. Geddes CC. Pathophysiology of renal anaemia. Nephrol Dial Transplant. 2019;34:921-2.
7. Eschbach JW. The anemia of chronic renal failure: pathophysiology and the effects of recombinant erythropoietin. Kidney Int. 1989;35:134-48.

8. Zadrazil J, Horak P. Pathophysiology of anemia in chronic kidney diseases: A review. Biomed Pap Med Fac Univ Palacky Olomouc Czech Repub. 2015;159:197-202.
9. Koury MJ, Haase VH. Anaemia in kidney disease: harnessing hypoxia responses for therapy. Nat Rev Nephrol. 2015;11:394-410.
10. Cases A, Puchades MJ, de Sequera P, Quiroga B, Martin-Rodriguez L, Gorriz JL, et al. Iron replacement therapy in the management of anaemia in non-dialysis Chronic kidney disease patients: Perspective of the Spanish Nephrology Society Anaemia Group. Nefrologia (Engl Ed). 2021;41:123-36.

CHAPTER 14

Tumor-like Lesions Associated with B-cell Predominance

Surbhi Mahajan, Swati Arora

■ INTRODUCTION

Amidst the spectrum of pathological variations, a group of conditions exists that mimics tumorous growth yet defies the typical characteristics of malignancy. Within this spectrum, a subgroup defined by an abundance of B-cells presents a diverse range of conditions that mimic neoplastic growth yet exhibit distinct biological behaviors. A recent addition to the WHO 'Blue Book' on hematolymphoid tumors introduces a classification, carving out a distinct category for tumor-like lesions primarily characterized by a prevalence of B-cells. This chapter embarks into the exploration of these distinctive tumor-like formations, aiming to highlight their specific cellular attributes and intricate diagnostic challenges.

The World Health Organization's "Blue Book" on hematolymphoid tumors (WHO-HAEM5) has recently introduced a new umbrella term of "tumor-like lesions associated with B-cell predominance." This new category includes five entities for the first time.[1]

1. Immunoglobulin G4-related disease (IgG4-RD)
2. Reactive B-cell predominant lymphoid proliferations that can mimic lymphoma
3. Unicentric Castleman disease (CD)
4. Idiopathic multicentric CD
5. KSHV/HHV8-associated multicentric CD.

■ IMMUNOGLOBULIN G4-RELATED DISEASE

Immunoglobulin G4-related disease is a chronic immune-mediated disorder characterized by the presence of tumefactive growths, fibrotic changes, and the accumulation of IgG4-positive plasma cells throughout different regions of the body.

The disease can manifest in multiple organs over time, leading to diverse clinical presentations.

Common presentations often involve the swelling of prominent salivary and lacrimal glands, orbital issues, autoimmune pancreatitis, retroperitoneal fibrosis, and tubulointerstitial nephritis.

The discovery of IgG4-RD can be traced back to the early 2000s when Japanese researchers, while investigating noninvasive biomarkers to differentiate sclerosing pancreatitis from pancreatic cancer, noticed elevated serum IgG4 levels and a prevalent IgG4-focused band in the beta-gamma segment of serum protein electrophoresis in patients with sclerosing pancreatitis. This finding led to the identification of abundant polyclonal IgG4 plasma cells in tissue samples from patients with autoimmune pancreatitis. The recognition of these unique features also linked several previously considered "idiopathic" and eponymous disorders, such as multifocal fibrosclerosis, Kuttner tumor, and Reidel thyroiditis, to the spectrum of IgG4-RD.[2.]

Immunoglobulin G4-related lymphadenopathy is a frequent occurrence in IgG4-RD and is observed in a substantial proportion of patients, ranging from 30 to 60% in significant cohorts.[3] It can be discovered incidentally during the removal of affected organs or with the use of medical imaging, and in some cases, it may precede the diagnosis of extranodal IgG4-related disease.

Immunoglobulin G4-related lymphadenopathy has been appropriately characterized as a condition that can be both underdiagnosed and overdiagnosed. Its underdiagnosis is due to the possibility of overlooking this entity during the diagnostic process, leading to missed cases. On the other hand, it can also be overdiagnosed when clinicians mistakenly attribute certain lymph node findings to IgG4-related disease without proper consideration of other potential causes such as Rosai–Dorfman disease and inflammatory vasculitis, which also show increased IgG4 plasma cells.

A lymph node biopsy might not always be the optimal approach for obtaining a histological diagnosis of IgG4-RD. Nonetheless, when dealing with patients who exhibit typical clinical features such as autoimmune pancreatitis or retroperitoneal fibrosis, a lymph node biopsy can serve as a suitable alternative when biopsying other affected organs is not feasible.[2]

Histopathological analysis plays a crucial role in diagnosing IgG4-RD. Key characteristics consist of a polyclonal, dense lymphoplasmacytic infiltrate that is enriched with IgG4-positive plasma cells, featuring an IgG4/IgG ratio exceeding 40%, as well as storiform fibrosis and obliterative phlebitis. Nevertheless, lymph nodes in individuals afflicted by IgG4-related ailment usually do not exhibit fibrosis or obliterative phlebitis. Instead, they display

- *Multicentric CD-like*: This pattern is characterized by hyperplastic follicles showing regressive changes and penetration by hyalinized blood vessels. Additionally, there is an increase in high endothelial venules and plasma cells in the interfollicular area.
- *Follicular hyperplasia*: This pattern demonstrates typical follicular hyperplasia, with increased plasma cells observed in the germinal centers and interfollicular zones.

- *Interfollicular expansion*: In this pattern, there are usually few, often atrophic follicles, and the interfollicular zone appears expanded. It contains high endothelial venules, small lymphocytes, immunoblasts, mature plasma cells, and eosinophils.
- *Progressive transformation of germinal centers (PTGC)*: This pattern presents enlarged follicles with PTGC amidst a background of follicular hyperplasia. There is an accompanying increase in plasma cells in germinal centers and interfollicular zones.
- *Inflammatory pseudotumor-like*: In this pattern, focal sclerosis of the lymph node parenchyma is observed, along with admixed lymphocytes, plasma cells, and eosinophils.

It is important to note that in these various patterns, there is an increase in plasma cells both within the interfollicular regions and germinal centers of reactive follicles.[4]

For an unsuspecting hematologist, it may be challenging to establish its diagnosis, given the potential overlap with disorders like plasma cell neoplasms, lymphoma, multicentric CD and hypereosinophilic syndrome.

When IgG4-RD is suspected, initial examinations such as serum protein electrophoresis and IgG subclass analysis can be informative, but a conclusive diagnosis necessitates histological confirmation in accordance with the International Consensus Criteria. These criteria encompass the presence of a concentrated lymphoplasmacytic infiltration, storiform fibrosis, and obliterative phlebitis, in conjunction with an elevated count of IgG4+ plasma cells and an IgG4/IgG plasma cell ratio exceeding 40%.[2]

Timely recognition and diagnosis are of utmost importance, as patients often exhibit favorable responses to early treatment with steroids or rituximab during the initial phases of the disease. If left untreated, fibrotic conditions and late complications, such as chronic pancreatitis, can progress to an irreversible stage.

Reactive B-cell rich lymphoid proliferations (RBRLPs), which can resemble lymphoma, encompass a range of conditions, including PTGC, florid reactive lymphoid hyperplasia/lymphoma-like lesions of the female genital tract, infectious mononucleosis (IM), and systemic lupus erythematosus (SLE).

While these lesions are frequently encountered or considered during lymphoma workup, it is important to note that various benign lymphadenopathies and related lesions can mimic lymphomas to some extent. Therefore, all possibilities should be thoroughly explored before reaching a final diagnosis.[1]

Progressive transformation of germinal centers is an innocuous response pattern in which follicles of different sizes, including some with prominent germinal centers, undergo infiltration by small mantle zone B-cells. The estimated prevalence of PTGC is approximately 3.5%.

Histologically, PTGC is usually observed as a limited occurrence, affecting less than 4–5% of follicles in over half of the cases. In instances of

PTGC-affected follicles, they appear notably enlarged; nearly, two to three times the size of a secondary follicle, with small lymphocytes from the mantle zone infiltrating the germinal center. In its early stages, the boundary of the germinal center begins to disintegrate, followed by a gradual breakdown of the germinal center due to an increased migration of mantle zone cells. In the later stages, one can observe collections of small lymphocytes within the germinal center, accompanied by remaining centrocytes and centroblasts interspersed throughout. The interfollicular area typically remains unaffected by these changes.

Immunohistochemistry examinations indicate that the small cells found within the germinal centers of PTGC consist of both B cells and T cells. The B cells exhibit an immunophenotype resembling mantle zone cells, expressing general B-cell markers, IgD, and BCL2, while not expressing CD10 and BCL6. On the other hand, the T cells show an immunophenotype of CD4 > CD8 and include numerous CD57$^+$ and PD-1/CD237$^+$ cells that are unusually evenly distributed throughout the germinal center. As PTGC progresses, the follicular dendritic cell networks gradually become disrupted, as revealed by CD21 or CD23 immunostaining. The native germinal center cells within PTGC follicles, similar to normal germinal centers, test positive for CD10 and BCL6 but negative for BCL2.[5]

Infectious mononucleosis is characterized by a collection of clinical and pathological findings associated with the swift onset of illness triggered by the Epstein-Barr virus (EBV). The traditional diagnostic trio of IM includes symptoms, such as lymphadenopathy, pharyngitis, and fever.

Laboratory examinations frequently uncover an increase in lymphocytosis and monocytosis. Within the realm of lymphocytes, a subset exhibits enlarged nuclei and an abundant pale blue cytoplasm, recognized as atypical lymphocytes (also known as Downey type 2 cells).

Although a lymph node biopsy is sometimes conducted to exclude the possibility of lymphoma, care is warranted, especially among younger individuals, due to the potential histopathological changes that can occasionally result in an incorrect lymphoma diagnosis.

The most distinguishing histological feature of IM involves the expansion of the interfollicular or paracortical regions due to a diverse infiltrate, which appears mottled under low-power magnification. Within this tissue infiltrate, one can observe a variety of cells, ranging from small to large lymphocytes, plasma cells, immunoblasts, and interdigitating dendritic cells. Initial indicators of an EBV infection include an increase in the size of follicles and scattered groupings of monocytoid B cells. Typical findings consist of isolated cell death or sporadic areas of tissue necrosis, along with prominently visible high endothelial vessels. The sinuses may appear enlarged and contain monocytoid B cells, small lymphocytes, and immunoblasts. Immunoblasts may display either a confined or widespread increase and could resemble the appearance of diffuse large B-cell lymphoma. Moreover, they can take on atypical or binucleated forms, resembling Hodgkin or Reed–Sternberg cells.

From an immunophenotypic perspective, hyperplastic follicles are marked by B-cell indicators, like CD20 or PAX-5, whereas germinal centers do not express BCL2. The paracortical area is predominantly occupied by T cells, with a higher prevalence of CD8$^+$ lymphocytes compared with CD4$^+$ lymphocytes. Immunoblasts exhibit CD30 expression, typically showing CD45/LCA positivity while lacking CD15. They can be associated with either B-cell or T-cell lineage, or in some instances, a combination of both may be observed.[6]

Systemic lupus erythematosus patients commonly experience localized or generalized lymphadenopathy, especially in younger individuals. Lymph nodes impacted by SLE often involve cervical, mesenteric, axillary, inguinal, and retroperitoneal regions. When examined under a microscope, these lymph nodes typically exhibit paracortical hyperplasia, with varying degrees of necrosis primarily concentrated in the paracortex. The viable lymph node tissue contains histiocytes, immunoblasts, and an abundance of plasma cells, sometimes including Russell bodies. Over time, necrotic areas become surrounded by granulation tissue and histiocytes.

Immunophenotypic analysis reveals a mixture of T-cells, with a predominance of CD8$^+$ cells over CD4$^+$ cells, alongside polytypic B cells and plasma cells.

Immunohistochemical examination indicates that SLE-related lymphadenopathy maintains a preserved organization of T-cell and B-cell compartments.[7]

Florid reactive lymphoid hyperplasia in the female genital tract represents a robust and extensive benign lymphoid reaction, which may prompt concerns about the possibility of malignant lymphoma.

The main histological features of florid RLH include marked lymphoid follicular hyperplasia, germinal center formation, and increased vascularity. It can occur in different locations within the female genital tract, such as the cervix, vagina, uterus, and ovaries.

The lesions consist of a diverse cellular infiltrate, comprising small and large lymphoid cells, including immunoblasts, along with admixed plasma cells and neutrophils. However, there is an absence of sclerosis. Lymphoma-like lesions affecting the cervix or endometrium are typically observed within a background of usual appearing chronic cervicitis or endometritis, respectively.

Immunohistochemistry reveals a mixture of B and T cells. Large cells are mostly CD20$^+$ B cells, and they may occasionally co-express CD30. Large B cells can form aggregates, sometimes resembling germinal centers. In the presence of germinal centers, they show positive staining for CD20, CD10, and BCL6, while being negative for BCL2, consistent with reactive follicles. The plasma cells show polytypic expression with a mixture of κ+ and λ+ cells.[8]

CASTLEMAN DISEASE

The nonclonal lymphoproliferative disorder known as CD is typified by systemic inflammation and is comprised of several conditions that exhibit common clinical and pathological manifestations.[9] CD was first described in the 1950s by Benjamin Castleman.[10] It is divided into unicentric CD (UCD), involving a single enlarged lymph node or region of lymph nodes, and multicentric CD (MCD), which involves multiple lymph node stations.[11,12] Recently, an intermediate subtype that affects a few lymph nodes and is generally thought to have a clinical course similar to that of UCD has been described. This subtype is known as "oligocentric CD" or "regional CD." Despite having enlarged lymph nodes in two or three nearby lymph node stations, these patients do not have enough clinical or laboratory abnormalities to meet the diagnostic standards for MCD.[13]

A new classification scheme has been proposed by the CD collaborative network (CDCN), which keeps the nomenclature used for UCD versus MCD but further divides MCD according to the etiological driver, for example, HHV8-associated MCD [HHV8-MCD] and POEMS-associated MCD [POEMS-MCD]. POEMS standing for polyneuropathy, organomegaly, endocrinopathy, monoclonal plasma cell disorder, skin changes; idiopathic MCD [iMCD] and within iMCD by phenotype, iMCD-TAFRO (thrombocytopenia, ascites, reticulin fibrosis, renal dysfunction, organomegaly) and iMCD–not otherwise specified (iMCD-NOS).[14]

UNICENTRIC CASTLEMAN DISEASE

Unicentric CD usually behaves in an indolent fashion. There is gradual enlargement of lymph nodes. Patients can be diagnosed at any age. Median age of diagnosis is 34 years. There is mild female preponderance.[13]

No known epidemiological factors have been identified to increase the risk of developing UCD. The estimated incidence of UCD in the US population is approximately 16–19 cases per million.[15] While UCD typically tests negative for RHV-8, there have been rare instances of positive cases documented in scientific literature. These instances should be classified as localized HHV-8-associated CD and treated accordingly.[16-19]

Patients who have underlying UCD may present with symptoms resulting from compression of vital structures (e.g., airways), or they may have iMCD-like inflammatory syndromes. The common sites of involvement are the neck, mediastinum, abdomen, and the retroperitoneum.[16] Other sites of involvement include axilla, inguinal regions, orbits, nasopharynx, and small bowel.[20-23] There is also increased risk of developing paraneoplastic pemphigus (PNP), AA amyloidosis, bronchiolitis obliterans (BO), vascular neoplasms (e.g., FDC sarcoma [FDCS]), and lymphomas.[13]

Paraneoplastic pemphigus: Life-threatening UCD linked to PNP frequently has progressive BO as well. The Asian population appears to have a disproportionately high frequency of this related condition. Typically, PNP and BO are found in the context of the HV histopathologic subtype of UCD, which is occasionally linked to stroma-rich characteristics. Patients with PNP with UCD should have complete surgical excision of UCD; this has been shown to frequently stop or reverse PNP. Despite therapy with a range of medications, either alone or in combination, such as corticosteroids, rituximab, cyclosporine A, and cyclophosphamide, BO has a significant fatality rate.

Follicular dendritic cell sarcoma: A rare kind of sarcoma called FDCS can co-occur with the HV histopathologic subtype of UCD and originate from FDCs. Differentiating UCD from lymphoma can be difficult. Patients with UCD have been found to have HD; nevertheless, the UCD plasmacytic-like histological alterations might just be reactive HD-related changes. Since UCD and HD are most commonly found in the same lymph node, surgical removal of the lesion is necessary. B-symptoms are present in many HD patients. Changes in PC UCD-like lymph nodes could be brought on by interleukin (IL)-6 and other cytokines that Reed–Sternberg cells produce. Sometimes, a distant lymph node has CD-like alterations, which can delay the diagnosis of HD. NHL is more frequently linked to UCD with HV histology than it is to HD. It has been reported that B- and T-cell lymphomas and UCD coexist. Follicular lymphoma (FL) with characteristics similar to HV UCD, an uncommon morphological variation of FL could make diagnosis challenging. According to van Rhee F, treatment for UCD and HD, or NHL should be predominantly determined by the lymphoma and involves excision, radiation, and chemotherapy.[13]

CLASSIC FEATURES OF UNICENTRIC CASTLEMAN DISEASE

The hyaline-vascular variant is the most common type of UCD, representing up to 65–75% of all cases. Hyaline-vascular UCD is characterized by abnormal follicles with small or atrophic germinal centers, sclerotic radial arterioles penetrating into germinal centers (so-called hyaline-vascular lesions or lollipop lesions), wide mantle zones with small lymphocytes arranged in linear arrays (so-called onion skin change), and interfollicular proliferation of stromal cells, often including many FDCs and small foci of hyperplastic plasmacytoid dendritic cells (PDCs).[15] Variation in the proportions of the follicular and interfollicular components can result in a wide spectrum of appearances,[13] ranging from predominantly follicular to stroma-rich presentations. Obliteration of the subcapsular and medullary sinuses is also commonly seen, and is often one of the earliest manifestations of UCD. Mixed/plasmacytic UCD represents 25–35% of all cases of UCD. This lesion is characterized by follicular hyperplasia and clusters or sheets of interfollicular plasma cells, with overall preserved nodal architecture, in contrast to hyaline-vascular UCD. The plasma cells are most often polytypic and show a range of cytologic features, usually mature but less often with mild atypia. Lymphoid follicles are generally hyperplastic in mixed/plasmacytic UCD, but a small subset of follicles often can show hyaline-vascular changes. Hybrid cases demonstrating features of both variants (hyaline-vascular and mixed/plasmacytic) can also be observed.[16]

Diagnosis and Evaluation of UCD

Unicentric Castleman disease is diagnosed after a lymph node biopsy to investigate patients presenting with solitary lymphadenopathy, having clinical suspicion of lymphoma. "Unlike MCD with its many overlapping conditions, few diseases other than UCD and lymphomas present with a solitary enlarged lymph node with CD-like histopathology. Thymomas, PTGC, unusual morphological variants of FL, and lymphoproliferations with regressive germinal centers, such as angioimmunoblastic T-cell lymphoma, can sometimes show histopathological features reminiscent of HV UCD. PC UCD-like histopathological features may be seen in many other conditions, such as infections, autoimmune diseases, primary or acquired immunodeficiencies, such as advanced phases of HIV-related lymphadenopathy, and malignancies, including Hodgkin lymphoma, but the lymphadenopathy is usually not unicentric" as cited by van Rhee F.[13]

It is unclear how UCD develops. Recent evidence points to the possibility that it is caused by a clonal expansion of lymph node stromal cells. It needs to be differentiated from other lymphoproliferative disorders that are common in children. These conditions include autoimmune and infectious diseases like autoimmune lymphoproliferative syndrome and IM, as well as other conditions such as Rosie–Dorfman disease and Kawasaki disease. For CD, there are no accepted treatment guidelines. Nonetheless, the cornerstone of UCD treatment continues to be surgery and total resection.[17]

Molecular lesions in the context of UCD are characterized by enrichment for genetic abnormalities within the interleukin signaling pathways (PDGFRB, FGFR3, NF1, PIM1, PTPN6, IL6ST, JAK1, HRAS, KRAS, NRAS, JAK2, AKT1, ERBB4, and JAK3) and MAPK pathway (FAS, PDGFRB, FGFR3, NF1, IL6ST, HRAS, KRAS, NRAS, ERBB4, JAK3, BRAF, and TGFBR2).[15]

IDIOPATHIC CASTLEMAN DISEASE

One-third and half of all cases of MCD are attributed to idiopathic MCD (iMCD). This rare but potentially fatal illness is characterized by multiple organ system involvement, polyclonal lymphocyte proliferation, generalized lymphadenopathy, and systemic inflammatory symptoms. The hyperinflammatory state brought on by dysregulated cytokine activity—often IL-6—is attributed to the symptomatology.

iMCD Diagnosis Criteria

Major and minor criteria are part of the proposed consensus diagnostic criteria. The diagnosis of iMCD necessitates the fulfillment of two major criteria (multicentric lymphadenopathy and characteristic lymph node histopathology), the exclusion of infectious, malignant, and autoimmune/autoinflammatory disorders that can mimic iMCD, as well as the fulfillment of at least two of the eleven minor criteria with at least one laboratory abnormality.[9]

Consensus diagnostic criteria for iMCD.[9]

I. *Major criteria (requires both)*:
   - Histopathologic characteristics of lymph nodes that align with the spectrum of iMCD. The following characteristics fall into the iMCD spectrum (needs grade 2-3 for either plasmacytosis or regressive GCs at minimum): Regressed, atrophic, or atretic germinal centers, frequently exhibiting enlarged mantle zones made up of lymphocytes arranged in concentric rings that resemble "onion skin," the prominence of follicular dendritic cells, hypervascularity with prominent endothelium in the interfollicular space and vessels that have "lollipop" appearance as these pierce the GCs. In the interfollicular space sheet-like and polytypic plasmacytosis (grade > 2), hyperplastic GCs.[9]
   - Enlarged lymph nodes in at least two lymph node stations (with a short-axis diameter of ≥1 cm).

II. *Minor criteria (must include at least one laboratory criterion among 2 of the 11 criteria)*:

    Laboratory criteria: (1) Increased ESR (>15 mm/h) or higher C-reactive protein (CRP) levels (>10 mg/L). (2) Anemia (hemoglobin <12.5 g/dL in men and <11.5 g/dL in women). (3) Platelet counts below 150 k/μL or above 400 k/μL, respectively, are referred to as thrombocytopenia or thrombocytosis. (4) Low albumin levels (<3.5 g/dL), (5) Proteinuria (10 mg/100 mL or 150 mg/24 h) or renal dysfunction (eGFR <60 mL/min/1.73 m^2), (6) Total gamma globulin or immunoglobulin G >1,700 mg/dL (polyclonal hypergammaglobulinemia).

    Clinical: (1) Constitutional symptoms—fatigue weight loss, fever (>38°C), or night sweats (≥2 CTCAE lymphoma score for B-symptoms). (2) A large liver or spleen. (3) Edema, anasarca, ascites, or pleural effusion, i.e., fluid accumulation. (4) Violaceous papules or eruptive cherry hemangiomatosis. (5) Lymphocytic interstitial pneumonitis.

III. *Exclusion criteria: Every illness that can resemble iMCD must be ruled out*: (1) HHV-8 (infection can be confirmed by blood PCR; positive LANA-1 staining by IHC is required for the diagnosis of HHV-8-associated MCD,

CHAPTER 14: Tumor-like Lesions Associated with B-cell Predominance

ruling out iMCD). (2) Clinical EBV-lymphoproliferative illnesses, such as persistently active EBV or IM (where a detectable EBV viral load is not always indicative of exclusion). (3) Other uncontrolled infections that result in inflammation and adenopathy (such as acute or uncontrolled CMV, toxoplasmosis, HIV, active tuberculosis).[9]

Autoimmune/autoinflammatory diseases (full clinical criteria must be met; the presence of autoimmune antibodies alone does not rule out a diagnosis).

(1) Systemic lupus erythematous. (2) The rheumatoid arthritis. (3) Adult onset still disease. (4) Juvenile idiopathic arthritis. (5) Autoimmune lymphoproliferative syndrome.[9]

Malignant/lymphoproliferative disorders (for these conditions to be excluded, they must be diagnosed concurrently with or before iMCD): (1) Lymphoma (both Hodgkin and non-hodgkin). (2) Primary lymphnode plasmacytoma. (3) FDCS. (4) Multiple myeloma. (5) POEMS syndrome.

Select additional characteristics that are helpful for the diagnosis but not necessary for it.

Increased levels of VEGF, IL-6, sIL-2R, IgA, IgE, LDH, and/or B2M. Bone marrow reticulin fibrosis (especially in TAFRO syndrome patients). Diagnosis of the following conditions associated with iMCD—inflammatory myofibroblastic tumor, autoimmune cytopenias, polyneuropathy (without the diagnosis of POEMS), glomerular nephropathy, PNP, and BO organizing pneumonia.[9]

Diagnostic criteria specific for iMCD-TAFRO were proposed in 2016 by Iwaki et al. and include histopathological and clinical criteria.[20]

In 2021, Iwaki et al.'s (2016) diagnostic criteria was updated to include the option of making a diagnosis without histological confirmation. TAFRO syndrome is divided into three categories by these authors. The following three scenarios have been described: (i) Possible iMCD-TAFRO: TAFRO syndrome without lymph node biopsy and without other comorbidities (autoimmune/autoinflammatory, infectious, or tumor pathologies). (ii) TAFRO syndrome with lymph node histopathology compatible with iMCD. (iii) TAFRO syndrome without iMCD or other comorbidities (TAFRO syndrome with lymph node histopathology not compatible with iMCD or other comorbidities).[21]

KSHV/HHV8-ASSOCIATED MULTICENTRIC CASTLEMAN DISEASE

The KSHV-MCD is an uncommon B-cell lymphoproliferative disorder that relapses and remits, typically affecting individuals living with HIV.[22] Elevated levels of cytokines, such as IL-10 and IL-6, as well as the generation of a KSHV-encoded IL-6 homolog known as viral IL-6 (vIL-6) are linked to this condition. Typically, patients have lymphadenopathy along with fever and night sweats, which are indicative of inflammation. Cytopenias, hypoalbuminemia, hyponatremia, and elevated CRP are examples of abnormalities in the laboratory.[22]

Diagnosis of KSHV-MCD requires pathological confirmation from an involved lymph node. If left untreated, KSHV-MCD can lead to multiorgan dysfunction and is fatal, with a two-year median survival rate. Patients may present with concurrent KS or PEL, or all three conditions (KS, KSHV-MCD, and PEL) in addition to KSHV-MCD. KSHV-infected, l-restricted plasmablasts are the main pathogenic cells in KSHV-MCD; these cells are typically found in the marginal zone or outer mantle zone of lymph nodes that are involved. In general, OCT2, BLIMP1, and IRF4/MUM1 are expressed by KSHV-infected plasmablasts; however, PAX5, BCL6, and CD13 are not.[22]

Follicle hyperplasia, NOS, HIV-associated lymphadenopathy, autoimmune disorders, HL, and plasmacytoma are among the conditions that morphologically overlap with MCD.[22]

■ DISORDERS AND CANCERS THAT COEXIST WITH KSHV-MCD[24]

KSHV-related Disorders

- *Kaposi sarcoma*: A neoplastic proliferation of endothelium that is exclusively linked to an infection with the Kaposi sarcoma herpesvirus (KSHV).
- *Primary effusion lymphoma (PEL; classic and solid variants)*: A third of patients with PEL also have Kaposi sarcoma. PEL an AIDS defining disease. Clinically, there is overlap between PEL, KSHV inflammatory cytokine syndrome, and KSHV MCD. In addition to being positive for LANA1, PEL tumor cells in both their classic and solid forms are also frequently positive for CD45, CD38, CD138, BLIMP1, VS38c, MUM1, CD30, and epithelial membrane antigen. They frequently test positive for small RNAs (EBERs) encoded by the EBV.
- *KSHV-positive diffuse large B-cell lymphoma*: A novel type of lymphoma that typically develops in conjunction with HIV infection and MCD. The tumor cells express markers of terminal B-cell differentiation, such as MUM1, and have plasmablastic characteristics. They are also typically positive for CD45 and CD20. They frequently test negative for EBER and/or EBV.
- *KSHV-positive germinotropic lymphoproliferative disorder*: Individuals are without immunodeficiency but localized lymphadenopathy is present. The clinical progression is indolent. The growth of plasmablasts is limited to enlarged germinal centers. Plasmablasts are positive for EBV and/or EBER, viral IL-6, MUM1, CD38, and cytoplasmic monotypic light chain.
- Reactive lymphoid hyperplasia that is KSHV-positive has been documented in HIV-positive individuals. There is follicular hyperplasia in the lymph nodes. Lymphoid cells express LANA1.

CHAPTER 14: Tumor-like Lesions Associated with B-cell Predominance

- *KSHV inflammatory cytokine syndrome*: The patients without KSHV-associated MCD have elevated serum levels of cytokines, high KSHV titers, and inflammatory symptoms. The outlook is not good.

HIV-related Illnesses

HIV-associated lymphadenopathies: these diseases are characterized by huge germinal centers and explosive follicular hyperplasia.

EBV-related illnesses

- *EBV infection*: Reactive hyperplastic lymphadenopathy with hyperplastic germinal centers is typically linked to the non-malignant pathological counterpart of EBV infection.
- *Hodgkin lymphoma*: Almost all cases of Hodgkin lymphoma in HIV-positive individuals are linked to EBV infection.

Two clinical criteria—one from the National Cancer Institute (NCI),[16] and the other one from the French ANRS (Agence Nationale de Recherche sur le SIDA)—have been developed for establishing a diagnosis of active MCD in KSHV/HHV8-MCD, a relapsing and remitting illness. According to the French ANRS definition; pyrexia, elevated serum CRP (in the absence of any other cause), and at least three of the twelve clinical characteristics must be present. The following are the prerequisites for the NCI scheme: elevated CRP in the serum, at least one clinical symptom, and one abnormality in the lab probably or definitely linked to MCD. The French scheme has a higher cut-off for serum CRP (>20 mg/L) than the US scheme (>3 mg/L).[24]

Potential treatment options for KSHV/HHV8-MCD are rituximab, etoposide, pegylated liposomal doxorubicin, anti-herpes virus therapies and tocilizumab, monoclonal antibody against IL-6 receptor **(Fig. 1)**.[24]

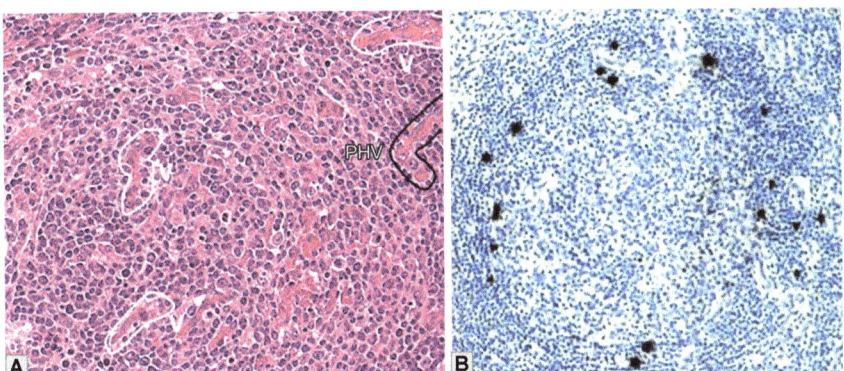

FIGS. 1A AND B: KSHV/HHV8-associated multicentric Castleman disease (MCD). (A) Depicting marked intrafollicular vascular proliferation (V). The lymphoid follicle also has typical penetrating hyalinized vessels (PHVs). (B) In the follicular mantle, some large atypical cells, consistent with plasmablasts, are positive for KSHV/HHV8 viral IL-6. Magnification ×20 (A and B).

Source: https://www.mdpi.com/hemato/hemato-02-00047/article_deploy/html/images/hemato-02-00047-g001.png

CONCLUSION

By delving into the complexities of B-cell-rich lesions masquerading as tumors, this discussion sheds light on their nuanced nature, guiding pathologists in their approach to their precise identification. The classification introduced by the WHO 'Blue Book' highlights the importance of recognizing these lesions as a separate entity, emphasizing the significance of accurate diagnosis and tailored management strategies. These lesions, mimicking tumorous growth yet exhibiting benign behaviors, challenge traditional diagnostic paradigms.

REFERENCES

1. Cree IA. The WHO Classification of Haematolymphoid Tumours. Leukemia. 2022;36:1701-2.
2. Chen LYC, Mattman A, Seidman MA, Carruthers MN. IgG4-related disease: what a hematologist needs to know. Haematologica. 2019;104:444-55.
3. Wallace ZS, Deshpande V, Mattoo H, Mahajan VS, Kulikova M, Pillai S, et al. IgG4-Related Disease: Clinical and Laboratory Features in One Hundred Twenty-Five Patients. Arthritis Rheumatol. 2015;67:2466-75.
4. Grimm KE, Barry TS, Chizhevsky V, Hii A, Weiss LM, Siddiqi IN, et al. Histopathological findings in 29 lymph node biopsies with increased IgG4 plasma cells. Mod Pathol. 2012;25:480-91.
5. Miranda RN, Medeiros LJ, Khoury JD. Atlas of Lymph Node Pathology. New York; Springer: 2013; pp. 87.
6. Anagnostopoulos I, Hummel M, Falini B, Joehrens K, Stein H. Epstein-barr virus infection of monocytoid B-cell proliferates: an early feature of primary viral infection. Am J Surg Pathol. 2005;29:595-601.
7. Kojima M, Motoori T, Asano S, Nakamura S. Histological diversity of reactive and atypical proliferative lymph node lesions in systemic lupus erythematosus patients. Pathol Res Pract. 2007;203:423-31.
8. Kurman RJ, Ellenson LH, Ronnett BM. Blaustein's Pathology of the Female Genital Tract. Boston; Springer: 2019; pp.1390-1.
9. Arikawa K, Williams DS. Organization of actin filaments and immunocolocalization of alpha-actinin in the connecting cilium of rat photoreceptors. J Comp Neurol. 1989;288:640-6.
10. Castleman B, Iverson L, Menendez VP. Localized mediastinal lymphnode hyperplasia resembling thymoma. Cancer. 1956;9(4):822-30.
11. Frizzera G, Banks PM, Massarelli G, Rosai J. A systemic lymphoproliferative disorder with morphologic features of Castleman's disease. Pathological findings in 15 patients. Am J Surg Pathol. 1983;7:211-31.
12. Weisenburger DD, Nathwani BN, Winberg CD, Rappaport H. Multicentric angiofollicular lymph node hyperplasia: a clinicopathologic study of 16 cases. Hum Pathol. 1985;16:162-72.
13. van Rhee F, Oksenhendler E, Srkalovic G, Voorhees P, Lim M, Dispenzieri A, et al. International evidence-based consensus diagnostic and treatment guidelines for unicentric Castleman disease. Blood Adv. 2020;4:6039-50.
14. Sager G. Effects of insulin on human beta-adrenoceptors. Br J Clin Pharmacol. 1990;30 (Suppl 1):139S-141S.
15. Frizzera G. Castleman Disease and related disorders. Semin Diagn Pathology. 1988;5(4):346-364.

16. González García A, Fernández-Martín J, Robles Marhuenda Á. Idiopathic multicentric Castleman disease and associated autoimmune and autoinflammatory conditions: practical guidance for diagnosis. Rheumatology (Oxford). 2023;62:1426-35.
17. Zhang J, Li C, Lv L, Yang C, Kong XR, Zhu J, et al. Clinical and experimental study of Castleman disease in children. Pediatr Blood Cancer. 2015;62:109-14.
18. Zhou T, Wang HW, Pittaluga S, Jaffe ES. Multicentric Castleman disease and the evolution of the concept. Pathologica. 2021;113:339-53.
19. Igawa T, Sato Y. TAFRO Syndrome. Hematol Oncol Clin North Am. 2018;32:107-18.
20. Nishimura Y, Fajgenbaum DC, Pierson SK, Iwaki N, Nishikori A, Kawano M, et al. Validated international definition of the thrombocytopenia, anasarca, fever, reticulin fibrosis, renal insufficiency, and organomegaly clinical subtype (TAFRO) of idiopathic multicentric Castleman disease. Am J Hematol. 2021;96:1241-52.
21. Ramaswami R, Lurain K, Peer CJ, Serquiña A, Wang V, Widell A, et al. Tocilizumab in patients with symptomatic Kaposi sarcoma herpesvirus-associated multicentric Castleman disease. Blood. 2020;135:2316-9.
22. Vega F, Miranda RN, Medeiros LJ. KSHV/HHV8-positive large B-cell lymphomas and associated diseases: a heterogeneous group of lymphoproliferative processes with significant clinicopathological overlap. Mod Pathol. 2020;33:18-28.
23. Carbone A, Borok M, Damania B, Gloghini A, Polizzotto MN, Jayanthan RK, et al. Castleman disease. Nat Rev Dis Primers. 2021;7:84.
24. Bower M, Carbone A. KSHV/HHV8-associated lymphoproliferative disorders lessons learnt from people living with HIV. Hemato 2021;(2)703-712.

Index

Page numbers followed by *b* refer to box, *f* refer to figure, *fc* refer to flowchart, and *t* refer to table.

A

Absolute neutrophil count 161
Adaptive immune system, parts of 118
Adeno-associated viral vectors 26, 35, 36
Adenosine deaminase deficiency 34
Adenovirus 17*f*, 20*f*, 21*f*
 vectors 19, 35
Aggressive natural killer-cell leukemia 81, 84
Agitation 130
Alanine aminotransferase production 60
Alkaline phosphatase 60
Allogenic hematopoietic stem cell transplant 118
Alpha-beta T cell 119
Alpha-hydroxybutyrate dehydrogenase 61
Alpha-retroviral vectors 38
Alveolar damage, diffuse 62
Amino acids 202
Amino actinomycin 51
Amyloidosis 136, 215
Anakinra 128
Anaplastic large cell lymphoma 82, 87, 88
 breast implant-associated 89
Anemia 61, 176, 180, 187, 199-201
 aplastic 108
 autoimmune hemolytic 49, 53, 61, 69, 73
 cancer-induced 184-186, 186*t*, 187, 189, 192
 chemotherapy-induced 190
 congenital hemolytic 69
 degree of 190, 190*t*
 evaluation of 200
 pathophysiology of 202
 severe 181
 treatment 206
  strategy of 205
Angiogenesis 148
Angiopoietin-like protein-1 148
Angiotensin-converting enzyme 68
 inhibitors 205
Antiangiogenic molecules 148
Anticoagulant 67
Antigen
 binding site 119
 escape 131
Anti-platelet autoantibodies 63
Anti-thymocyte globulin 108
Aphasia 130
Apoptosis 149
Apoptotic, modulation of 148
Arteriovenous malformation 176-178
Aspartate aminotransferase production 60
Ataxia telangiectasia 96
Autoantibody 54
Autoimmune disorders 127
Autologous transplantation 34
Auxiliary genes 27
Avapritinib 164
Axicabtagene ciloleucel 124, 126
Azurophilic granule pattern 65*f*

B

Basic fibroblast growth factor 141
B-cell
 activated 144
 acute lymphoblastic leukemia 33
  genetics of 97
 admixed 84
 maturation 144
 predominance 210
 prevalence of 210

Bleeding, gastrointestinal 176
Blinatumomab 102
Blood
  bank
    quality control in 55
    technology 6
  cell
    lineages 13
    production of 12
  components 50
    contamination of 49
    quality control of 49, 50
  forming cells 40
  group 1
  pressure, low 31
  quality control of 49
  transfusions 5
  typing 5
B-lymphocytes 118
Body mass index 189
Bone marrow 62, 71, 107-109, 111, 139, 141
  cellularity 107
  mastocytosis 112
  microenvironment
    modulation of 147
    role of 141
  smear 67
Bortezomib 148, 149
Bosutinib 171, 172
Breast cancer 190
Breathing problems, acute 58
Brexucabtagene autoleucel 124
Bronchiolitis obliterans 215
Bruton tyrosine kinase 125
Burst forming unit erythroid 202

C

Cancer 184
  breast 190
  colorectal 191
  diagnostics 158
  genomics 158
  ovarian 190, 191
  stem cells 149
  type 190, 190t
Cancer-induced anemia 184-186, 186t, 187, 189, 192
  pathogenesis of 184, 185
  prevalence of 184

Capsid
  majority of 20
  protein precursors 20
Cardiac markers 61
Cardiac troponin 61
Cardiovascular risk reduction 206
Castleman disease 215
  idiopathic 217
Celiac disease 87
Cell
  cycle signaling pathways 148
  enumeration 49
  expansion 30
  leukemic 167
  multiple clones of abnormal 170
  nucleus of 17f
  selection 40
  surface molecule 31
    ligand for 29
Central nervous system 101, 179
  toxicity, frequency of 128
Cerebral edema 130
Cerebriform nucleus 84
Chemotherapeutic drugs 190, 190t
Chemotherapy 31
  lymphodepleting 128
  pathogenesis of 184
Chemotherapy-induced anemia 190
  management of 191
Chest syndrome, acute 70
Childhood myelodysplastic neoplasms 109, 109t
Chimeric antigen receptor-T cell 102, 118
  associated neurotoxicity 128
  construct, cartoon depiction of 119f, 121f
  manufacture of 120
  product 124
  production process 122t
  therapy, origin of 118
  toxicity 127, 127t
Chromatin 64
Chromosomal analysis 154
Chromosomal banding analysis 155, 167
Chromosomal microarray 156, 159
Chromosomal ploidy, determination of 156
Chromosomal translocations 97, 157

Chromosome 140
  banding analysis 155
Chronic granulomatosis disease 34
Chronic kidney disease 199, 200, 202, 203, 205
  monitoring of 201
  stages of 200
Chronic lymphoproliferative disorder 81, 83
Ciltacabtagene autoleucel 125
Circulatory system 4
Classical myeloproliferative neoplasms 163
Clinical molecular pathology analysis 155
Clonal cytogenetic, acquired 111
Clonal cytopenia 11, 14, 108, 161
Clonal diseases 12
Clonal hematopoiesis 11, 12, 14, 108, 161, 162
Clonal plasma cells 136, 147
Clonal T-cells 164
Colony forming unit erythroid 202
Complete blood count 14, 180, 200
Complex cytogenetic patterns 161
Comprehensive genomic methods 159*t*
  clinical applications of 159*t*
  limitations of 159*t*
Conventional molecular methods 155
Copy number variations 159
Cord blood 97
Core binding factor 166
Core protein genes 27
Coronary damage, acute 58
Coronavirus disease 2019 (COVID-19) 58, 59, 61, 66, 67, 69, 70, 72
  attenuation of 72
  bone marrow effects in 71
  effect of 71
  hematological abnormalities in 68
  infection 58, 70, 71
  lower incidence of 69
  severe acute 72
  severity of 62
Corticosteroids 122
Coughing 59
C-reactive protein 60, 218
  serum 201
Creatine kinase 61
Cryoprecipitate 50

Cryptic copy number alterations 156
Cutaneous anaplastic large cell lymphoma 85
Cyclophosphamide 191
Cystic fibrosis transmembrane regulator gene 26
Cytarabine 122
Cytogenetic 155, 159
  abnormalities 140
  criterion 106
  irregularities 140
Cytokine
  cocktail 122
  release syndrome 122, 127-129
    management 128
  storm 61, 62
Cytopenia 11, 73, 127, 131, 158, 161
  idiopathic 13, 14, 161
  persistent 158, 161
Cytoplasmic granule content 48
Cytosine phosphate-guanine dinucleotides 142
Cytotoxic T-lymphocyte response 24
Cytotoxicity 39

D

D antigen, quantification of 49, 53
Dasatinib 172
Degranulation 55
Delirium 130
Dendritic cells 141
Dexamethasone 148, 149
Diffuse large B-cell lymphoma 125, 126
Digital signal's intensity 48
Direct antiglobulin test 6, 53
Disseminated intravascular coagulation 54
Divalent metal transporter 203
DNA
  binding proteins, modifications of 142
  methylation 142, 157
  methyltransferases 142
Donor units, selection of 6
Doughnut cells 88
Down syndrome 96, 109
Downey cells 65*f*
Doxorubicin 191
Dysplasia 11, 111, 161
Dyspnea 59

E

Electroporation 121
Empirical antibiotics 128
Enasidenib 171, 172
Encephalopathy 130
   immune effector cell-associated 130
   syndrome 127
Endosomal disruption 23
Endothelial cells 62
Enteropathy-associated T-cell
   lymphoma 82, 87
Enzymatic activity 55
Enzymatic digestion 156
Enzyme-linked immunosorbent
   assay 83
Eosinophilia 111, 112, 113b, 160, 164
Eosinophilic neoplasm 163
Epidermis 84
Epigenetic 158
   mechanism 142
   modification 142
      forms of 142
   mutations 166
   phenomena 147
Epistaxis 179
Epithelial cells, surface of 60
Epstein–Barr virus 91, 213
Erythrocytes
   diagnose genetic disorders of 49
   genetic disorders of 53
   sedimentation rate 60, 180
Erythrocytosis 163
Erythroferrone 203
Erythroid
   leukemia, acute 103
   precursors 185
Erythrophagocytosis 90
Erythropoiesis
   related molecules 203f
   stimulating agents 192, 199
Erythropoietin 184, 203, 205
Estrogen receptor antigen 1
Etanercept 128
Etoposide 191
European Committee on Blood
   Transfusion 50
Ex vivo gene therapy 18, 41
Excessive cytokines 73
Exocytosis 55
Exome sequencing 159

Extracellular matrix 141
Extramedullary multiple myeloma 136

F

Fast breathing 59
Ferritin 180
   levels 180
Ferroportin 203
Fetal erythrocytes 49, 52
Fever 31, 54
Fibrin degradation products 58
Fibroblasts 141
Flow cytometry 48, 54, 66
   role of 48
Fludarabine 122
Fluorescence in situ hybridization 100,
   140, 154, 156, 159
Folate levels 201
Follicular
   dendritic cell
      meshwork 90
      sarcoma 216
   hyperplasia 211
   T-cell lymphoma 82
Fragment
   antigen binding region 119
   crystallizable region 119
   variable region 119
Free fatty acids 187
Fresh frozen plasma 50

G

Gamma-glutamyl transferase 60
Gamma-retroviral vectors 36, 37, 120
Ganciclovir 32
Gastrointestinal symptoms 180
Gastrointestinal tract 81, 86
   indolent T-cell lymphoma of 86
Gemtuzumab ozogamicin 171
Gene
   addition 18
   delivery, vector platforms for 19
   editing 18, 39
      techniques 28, 39, 40
   expression 157
      profiling 90
   fusions 157, 167
   harboring germline 97
   mutations 177

Index

products, late-phase 19
replacement 18
silencing 18
therapy 16, 17f, 20f, 27, 28
  ex vivo 40
  viral vector systems for 19
Genetic
  abnormalities 108, 113b
  alterations 98t
  complexity 169
  diseases 18, 23, 40
  disorders 18, 23, 40, 53
  mutation 178
    testing 180
  tumor syndromes 113
Genital tract, female 212
Genome 25
Genome-wide association studies 97
Genomic
  analysis 162
  explosion changes 154
  profiling 154, 155
  role of 162
  sequencing 157
  signature analysis 84
  technologies 157
  testing 161, 165
Germinal centers, progressive
  transformation of 212
Gilteritinib 172
Glasgow prognostic score 189
Glomerular filtration rate 199
Glucose metabolism, abnormal 73
Glycoprotein 53
Glycosylphosphatidylinositol 53
Graft-versus-host disease 29, 50, 127
Granulocyte 55
  function, analysis of 55
  macrophage colony-stimulating
    factor 29, 33, 131
  reactive oxygen species 55
Growth hormone 186

H

Harvest sufficient peripheral blood
  progenitor cells 55
Head and neck cancer 190, 191
Hematologic
  abnormalities 72
    cutoff values 59
  autoimmune diseases 73
  cancers, classification of 96
  malignancies 11, 154, 172
    treatment of 118
  neoplasm 112, 170
Hematolymphoid tumors, classification
  of 80
Hematopoiesis, ineffective 109
Hematopoietic
  cells 40
  lineage, cells of 111
  microenvironment 62
  stem cell 53, 108
    transplantation 33, 49, 55, 122
Hemoglobin 199
  correction of 206
Hemoglobinopathies 70
Hemolytic crises 69
Hemolytic disease 5, 6
Hemophagocytic lymphohistiocytosis
  73, 122
Hemophagocytosis 71
Hemophilia 70
Hemorrhage, fetomaternal 49, 52
Hepatic symptoms 180
Hepatosplenic T-cell lymphoma 82, 90
Hepcidin 204
Herpesvirus 220
Heterozygosity
  copy neutral loss of 107, 163
  loss of 156, 159, 165
Hexon 20
High transduction efficiency 23
Histone
  deacetylase 100
  modifications 142
Hodgkin's lymphoma 221
Homozygosity 87
Host cell 20
  cytoplasm 23
Host immune response 24
Howell-Jolly bodies 64
Human genome project 157
Human leukocyte antigen
  crossmatching 49, 55
  markers 38
Human platelet antigens 54
Hyaline vascular lesions 216
Hydroa vacciniforme
  lymphoproliferative disorder 82, 91

Hydroxycarbamide 72
Hyperbasophilic cytoplasm 65f
Hyperdiploidy 98, 102, 140
Hyperferritinemia 58, 72, 73
Hyperparathyroidism, secondary 205
Hyperplastic plasmacytoid dendritic cells 216
Hyper-segmented nuclei 64
Hypersplenism 199
Hypodiploid, low 98
Hypogammaglobulinemia 127
Hypotension 31
Hypoxia
  inducing factor, role of 203f
  response element 203

I

Icosahedral vertices, apex of 20
Idecabtagene vicleucel 125
Ileum 87
Imatinib 171, 172
Immune
  receptors, biology of 119
  responses 28
  thrombocytopenia 73
Immunity 36
Immunogenicity 37
  low 36
Immunohematology 51
Immunohistochemistry 165
Immunomodulatory drugs 125
Immunosuppressive microenvironment 132
In vivo gene therapy 18
Indolent natural killer-cell lymphoproliferative disorder 81
Indolent systemic mastocytosis 112
Infections 127, 131
  signs of 128
Inflammation 205
Inflammatory cytokine levels 60
Inflammatory markers 61
Inner icosahedral shell 23
Innovative immune cell receptors 29
Inotuzumab ozogamicin 102
Insulin-like growth factor 186
Interfollicular expansion 212
Interleukin 186

International Consensus Classification 10
  of Mature Lymphoid Neoplasms 137
Intestinal T-cell lymphoma 82, 87
Intracellular calcium 55
Intradermal vaccine 38
Intrafollicular vascular proliferation 221f
Intravascular hemolysis 53
Iron
  balance, regulation of 204f
  deficiency 203
    absolute 204
    anemia 181
    functional 204
    homeostasis 187
    supplementation 192
Ischemic hypoxic reperfusion injury 60
Ivosidenib 172

J

Janus kinase 2 202
Jejunum 87

K

Kaposi sarcoma 220
  herpesvirus
    inflammatory cytokine syndrome 221
    positive diffuse large B-cell lymphoma 220
    positive germinotropic lymphoproliferative disorder 220
Kidney
  disease, chronic 199, 200, 202, 203, 205
  function 61
Kinase driven subtypes 100
Kleihauer–Betke test 52

L

Lactic dehydrogenase 60
Lentivirus
  particles encapsulate 27
  vectors 19, 20f, 27, 120
Leptin 189

Lethargy 130
Leucovorin 191
Leukemia 49, 82, 160*t*
  acute 154, 170
    basophilic 103
    lymphoblastic 96, 98*t*, 100-102,
      102*f*, 118, 122, 125, 159, 160, 167
    megakaryoblastic 103
    monocytic 103
    myeloid 10, 11, 72, 103, 103*b*, 104,
      108, 159, 160, 165
    myelomonocytic 103
    promyelocytic 103, 104
  adult T-cell 83
  B-cell acute lymphoblastic 33
  childhood 97
  chronic
    eosinophilic 105
    lymphocytic 31, 118, 126, 143
    myeloid 105, 164
    myelomonocytic 72, 110, 111*b*
    neutrophilic 105, 163
  core binding factor 104
  juvenile myelomonocytic 105, 106
  mixed-phenotype acute 100
  pediatric 96, 100
    acute lymphoblastic 96, 101*t*
    acute myeloid 103
  prenatal origin of 97
  subtype 169
  T-lymphoblastic 112
Leukemoid reactions 72
Leukocyte subpopulation analysis 49
Leukodepleted cellular blood products
  49, 50
Light beam measures
  forward scatter 48
  side scatter 48
Lisocabtagene maraleucel 124
Lollipop lesions 216
Lymph nodes 85
Lymphadenopathies, HIV-associated
  221
Lymphocytes 62, 63
  abnormal 65*f*
  atypical 65*f*
  large 84
Lymphoid
  follicle 221*f*
  neoplasms 111, 112, 113*b*

Lymphoma 80, 81, 83, 84, 86, 91, 112,
  154, 190, 191, 210
Lymphomatoid
  gastropathy 86
  papulosis 85
Lymphopenia 31, 72
  causes of 62
Lymphoproliferative disorder 84, 85,
  136, 219

M

Macrophage 71
  activation syndrome 73, 122
  tumor associated 188
Maculopapular cutaneous
    mastocytosis 112
Malignancy 71
  second 127
  solid 126
Malignant
  cells 12
  disorders 219
Malnutrition 189, 205
Mantle cell lymphoma 125
Mast cell
  leukemia 112
  neoplasms 163
  sarcoma 112
Mastocytoma
  cutaneous 112
  isolated 112
Mastocytosis 110
  aggressive systemic 112
  cutaneous 110, 112
  diffuse cutaneous 112
  subtypes 112*b*
  systemic 164
  types 112*b*
Mature natural killer cell neoplasms 80
Mature T-cell neoplasms 80
Mechlorethamine 191
Melphalan therapy 149
Membrane-associated accessory
    protein 26
Mesenchymal stem cells 62, 141
Metagenomics 158
Methotrexate 191
Microorganisms
  degradation of 55

intracellular killing of 55
phagocytosis of 55
Midostaurin 164, 171
Minimal residual disease 101
Mitotic entry, stimulation of 28
Molecular genetic features 80
Molecular international prognostic scoring system 155, 162
Molecular remission, confirmation of 163
Molecular technologies 157
Monoclonal gammopathy 136, 145
Monoclonal immunoglobulins, production of 137
Monocytes 55*f*
function, analysis of 55
Monocytosis 111
Monomorphic epitheliotropic intestinal T-cell lymphoma 82, 87
Mononucleosis, infectious 212
Monosomy 106
Morphologic dysplasia 111
Mosquito bite allergy, severe 82, 91
Multicentric Castleman disease 211, 219, 221*f*
Multicolor flow cytometry 170
Multigene expression 28
Multilocalized mastocytoma 112
Multiple myeloma 126, 136, 138, 145, 147, 148
Multiplex ligation-dependent probe amplification 168
Mycosis fungoides 81, 85
Myelodysplastic
neoplasms 106, 107*t*, 109, 110*b*, 160
syndrome 11, 108, 155, 158, 161
Myeloid 111, 112, 113*b*
cells, recruitment of 128
growth factors 131
leukemia 72
malignancy 11
neoplasia 113
neoplasm 14, 160*t*, 162, 170
therapy-related 104
precursor conditions, management of 13
Myelopoiesis, transient abnormal 104
Myeloproliferative neoplasms 105, 105*b*, 106, 110*b*, 111, 159, 160, 162
Myoglobin 61

N

Natural killer-cell
enteropathy 86
lymphoid proliferations 80
Neoplasms 80, 164
Neurological signs 58
Neurotoxicity 127, 130
Neurotoxicity syndrome, immune effector cell-associated 122, 127, 129, 130
Neutropenia 83, 122
Neutrophils 64, 65
Next-generation sequencing 154, 157, 158
Nilotinib 171, 172
Nodal peripheral T-cell lymphoma 82
Nodal T-follicular helper cell lymphoma 89, 90
Nonhemolytic febrile transfusion reaction 50
Non-Hodgkin's lymphomas 80, 126, 127
Noninvasive prenatal testing 7
Non-small cell cancer 190*t*
Novel plasmid-based integration system 120
Nuclear
abnormalities 64
hyposegmentation 64
pseudoinclusions 88
structure 48

O

Onion skin change 216
On-target off-tumor 132
Optical genome mapping 156, 159
Optimal transplantation protocols 35
Osler–Weber–Rendu
disease 181
syndrome 176
Osteoblasts 141
Osteoclasts 141
Oxidative metabolism 55

P

Pancytopenia 53
Paraneoplastic
pemphigus 215
syndrome 139

Paroxysmal nocturnal hemoglobinuria 49, 53, 108
Pediatric delirium, Cornell assessment of 130
Peripheral blood 107, 109, 136
  leukocytes 112
  smear 63, 65f, 84
Peripheral T-cell lymphoma 82, 90, 91
Phagocytes, regulatory molecules of 55
Philadelphia chromosome 101
Photomultiplier tubes 48
Plaque 85
Plasma 50
  cell 71, 136, 139, 141, 144
    abnormal 144
    dyscrasias 136, 137, 138t, 139f, 140, 141f, 142-144, 145f, 146-148
    leukemia 136, 139
    myeloma 138
    neoplasms 139
    normal 144, 145
  concentrations 204
Platelet 49, 50, 66
  agonists 54
  antibodies 49, 54
  crossmatching 49, 54
  derived growth factor 202
  function 54
  immunology 49, 54
  refractoriness 54
  units 54
Pleomorphic megakaryocytes 71
Pluripotent stem cells 34
Pneumonia symptoms 59
POEMS syndrome 139
Polycythemia vera 105
Polymerase chain reaction 72, 154, 156
Polyposis, juvenile 178
Ponatinib 171, 172
Post-acute coronavirus disease 2019 (COVID-19) syndrome 72
Postmitotic cells, transduction of 28
Post-transplant cyclophosphamide 72
Potential disease progression 133
Precursor myeloid
  lesions 14
  neoplasms 10
Prednisone 191
Primary amyloid light chain 136

Primary cutaneous
  anaplastic large cell lymphoma 85
  lymphomas 85
  peripheral T-cell lymphoma 86
  T-cell lymphoid proliferations 84
Primary effusion lymphoma 220
Primary mediastinal B-cell lymphoma 125
Primary myelofibrosis 105
Primary plasma cell leukemia 136
Procalcitonin 61
Procarbazine 191
Prohormone brain natriuretic peptide, N-terminal of 61
Proinflammatory cytokines 186
  role of 185, 186t
Prolylhydroxylase domain 203
Propidium iodide 51
Protein 136
  capsid 19
Pseudo-Pelger-Huët anomaly 64

Q

Quantitative polymerase chain reaction 145
Quiescent cells 28
  transduction of 28

R

Raised D-dimer levels 58
Random donor platelets 50
Reactive B-cell predominant lymphoid proliferations 210
Red blood cell 5, 184, 199
  alloantibodies 1
  characterization 49
  distribution 61
  immunology 49, 51
Red cell
  antigen, semiquantification of 49, 51
  autoantibody 49
    characterization of 53
    diagnosis of 53
  concentrate 49, 50
  distribution width 12
  membrane encoding 70
  phenotyping 49
  survival, estimation of 49, 52
  transfusion 6

Refractory cytopenia 109
Renal anemia 205
Renal insufficiency 206
Replication-competent adenovirus generation 24
Residual white blood cells, quantification of 49, 50
Reticulocyte count 180
Retroviruses 19, 27
Rituximab 70

S

Sanger sequencing 156
Scalable production systems 23
Seizures 130
Sepsis 54
Severe acute respiratory distress syndrome 128
Severe acute respiratory syndrome coronavirus 2, infection of 62
Sezary
  cells 84
  syndrome 81, 84
Siltuximab 128
Single cell level studies 170
Single nucleotide variant 157, 159
Single-chain variable fragment 29
Sleeping beauty transposon system 120
Small-cell lung cancer 190
Smoldering systemic mastocytosis 112
Solitary plasmacytoma 139
Somatic mutations 11
Spetzler–Martin grading scale 181
Spherocytosis, hereditary 70
Stem cell 63
  grafts 49
Steroids, larger dosages of 70
Stringent blood typing 6
Stromal cells 141
Suicide strategies, limitation of 133
Systemic lupus erythematosus 212
Systemic mastocytosis, well-differentiated 112

T

Target antigen 124, 125
Target cancer cell 29
Target gene, genetic information for 32

T-cell
  acute lymphoblastic leukemia, genetic basis of 100
  based therapy 102
  collection 30
  isolation 30
  large granular lymphocytic leukemia 81
  lymphoid proliferations 80
  lymphoma 85-87, 91
  lymphoproliferative disorder 84, 85
  mediated immune attack 108
  production methods 30
  prolymphocytic leukemia 81
Telangiectasia, hereditary hemorrhagic 176-178, 181
Telangiectasis 179
Therapeutic transgene therapy 16
Therapy, abrupt loss of 133
Thrombocythemia, essential 105
Thrombocytosis, hereditary 163
Thrombopoietin receptor agonist 70
Thrombotic events 53
Thymic stromal lymphopoietin receptor 102, 167
Thymidine kinase gene 32
Tissue factor pathway inhibitor 60
T-large granular lymphocytic leukemia 83
T-lineage
  acute lymphoblastic leukemia 99
  transcription factor, deregulation of 169
T-lymphocytes 118, 141
Tocilizumab 128
Toll-like receptors 38
Total iron-binding capacity 180
Toxicity, grade of 127
Transcription activator-like effector nucleases 39
Transduction rates 37
Transferrin saturation 200
Transformed follicular lymphoma 125
Transforming growth factor-beta 177
Transfusion
  dependent beta-thalassemia 35
  medicine 48
  reactions 5
Transgene 19
  capacity 24

Tremors 130
Trisomy 91
Tumor 85, 205
  cell
    medium-to-large clear 90
    vaccines 29
  load, estimation of 166
  lysis syndrome 31, 127, 130
  necrosis factor 185, 186
Tyrosine kinase gene fusions 111, 112, 113*b*

U

Unfractionated heparin 69
Unicentric Castleman disease 210, 215
  classic features of 216
Uremic toxins 205
Urine protein electrophoresis 201
Urticaria pigmentosa 112

V

Vascular endothelial growth factor 141, 202, 203
Vector
  genome cloning 26
  types of 16
Vemurafenib 172

Venetoclax 169
Versatile testing technique 48
Vincristine 191
Viral genes 19
Viral genome 23
Viral vector
  amplification, process of 24
  based gene therapy 16
  delivery 35
  encapsulate, envelope of 19
von Willebrand disease 70

W

Waldenström's macroglobulinemia 136
Weight loss 189
Western blot 83
White blood cell 68, 101, 122
Whole genome sequencing 165, 169
Wiskott–Aldrich syndrome 34

X

X-linked severe combined immunodeficiency 34

Z

Zinc-finger nucleases 39

EU GSPR Authorised Reprsentative
Logos Europe, 9 rue Nicolas Poussin
1700, La Rochelle, France
Phone: +33 (0) 6 67 93 73 78
E-mail: contact@logoseurope.eu

www.ingramcontent.com/pod-product-compliance
Ingram Content Group UK Ltd.
Pitfield, Milton Keynes, MK11 3LW, UK
UKHW050428150426
5217IPUK00019B/1289